AF556843

Topical Reviews in

Vascular Surgery

Volume 1

EDITED BY

J. G. Pollock MB ChB, FRCS(Edin), FRCS(Glas)

Consultant Surgeon, Glasgow Royal Infirmary

With the assistance of

A. J. McKay MB ChB, FRCS(Glas)

Senior Surgical Registrar, Glasgow Royal Infirmary

with a Foreword by

H. H. G. Eastcott MS, FRCS

WRIGHT · PSG

Bristol London Boston

1982

Published by

John Wright & Sons Ltd, 823–825 Bath Road, Bristol BS4 5NU, England.
John Wright PSG Inc., 545 Great Road, Littleton, Massachusetts 01460, USA.

British Library Cataloguing in Publication Data

Topical reviews in vascular surgery.—Vol. 1
1. Vascular surgery—Periodicals
I. Pollock, J. G. II. McKay, A. J.
617'.414'05 RD598.5

ISBN 0 7236 0575 0

Library of Congress Catalog Card Number: 82-50072

Typeset and printed in Great Britain by
John Wright & Sons (Printing) Ltd at The Stonebridge Press, Bristol.

Preface

Within the past 30 years vascular surgery has moved from the phase of animal experiments to routine surgical practice. Inevitably, when reliable arterial conduits became available, there was an understandable but, in retrospect, inappropriate period of unbounded surgical enthusiasm. However, as the natural history of patients with peripheral vascular disease has become more apparent, so the selection of patients who will most benefit from surgery has become more accurate. This book attempts to review certain selected topics which currently challenge vascular surgeons world wide. While it is not intended to be a detailed surgical textbook, specific points of relevant technique are emphasized by each of the contributors. For the experienced vascular surgeon it will serve as a review and bibliography. For the general surgeon with an interest in vascular surgery it will provide an insight into the results that are attainable by acknowledged experts. For the surgical trainee it will provide a reference text which places the modern practice of vascular surgery in perspective.

Reconstructive surgery for occlusive aorto-iliac disease is not covered in this book, which deliberately dwells on the newer and, in some instances, pioneer areas of the specialty. The importance of the vascular laboratory in affording the surgeon accurate preoperative information is emphasized. Two important chapters have been written by physicians dealing with haematological factors and the medical management of patients with peripheral vascular disease.

The editors are grateful to each of the contributors whose practice of vascular surgery in both the United States and the United Kingdom has rightly earned them an international reputation.

As vascular surgeons, we must critically and continually analyse our results and it is hoped that this book will serve to provide a standard against which we should all judge ourselves.

J. G. Pollock
A. J. McKay

Contributors

D. Annis MD, ChM, FRCS
Consultant Surgeon, Royal Liverpool Hospital; Director, Biomechanics and Medical Physics Unit, University of Liverpool

Roger N. Baird ChM, FRCS, FRCS(Edin)
Consultant Surgeon, Bristol Royal Infirmary and Cossham Hospital, Bristol

R. M. Clarke MSc
Research Assistant, Biomechanics and Medical Physics Unit, University of Liverpool

Herbert Dardik MD, FACS
Chief, Vascular Surgical Service, Englewood Hospital, New Jersey; Clinical Associate Professor of Surgery, New Jersey Medical School, University of Medicine and Dentistry of New Jersey

Edward B. Diethrich MD
Section of Cardiovascular Surgery, Arizona Heart Institute, Phoenix, Arizona

Sushil K. Gupta MD
Assistant Professor, Division of Vascular Surgery, Montefiore Hospital and Albert Einstein College of Medicine, New York

Crawford Jamieson MS, FRCS
Consultant Surgeon, St Thomas's Hospital and Hammersmith Hospital, London

G. D. O. Lowe MB ChB, MRCP
Lecturer in Medicine and Honorary Senior Registrar, Department of Medicine, Glasgow Royal Infirmary

John Lumley MS, FRCS
Professor of Vascular Surgery/Assistant Director, Surgical Professorial Unit, St Bartholomew's Hospital Medical College, London

A. J. McKay MB ChB, FRCS(Glas)
Senior Surgical Registrar, Glasgow Royal Infirmary

G. P. Noon MD
Professor, Cora and Webb Mading Department of Surgery, Baylor College of Medicine, Houston, Texas

J. G. Pollock MB ChB, FRCS(Edin), FRCS(Glas)
Consultant Surgeon, Glasgow Royal Infirmary

C. R. M. Prentice MD, FRCP
Reader in Medicine, University of Glasgow; Honorary Consultant, Glasgow Royal Infirmary

D. Short MD
Cora and Webb Mading Department of Surgery, Baylor College of Medicine, Houston, Texas

Martin Thomas MS, FRCS
Senior Registrar, St Thomas's Hospital, London

Frank J. Veith MD
Chief of Vascular Surgery, Montefiore Hospital and Albert Einstein College of Medicine, New York

Contents

Foreword xi

1 **Measurement in Vascular Surgery** 1
Roger N. Baird

2 **Haemostatic and Haemorheological Factors in Peripheral Vascular Disease** 25
G. D. O. Lowe and C. R. M. Prentice

3 **Modern Vascular Prosthetic Materials**
I. Dacron 49
J. G. Pollock and A. J. McKay
II. Role of Expanded Polytetrafluoroethylene (PTFE) Grafts 57
Frank J. Veith and Sushil K. Gupta
III. The Glutaraldehyde Stabilized Umbilical Vein Graft: Experience with Lower Extremity Revascularization 63
Herbert Dardik
IV. The Need for Compliance in Prosthetic Arterial Replacements 82
D. Annis and R. Clarke

4 **Surgery of the Branches of the Aortic Arch** 88
Edward B. Diethrich

5 **Carotid Artery Surgery in Patients with the Stroke Syndrome** 112
John Lumley

6. **Abdominal Aortic Aneurysm** 135
J. G. Pollock and A. J. McKay

7 **Reoperation For Recurrent Arterial Occlusive Disease of the Lower Extremity** 161
G. P. Noon and D. Short

8 **Limb Salvage** 188
Crawford Jamieson and Martin Thomas

9 **Medical Management of Peripheral Arterial Disease** 211
G. D. O. Lowe and C. R. M. Prentice

Index 225

Foreword

by **H. H. G. Eastcott**
Consultant Surgeon, St Mary's Hospital, London

Events during the late 1960s brought an end to empiricism in vascular surgery and soon transferred it from a craft to a science. Travel between Europe and North America came within the reach of young postgraduates as well as the elder statesmen who had forged the earlier links. We have entered a more critical and progressive phase; our search is now for reasons as much as for remedies. This clearly has guided the Editor of this timely new book in the choice of his fellow contributors, all of whom belong to the second generation of eminence in this large and growing specialty. In the modern style, the outlining of the text rests more upon the strict examination of methods and results than seniority of long experience, though as a group the authors are old in wisdom and have learned well in the hard school of practice. Yet, they can still see that change is inevitable, indeed essential, in both the operating theatre and laboratory. Each of the chapters is concerned with a familiar area, though viewed with a new perspective which is both refreshing and invaluable. The book should help equally those whose whole work is in vascular surgery and the still larger number of general surgeons whose skills and inclinations take them often into this fascinating field.

Roger N. Baird

1 Measurement in Vascular Surgery

INTRODUCTION

A definition of the word measure is 'to ascertain extent by comparison with a standard'. In vascular surgery measurements are used to define the extent of disease before and after treatment. Symptoms and their relief are the most common measurements and tend to be subjective in nature, e.g. intermittent claudication or a transient ischaemic attack. Physical signs are usually more reliable, as with venous guttering and dependent rubor in severe lower limb ischaemia. Other clinical features are more variable. Arterial pulses and bruits can be felt or heard on one occasion and not another, and an ischaemic foot may be deceptively warm in the ward environment. Nevertheless, clinical features are the most important measurements so far as the patient is concerned. This chapter is concerned with methods for detecting disordered structure and function of the arterial system. Ultrasonic investigation now plays an important role in the diagnosis of lower limb arterial ischaemia and extracranial carotid artery disease. The use of Doppler flowmeters and real-time B-scanners will be considered, as well as invasive and non-invasive pressure measurements and pulse volume recordings. Contrast arteriography is the standard against which most methods are tested and will be discussed first.

ARTERIOGRAPHY

Arteriography is *the* definitive preoperative investigation and precedes almost every arterial operation. In skilled and experienced hands, irregular, narrowed and occluded segments are outlined with great clarity, and an unrivalled survey is provided of arterial morphology over a wide area. An inevitable drawback is the loss of a dimension in representing a tubular structure in only two dimensions on X-ray film. Theoretically a large number of multiplanar views are required to make an accurate image of a diseased artery, but in practice two or three projections are sufficient. Reliance on a single projection can result in an underestimate of arterial stenosis of up to 38 per cent diameter loss, according to a recent study. Oblique views are especially helpful in defining lesions of the iliac, profunda femoris (*Fig. 1.1*) and renal

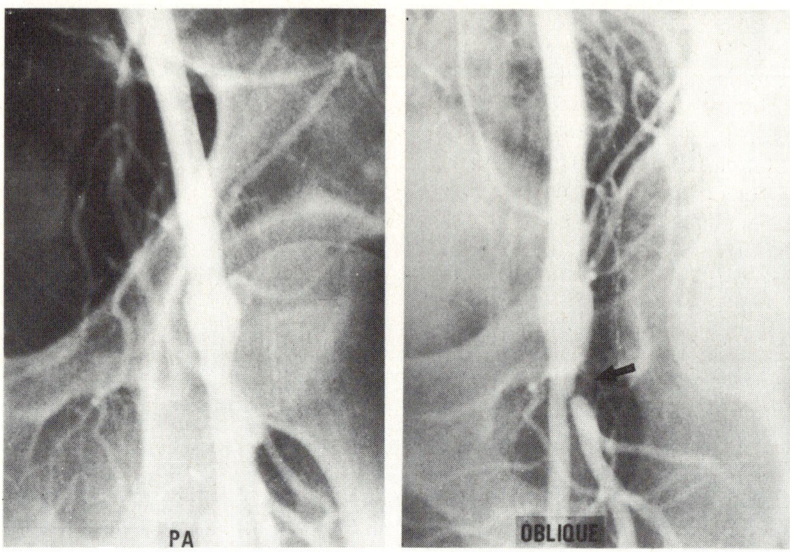

Fig. 1.1. Posteroanterior (PA) and oblique views of a Dacron arterial graft implanted to the common femoral artery. Note that the tight stenosis of the origin of the profunda femoris artery seen on the oblique view is not visible on the PA projection.

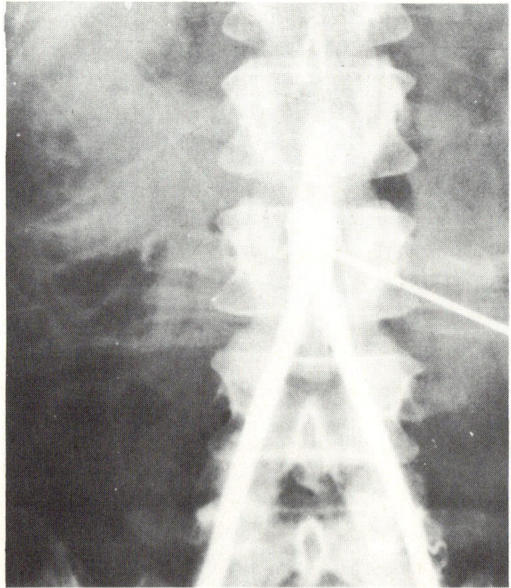

Fig. 1.2. Translumbar aortogram. The needle has been inserted below a complete occlusion of the aorta. Note the high aortic bifurcation and small vessels of a middle-aged female patient.

arteries; the origins of the mesenteric and internal carotid arteries are most clearly defined in lateral views. Other points of radiographic technique include the volume, concentration and type of contrast material and the timing of exposures following injection. Errors can lead to over-, under- or non-filling of patent vessels. Care must also be taken not to inject distal to a stenosis, as with aortic stenosis at the level of the inferior mesenteric artery (*Fig. 1.2*). Further, direct puncture studies of the carotid artery in the neck may fail to show narrowing at the origin of the common carotid artery.

Arteriographic grade is derived from the diameter ratio of the narrowest segment to the nearest normal artery. Difficulties arise at the origin of the internal carotid artery as the normally distensible carotid bulb is 150 per cent larger than the distal internal carotid artery (*Fig. 1.3*).

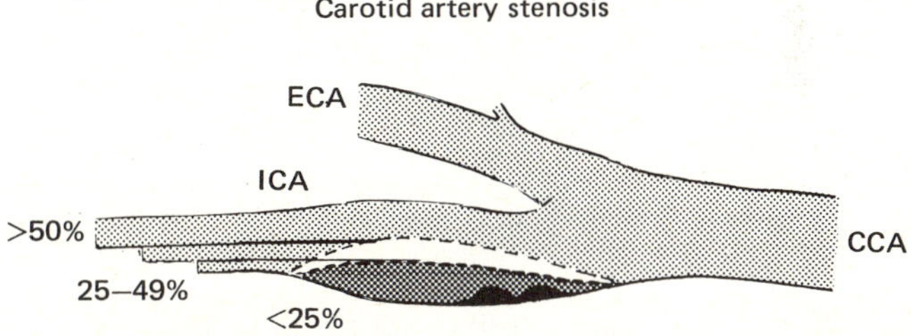

Fig. 1.3. Diagram of various percentage stenoses of the normally dilated carotid bulb compared with the distal internal carotid artery (ICA).

Subject to the foregoing, measurements of arteriographic diameter and percentage stenosis are the best available parameters of disordered arterial morphology.

LOWER LIMB ISCHAEMIA

Exercise-related Leg Pain

A diagnosis of intermittent claudication is normally made on the clinical findings alone. Problems arise where there is a good description of exercise-related leg pain and, surprisingly, the pedal pulses are palpable. In other circumstances, the pain is atypically constant in nature with paraesthesia and numbness suggestive of spinal stenosis. If, in addition to neurological features, the distal limb pulses are impalpable, the contribution of vascular impairment to the overall clinical picture is best quantified by ankle systolic pressure measurements using a Doppler probe.

Doppler Systolic Ankle Pressure (DSAP)

Measurement of calf or ankle systolic pressure was first proposed by Winsor and popularized in the late 1960s by Strandness, Carter and by Yao, who used a Doppler probe to insonate the pedal arteries (*Fig. 1.4*). The technique has since gained widespread acceptance and has supplanted the oscillometer in the consulting rooms of most vascular surgeons. In normal subjects the resting DSAP equals or exceeds the arm systolic pressure. A DSAP of <100 mmHg indicates severe arterial ischaemia. Pressures of 70 mmHg or less point to ischaemic rest pain and incipient gangrene.

In patients with incomplete stenosis of the iliac arteries or the popliteal entrapment syndrome resting ankle pressures may be normal.

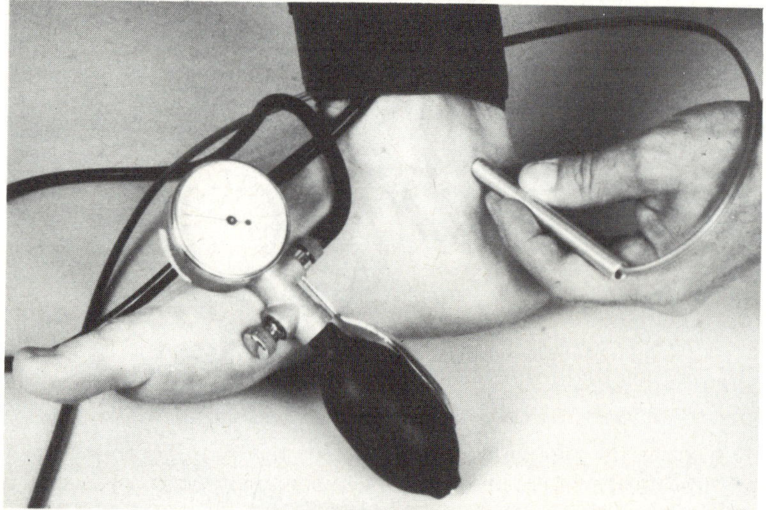

Fig. 1.4. Ankle systolic pressure measured with a Doppler probe.

In these circumstances, stress testing may reveal an arm/ankle pressure gradient. This useful test is performed using treadmill exercise, step-ups on to a bench or simply by walking; otherwise blood flow in the limb is augmented by cuff-induced hyperaemia or following injection of papaverine. Sometimes the systolic pressures are expressed as a ratio known as the ankle/brachial pressure index. Problems arise in the presence of increased arterial wall stiffness due to diabetes or vessel wall calcification, resulting in erroneously normal or elevated pressure readings.

Clinically, DSAP is a virtually indispensable measurement, but it may fail to correlate with the restriction in walking distance and several refinements have been proposed. These include detection at toe level of blood flow using an air-filled cuff or mercury strain gauge recorder, standardizing work done in the exercise test, and measuring the pattern of fall in ankle pressure and its subsequent return to resting values following exercise or hyperaemia.

Ankle Doppler Velocity Measurements

Damping of the Doppler velocity time signal from a pencil probe used to insonate the posterior tibial or dorsalis pedis artery is a sensitive indicator of arterial disease (*Fig. 1.5*). Changes in the audible or recorded Doppler signal can be detected easily in complete arterial

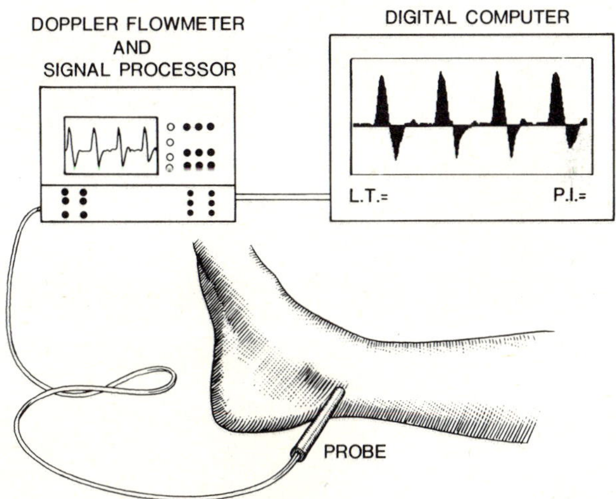

Fig. 1.5. Diagram of Doppler signals from the posterior tibial artery analysed as Laplace transform damping (LT) and pulsatility index (PI).

occlusions and in poorly collateralized stenoses. In milder disease states, numerous analytical techniques have been proposed to measure the loss of pulsatility. The height (or amplitude), acceleration time (or upward slope) of the wave form and crest time (or initial deceleration time) are the best manually derived discriminators of early disease. Waveform amplitude is affected by the angle of the Doppler probe with the insonated vessel and is somewhat variable even though the probe is always positioned to obtain a maximal signal. Computer-assisted frequency analysis of the shape of the Doppler signals is independent of probe position and can be used to derive pulsatility index (*Fig. 1.6*), Laplace transform damping (*Fig. 1.7*) or principal component analysis. These techniques for describing the waveform shape have produced

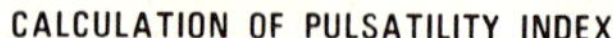

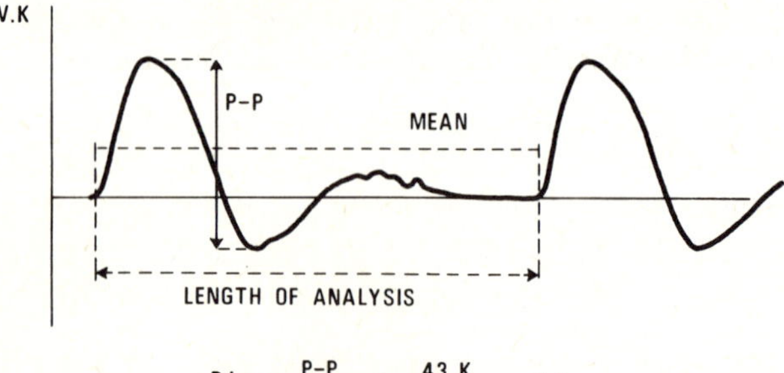

$$\text{P.I.} = \frac{\text{P–P}}{\text{MEAN}} = \frac{43\ \text{K}}{7\ \text{K}} = 6.1$$

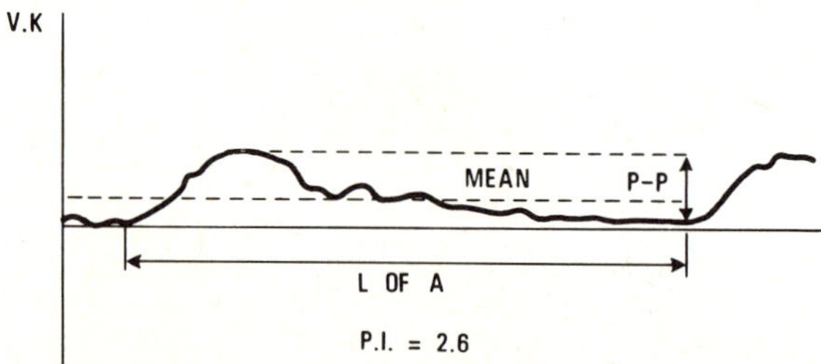

Fig. 1.6. Pulsatility index is the ratio of peak-to-peak to mean waveform amplitude. It is independent of the position or angle of the probe on the artery.

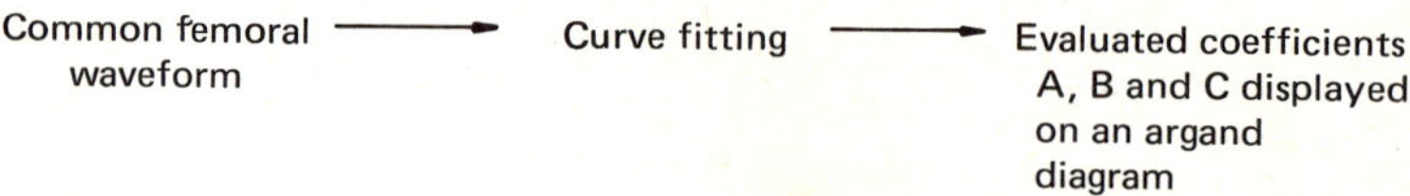

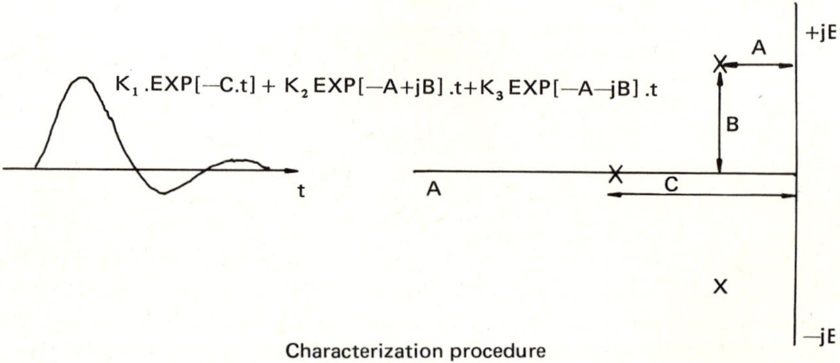

Fig. 1.7. Laplace transform damping is derived from a curve-fitting equation of the Fourier transform of the Doppler waveform shape. The relationships are expressed graphically on an Argand diagram.

encouraging results in preliminary studies from vascular laboratories in Bristol, Leicester and Southampton and from Guy's Hospital and King's College Hospital in London, as well as from Dutch and American investigators. Initially, analyses were used of sonograms from single waveforms. More recently, five consecutive waveforms have been averaged to minimize the effects of beat-to-beat variability of the pulse wave. More accurate waveforms obtained by maximum frequency following are superseding the earlier zero-crosser systems (*Fig. 1.8*). The signal processing equipment is at present bulky and complex, but technology is developing rapidly and a ready market awaits the successful manufacturer of a portable arterial waveform analyser for routine clinical use.

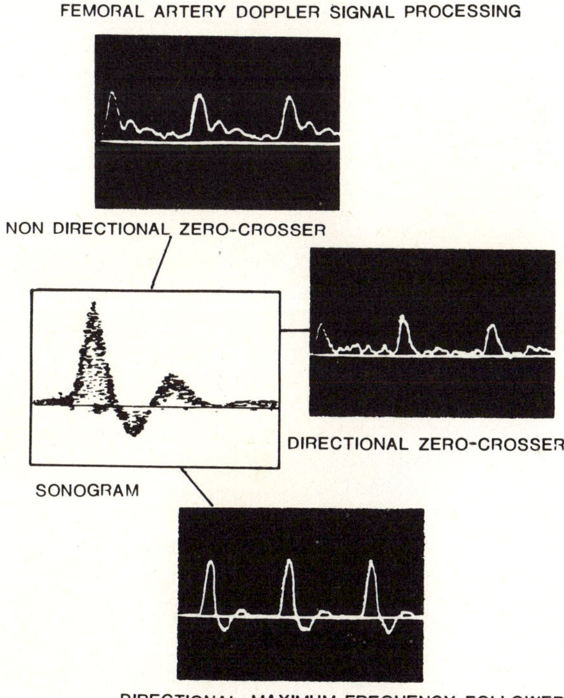

Fig. 1.8. Maximum frequency follower signal processing of the sonogram, showing increased accuracy compared with zero-crosser techniques.

Other Measurements in Early Arterial Disease

In the early stages of atherosclerosis there is thickening of the arterial intima. The elastic tissue of the media becomes fragmented with calcific deposits and increased collagen deposition. These early changes result in a loss of arterial distensibility, leading to the Doppler velocity waveform changes referred to above. The pulse wave velocity and its increase with stiffening of the arterial wall has been calculated from transit time recordings measured by simultaneous recordings from probes placed at a known distance apart. The time delay of the pulse wave to the arteries of the foot is delayed when vessels are completely occluded but not in early disease, whether the proximal recordings are from the heart (R wave of ECG) or from insonating probes placed in the suprasternal notch, abdomen or groin.

The relationship between tobacco smoking and the development of peripheral arterial disease is well established. However, only a small proportion (5–10 per cent) of habitual smokers—who at present comprise more than 40 per cent of the adult population—develop intermittent claudication. It is likely that some individuals are particularly susceptible to the effects of cigarette smoking. Patients with arterial occlusive disease exhibit an acute vasoconstrictor response to the inhalation of tobacco smoke (*Fig. 1.9*) which is not seen in most normal subjects. Repeated exposure to these acute changes will inevitably cause permanent arterial damage in susceptible individuals.

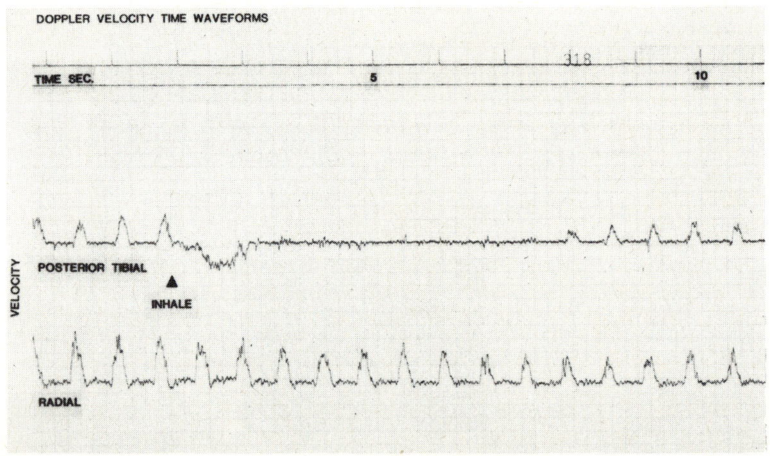

Fig. 1.9. Effects of smoking. An abolition of pulsatile blood flow in the posterior tibial artery after inhalation of cigarette smoke in an arteriopath, with reduction in radial artery amplitudes.

There are many abnormalities other than arterial pressure and flow velocity in patients with peripheral arterial disease. These include the following:

Blood Lipids

The relation of serum cholesterol level to intermittent claudication is much weaker than for other risk factors, particularly cigarette smoking. In the Framingham study, those with the highest cholesterol levels were at greatest risk of intermittent claudication, but otherwise no consistent gradient was observed. The high-density lipoprotein (HDL) cholesterol fraction may be protective, since it is inversely related to coronary heart disease development. In the Framingham population, high average cholesterol levels were ascribed to a diet containing a preponderance of animal fat and cholesterol, resulting in an increased frequency of obesity and atherosclerosis. The hypothesis that reducing the animal fat and cholesterol content of the diet with restriction of calories will maintain an ideal weight remains unproved. Nevertheless, the evidence is sufficiently convincing for many clinicians to give dietary advice to those at increased cardiovascular risk.

Haemorheology

Most patients with lower limb atherosclerosis are habitual smokers and show widespread haemorheological changes including polycythaemia, increased blood viscosity, hypercoagulability and reduced red cell deformability. Dormandy has drawn attention to the beneficial effects of haemodilution and plasmapheresis, as well as the use of pharmacological agents to decrease red cell aggregation and to increase the compliance of the red cell envelope (*see also* Chapter 2).

Sequential Arteriograms

These have been used to show progression and regression of non-occlusive arterial plaques. The measurements are fraught with difficulties and minor positional changes can substantially affect the appearances of follow-up arteriograms.

At present prevention is the main hope for those at risk, stemming the progression of early disease to advanced atherosclerosis by correcting cardiovascular risk factors. Disease of the blood vessel wall is the primary cause of death in over half of the population of developed countries, and is only exceeded in magnitude as a world problem by malaria and malnutrition. All too often the first manifestation of atherosclerosis is a stroke, myocardial infarct or ischaemic limb. These crippling cardiovascular events are of sudden onset and treatment frequently comes too late to be effective. Therein lies the importance of detecting arterial disease at an early and often asymptomatic stage.

Severe Lower Limb Ischaemia

There are few surgical procedures more rewarding than a timely arterial reconstruction which cures ischaemic rest pain and results in healing of ischaemic ulceration or gangrene. Most patients with severe limb ischaemia have widespread atheroma and an aggressive surgical approach is justified since the alternatives are to leave the ischaemic pain unrelieved or to amputate.

In most patients with chronic limb ischaemia the superficial femoral artery is occluded. The onset of worsening claudication, ischaemic rest pain, digital gangrene or an unhealed ulcer results from extension of occlusive or embolic atherosclerosis to include some or all of the aorta, common and external iliac arteries, common femoral and profunda femoris arteries and the calf vessels. The decision to do a proximal or distal reconstruction depends on the severity of aorto-iliac disease.

Disease above the Inguinal Ligament

Complete occlusion of the aorta or iliac arteries is readily diagnosed clinically by reduction or absence of the femoral pulse. The arteriogram serves to localize the level of occlusion and define any involvement of patent arteries on either side.

Difficulties can arise in the assessment of *incomplete* stenoses of the iliac arteries. The main treatment options are aortofemoral bypass, endarterectomy, extra-anatomical bypass and balloon (Grünzig) catheter dilatation. As mentioned earlier, the superficial femoral artery is usually occluded, and an additional factor is that the orifice of the profunda femoris artery is often narrowed. The aim of successful treatment is to improve arterial perfusion of the profunda femoris artery. If the degree of upstream stenosis is haemodynamically minor, a proximal reconstruction will fail to improve blood flow into the profunda femoris artery. On the other hand, some femoro-distal bypass operations will fail because of iliac artery stenosis of unrecognized severity. How can the risk of selecting the wrong treatment option be minimized? Good quality arteriograms are an essential first step, augmented by the pressure and flow measurements outlined below.

Arterial Pressure Gradient

The presence of a resting systolic pressure gradient is one of the most important parameters in deciding upon the significance of incomplete stenoses of the cardiovascular system. Iliac artery pressure measurements are most readily made by a catheter introduced from the femoral artery (*Fig. 1.10*). A pressure drop across a stenosis of 10 mmHg or more is usually regarded as significant. The effect of a stenosis on distal systolic pressure is magnified if flow through the iliac vessels is

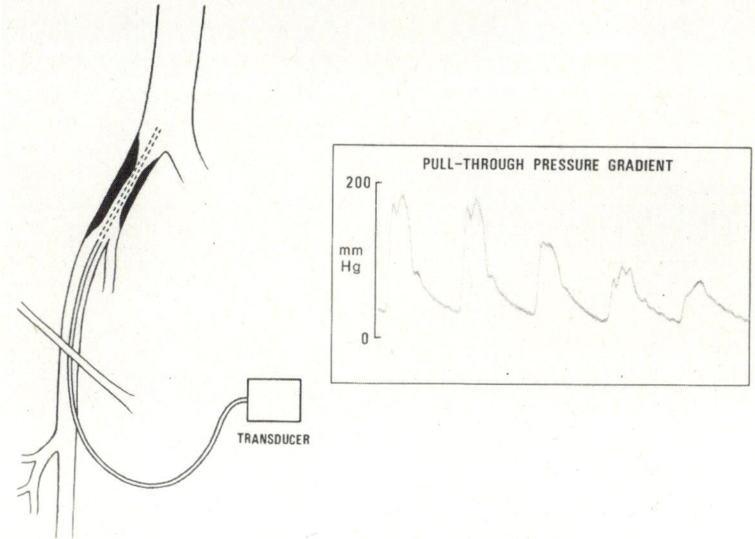

Fig. 1.10. Diagram of the measurement of arterial systolic pressure gradient across an iliac artery stenosis using a catheter 'pull-through' technique.

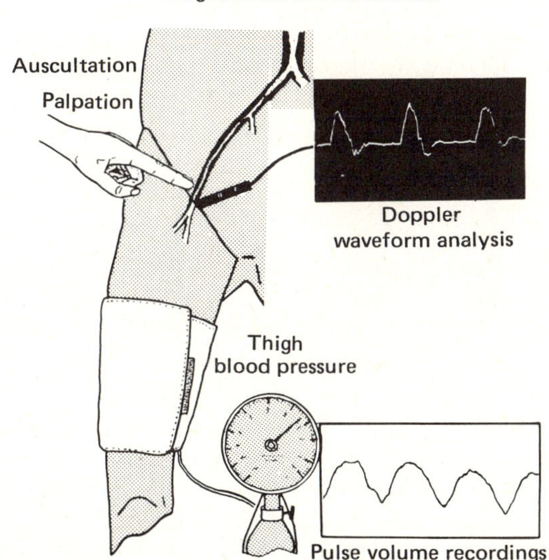

Fig. 1.11. Diagram illustrating the use of a Doppler probe on the femoral artery and also an air-filled thigh cuff in the diagnosis of iliac artery stenosis.

augmented by papaverine or cuff-induced hyperaemia. The pressure gradient across the aorto-iliac segment can also be measured at the time of translumbar aortography by recording the arterial pressures from the aortogram needle with a recording needle placed synchronously in the femoral artery.

Indirect pressure measurements are available in which the systolic pressure of an air-filled sphygmomanometer cuff applied to the thigh (*Fig. 1.11*) is compared with the brachial artery systolic pressure. Thigh/brachial pressure measurements have the advantage of being non-invasive, but reflect the state of the iliac arteries less precisely than direct aortofemoral recordings for two main reasons. First, segmental limb pressures of the wide tapering thigh are subject to a cuff artefact which makes them less accurate than cuff pressure measurements elsewhere in the limbs. In addition, thigh cuff pressure is reduced by atherosclerosis of the profunda femoris artery as well as disease of the common and external iliac arteries, and this can result in an over-estimate of iliac artery disease.

Femoral Artery Doppler Flow Velocity Signals

It is now possible to analyse Doppler signals from the femoral artery instantaneously to provide a numerical value that corresponds to the degree of iliac artery stenosis. Damped femoral artery Doppler signals in poorly collateralized severe disease are easily recognized both audibly and on the oscilloscope screen (*Fig. 1.12*), just as weak or absent femoral pulses are clinically obvious. In incomplete iliac artery stenoses Doppler waveform changes are not obvious audibly or

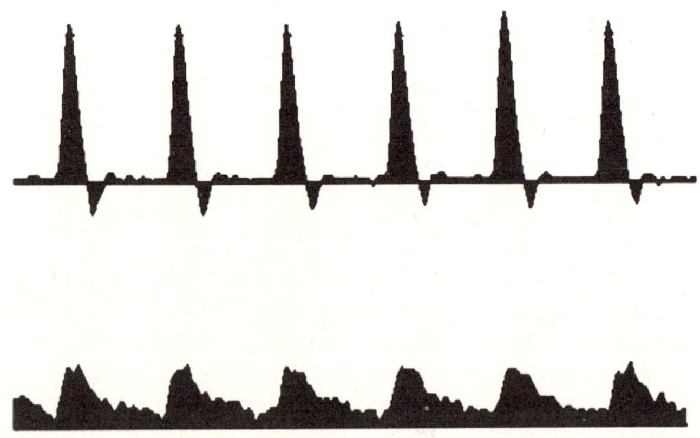

Fig. 1.12. Blood velocity/time waveforms of the femoral artery in a normal subject (*above*) and a patient with severe iliac artery stenosis.

visually but can be quantified as pulsatility index, Laplace transform damping and principal component analysis as described earlier. These numerical analyses of waveform damping provide useful corroborative evidence in deciding whether distal limb perfusion will be improved by a proximal reconstruction.

Care has to be taken that the Doppler probe insonates the common femoral artery, and not the superficial femoral artery, profunda femoris artery or other arterial branch. A second potential source of error concerns the degree of opposition to arterial flow distal to the probe. If this distal impedance is high, as in severe combined disease of the superficial and profunda femoris arteries, then pulsatile waves are reflected backwards along the arteries proximal to the high-impedance zone and can suggest upstream disease where none is present.

Disease above the inguinal ligament is generally amenable to arterial bypass. Proximal reconstructions result in excellent immediate and long term graft patency. In consequence, the indications for operation can be extended to include less severe degrees of incapacity provided that the patient is motivated towards a reconstruction and his general health is satisfactory. These last variables are difficult to measure and are often insufficiently acknowledged when defining the risk-benefit ratios of arterial operations.

Femoro-distal Bypass

A successful femoro-distal bypass depends on the arterial input to the graft at the common femoral artery being unimpeded by upstream disease. The femoral pulse must be of good volume on palpation and the aortogram should show that the input vessels are patent and of adequate diameter. Using the Doppler techniques for detecting aorto-iliac disease described above, Charlesworth's group from Manchester have shown an increased failure rate of femoropopliteal grafts if the pulsatility index at the common femoral artery is less than five.

The adequacy of the outflow tract is likewise a key factor. There is no substitute for expert arteriography to show the popliteal and calf vessels and the pedal arch. Not infrequently the vessels are inadequately opacified or overlie the dense cortical bone of the tibia. A repeat arteriogram by femoral puncture, injecting a larger volume of dilute contrast medium, can show a previously unsuspected patent peroneal artery (*Fig. 1.13*). In the example illustrated, a femoroperoneal graft resulted in the healing of digital gangrene.

The popliteal and distal arteries can also be opacified by direct needle puncture, either pre- or intraoperatively. Other imaging techniques, including intravenous isotope angiography, ultrasound imaging and intravenous xero-angiography, demonstrate arterial morphology less well. The results of digital subtraction angiography of this area are not

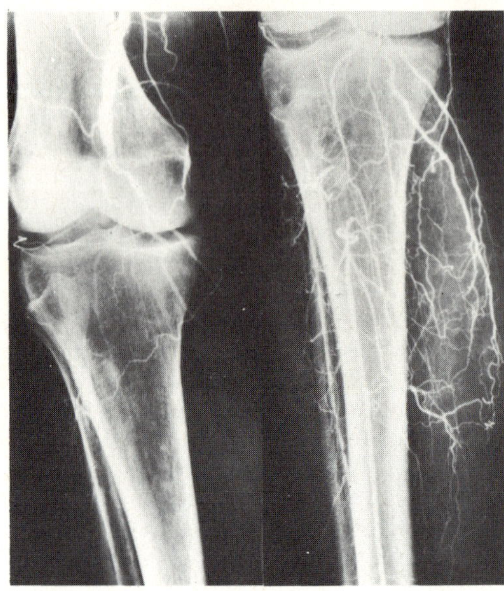

Fig. 1.13. Arteriogram showing absence of filling of calf vessels (*left*). Repeat study demonstrated a patent peroneal artery (*right*) to which an arterial graft was successfully attached.

yet available. Preoperatively the fall in systolic pressure from thigh to calf has been correlated with graft patency by Buth from Eindhoven, Holland. He found that large thigh/calf pressure gradients are associated with increased graft failures.

The degree of resting ischaemia at calf level can be measured by transcutaneous or intramuscular electrodes as low pH, low $P\text{O}_2$ and high $P\text{CO}_2$ levels. However, the practical value of these research techniques has not yet been established.

Amputations of the Ischaemic Leg

Selection of an appropriate level for amputation is of cardinal importance. Reliable measurement techniques are badly needed to judge whether healing is likely at the chosen level. It comes as no surprise that arteriography is unhelpful since arterial structure is shown but not the blood supply of the skin at the level of amputation. The simplest and most popular technique employs a portable Doppler probe to detect blood flow signals in the posterior tibial and dorsalis pedis arteries and to measure the systolic blood pressure below the knee.

There is a safe clinical rule for amputating just below the most distal palpable pulse. This rule will, if slavishly followed, result in an excess of above-knee amputations. Amputations at this level are associated with a high hospital mortality and a poor prospect of becoming mobile on a prosthesis. A Doppler probe can be used to identify the circumstances in which a below-knee amputation may heal even if the popliteal pulse is impalpable, as follows.

If Doppler signals cannot be detected at the ankle, or the calf systolic pressure is less than 40 mmHg, a below-knee amputation will invariably fail. However, below-knee amputations almost always heal where the calf systolic pressure is in excess of 70 mmHg, according to several published series. Some experienced surgeons can achieve healing below the knee with the preoperative calf pressure in the 40–70 mmHg range. However, a failed amputation subjects the patient to the risk of another operation and more than doubles his already long hospital stay.

Attempts to refine Doppler segmental pressure measurements by recording skin blood pressure have not achieved widespread success. Measurements by a radioactive probe of skin blood flow as a washout rate following the intradermal injection at tibial level of xenon-133 suggest that the critical rate for healing is 2·6 ml/100 g of tissue/min. These and other research techniques have yet to become accepted into routine clinical practice. Furthermore, there are many variables to be considered other than the state of the arterial circulation in the calf. For example, an established deep vein thrombosis is a serious adverse factor. Also, for a below-knee amputation to succeed, it is essential that the patient can and will extend the knee joint fully. Diabetics present special problems since neuropathic and septic foot lesions are frequently associated with a microangiopathy as well as atherosclerosis of the main leg arteries. Finally, operative technique is particularly important, and substantially better results are obtained by a committed team such as Robinson's at Queen Mary's Hospital, Roehampton, London, than if the amputation is routinely delegated to unsupervised surgical trainees.

CEREBROVASCULAR DISEASE

The use of carotid endarterectomy for the treatment of transient cerebral ischaemia and prevention of cerebral infarction is only possible if X-ray contrast arteriography shows an operable lesion. Arteriography is indicated if the clinical presentation is clear-cut, as is frequently the case, for both hemispheric transient ischaemic attacks (TIAs) and amaurosis fugax, especially if the ischaemic episodes are typical and recur at frequent intervals.

Arteriography

At Bristol Royal Infirmary carotid angiography is performed by percutaneous puncture of the femoral artery followed by selective catheterization of the aortic arch branches. Films of each carotid bifurcation are obtained in three projections, together with biplane views of the intracranial vessels and single views of each subclavian artery to show the vertebral arteries and their origins. Even in expert hands, these essential preoperative studies are not without a small risk of inducing a hemiparesis, and this has to be balanced against the probability of demonstrating an operable lesion. Other techniques have therefore been developed for use in patients whose clinical features are worrying and in whom evidence of carotid disease is required prior to arteriography.

Ultrasound and Related Techniques

There are four types of ultrasound instrument used to investigate the carotid arteries. These are the Doppler flowmeter, the Doppler scanner, the B-scanner and the Duplex scanner. Two related techniques, phonoangiography and oculoplethysmography, are also described.

Doppler Flowmeter

The basic Doppler instrument emits ultrasound waves continuously. Back-scattered waves are received by a transducer in the probe adjacent to the emitting transducer, and the instantaneous frequency difference between the emitted and received waves is measured (*Fig. 1.14*). *No depth information is available.*

The simplest application of this Doppler probe is in the periorbital artery occlusion test. In this test the supraorbital artery is insonated before and after digital occlusion of the superficial temporal and facial arteries. Occlusion of these branches of the external carotid artery in a normal individual results in augmentation of orthodirectional flow in the supraorbital artery. This response in the supraorbital artery is mediated via the ophthalmic branch of the internal carotid artery. If there is occlusion of the internal carotid artery or a poorly collateralized stenosis, supraorbital flow is reduced, abolished or reversed upon compression (*Fig. 1.15*). The test is simple to perform and an abnormal response is a good predictor of a tight stenosis. A normal response, however, does not rule out lesser degrees of stenosis or atheromatous ulceration.

Insonation of the carotid arteries in the neck using a Doppler pencil probe provides blood velocity/time waveforms in the region of the carotid bifurcation. Atheromatous plaques result in turbulence and disorganization of laminar flow which is seen as increased amplitudes in the lower frequency range of the Doppler sonogram. This change was described by Strandness as *spectral broadening*. Other waveform analyses have been used. Gosling's group at Guy's Hospital, London,

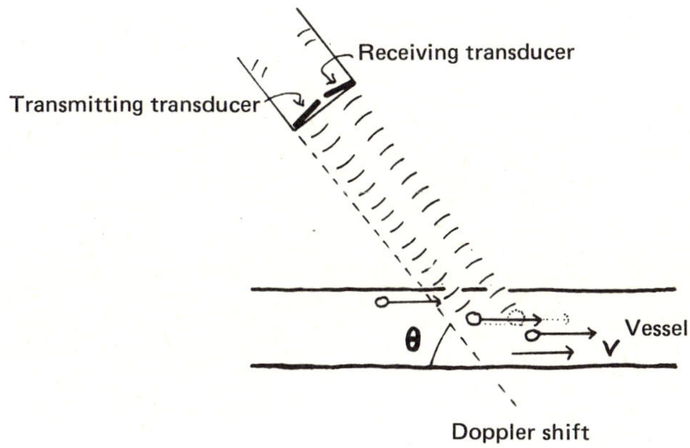

Fig. 1.14. Diagram of a continuous wave ultrasonic Doppler frequency shift detector.

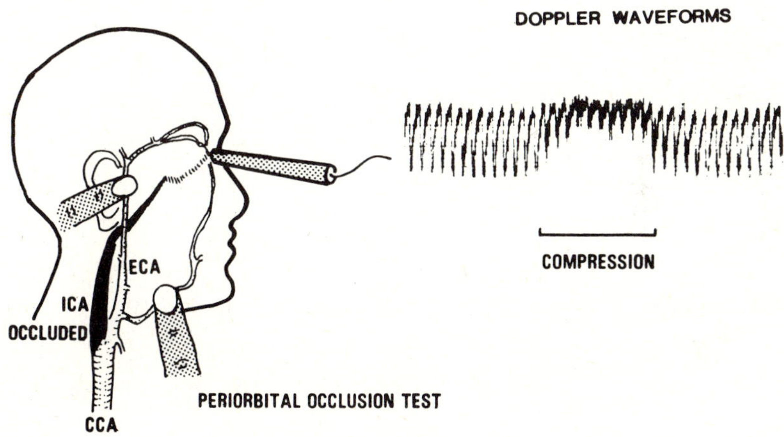

Fig. 1.15. Periorbital occlusion test. Changes in collateral blood flow patterns in a patient with an occluded internal carotid artery. Digital compression of the temporal and facial arteries results in diminution of blood flow in the supraorbital branches of the internal carotid artery (via the ophthalmic artery).

have expressed the increased diastolic flow component in the internal carotid artery in diseased states as the A/B ratio; Planiol and Pourcelot have used a resistance index, and so on. These changes in the Doppler spectrum help to detect stenoses of greater magnitude than mild wall irregularity. The accuracy of these techniques is greatly improved if an imaging system is used to localize the insonated vessel, as described below.

Phonoangiography

Auscultation by stethoscope of a localized bruit at the carotid bifurcation points to the presence of an atheromatous plaque. Lees, of Massachusetts Institute of Technology, Boston, has pioneered the analysis of the spectral content of carotid bruits to show a correlation with the degree of carotid stenosis on arteriograms. Analysis of sounds obtained from a microphone placed on the skin overlying the vessel as a frequency/intensity spectrum shows that the frequency beyond which the amplitude falls sharply—the break frequency—is directly related to the residual lumen diameter of the stenosis in millimetres. Although this technique may not separately identify disease of the internal from the external carotid artery, and will not detect complete arterial occlusion in the absence of a bruit, the residual lumen diameter can be predicted accurately and the technique is simple to perform. Again, the microphone can be more accurately placed at the carotid bifurcation if an imaging system is used.

Oculoplethysmography

The presence of a poorly collateralized carotid stenosis or occlusion results in reduced arterial pressure and delay in transmission of the pulse to the upper reaches of the internal carotid artery. These changes are detectable in the eye, since the ophthalmic artery is the first branch of the internal carotid artery within the skull. Reduced ophthalmic artery pressure can be usefully assessed by oculopneumoplethysmography (OPG). This method involves the application of suction to a small plastic cup placed on the sclera of the eye, resulting in increased intraocular pressure above systolic pressure and the abolition of ocular pulsations. Next, the vacuum applied to the eye cup is depleted until the arterial pulse is detected by a transducer connected to the eyecup. The degree of vacuum at which arterial pulsations return gives a measure of systolic arterial pressure within the ophthalmic artery and hence the intracranial internal carotid artery. Both eyes are tested synchronously and the side with reduced pressure is abnormal if (*a*) the ophthalmic artery pressures differ by 5 mmHg or more *or* (*b*) the sides differ by 1–4 mmHg and ophthalmic pressure is less than 66 per cent of the brachial systolic pressure. If this ratio is less than 60 per cent, the result is invariably abnormal even though the pressure on both sides is equal. Using this technique, Machleder's group in Los Angeles, California, have shown that at 5 years patients with a haemodynamically significant carotid stenosis treated non-operatively have a greater risk of cerebrovascular death, stroke and transient ischaemic attack than patients treated with carotid endarterectomy. Those with a normal test fared well without operation.

Doppler Scanning

Two Doppler scanners are currently available: both employ pulsed range-gated Doppler flowmeters which emit pulses of ultrasound of teardrop shape (*Fig. 1.16*). Reflected Doppler-shifted signals from moving blood within acoustic sample volumes each 1 mm^3 in size are received following a time delay which is proportional to the depth of

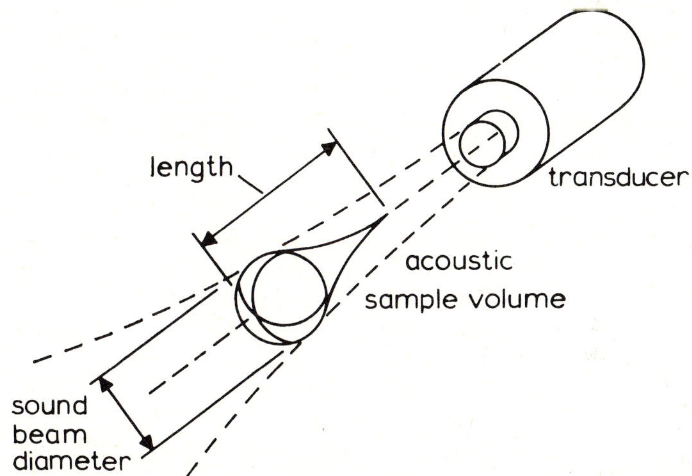

Fig. 1.16. A diagram representing the 'teardrop' acoustic sample volume of a pulsed Doppler, range-gated instrument.

the moving blood below the surface. This system provides depth information which is not available with continuous wave instruments (*Fig. 1.14*). By moving the transducer across the skin, an image of the moving column of blood is built up on a storage oscilloscope. The MAVIS instrument, developed by Fish, is a sophisticated 30 channel, 5 MHz system which produces images in anteroposterior, lateral and

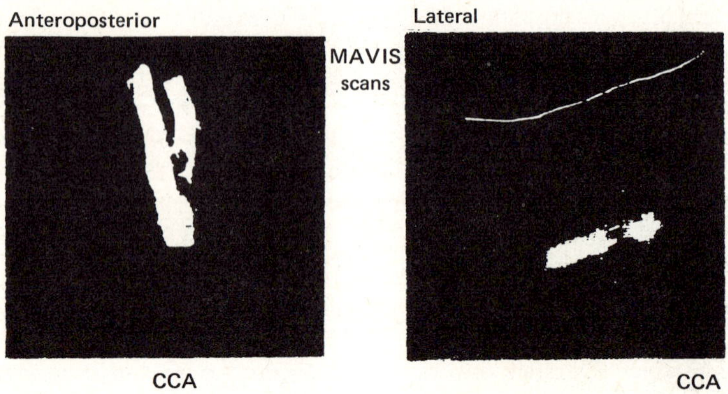

Fig. 1.17. MAVIS scans showing stenosis at the origin of the internal carotid artery (CCA, common carotid artery).

cross-sectional planes (*Fig. 1.17*). Resolution is of the order of 1 mm. The instrument has the facility for calculating volume blood flow from Doppler velocities and measurements of the diameter of the arterial lumen. A simpler, cheaper instrument developed by Hokanson is useful but less versatile than MAVIS.

B-scanning

Orthodox ultrasound B-scanners are currently in widespread use for displaying anatomical structures within the body. Abdominal aortic aneurysms are well shown. Sometimes occluded arteries appear to be patent because thrombus within the arterial lumen fails to reflect ultrasound waves, and Doppler sampling is necessary to establish patency.

Duplex Scanning

Duplex scanners are a combination of a real-time B-scanner and a direction-resolving pulsed range-gated Doppler flowmeter. Several instruments are now available, and can be used for a variety of purposes. For carotid artery studies a 5 MHz scanning head is used. The B-scanner demonstrates the arteries and Doppler flow signals are obtained from points of interest within the vessel lumen. Increased turbulence can be accurately localized adjacent and distal to vessel wall irregularities and narrowed segments. Atheroma at the carotid bifurcation can be studied before and after carotid endarterectomy (*Fig. 1.18*).

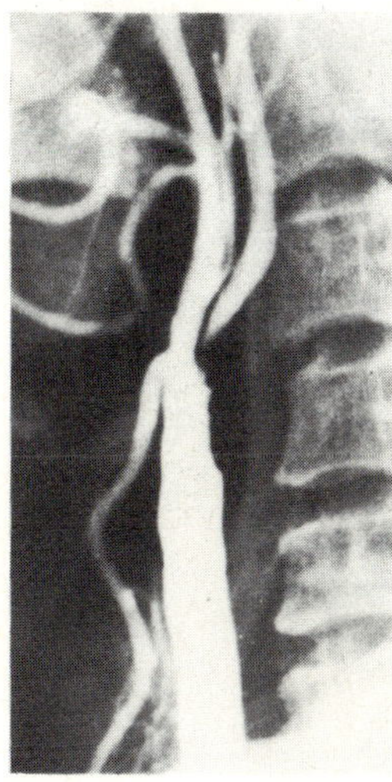

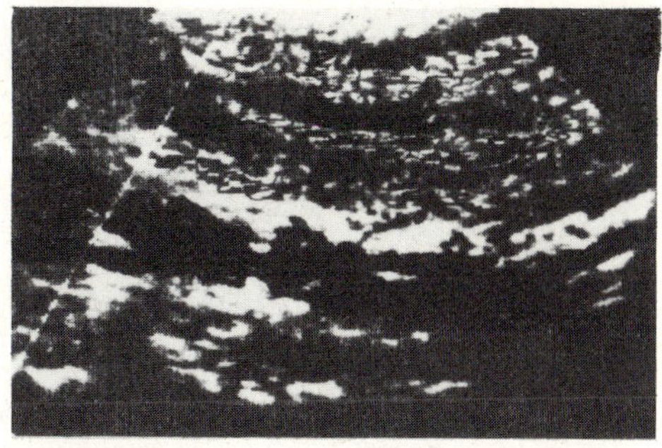

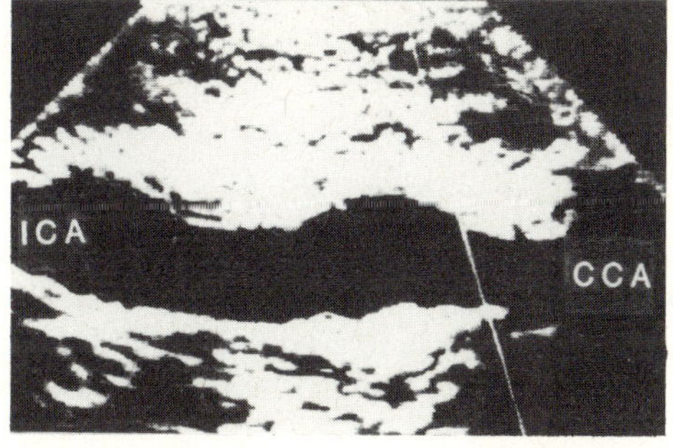

Fig. 1.18. Left, Arteriogram showing tight stenosis at the origin of the internal carotid artery (ICA), seen also preoperatively (*top right*) on real-time B-scan image of a Duplex carotid scan. The postoperative scan (*bottom right*) shows a widely patent lumen.

ABDOMINAL AORTIC ANEURYSMS

The abdominal aorta can be outlined from the level of the diaphragm and the common iliac arteries can be shown to the brim of the pelvis using B-scan at frequencies in the range 1-MHz. The extent of an aortic aneurysm is best seen on longitudinal scans and its diameter is measured from transverse scans. The ultrasonic outline of the vessel wall is unaffected by the presence of thrombus and is therefore more accurate than contrast aortography. Serial measurements will detect expansion in the size of an aneurysm, indicating an increased risk of rupture. CT scanning also demonstrates aneurysms well, and a left iliac aneurysm is shown in *Fig. 1.19*.

INTRAOPERATIVE MONITORING

The case for intraoperative monitoring rests on the elimination of early graft failures which are usually due to poor patient selection, errors in

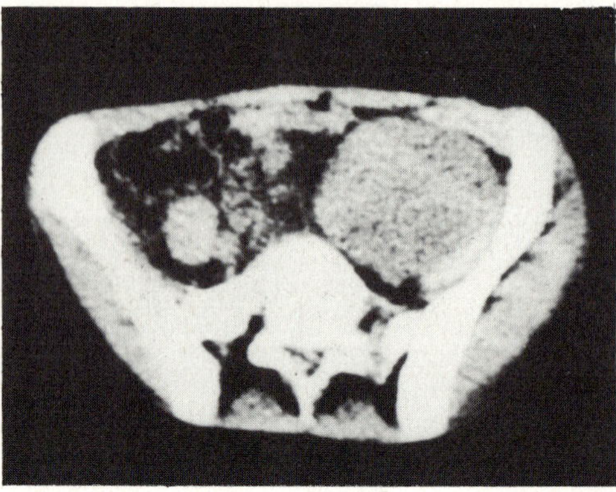

Fig. 1.19. CT scan of an aneurysm of the left common iliac artery. Note that the right common iliac artery is slightly dilated.

surgical technique or adverse operating conditions. Occasionally, a low flow graft may occlude in the early postoperative hours because of the combined effects of hypercoagulability and low cardiac output.

When, upon completion of a haemostatic anastomosis, the vascular clamps are released, the surgeon tests its success by palpating the distal host vessel to ensure that strong arterial pulsations are propagated well beyond each anastomosis. This qualitative test is restricted by limited access to distal arteries within the surgical incision. Pedal pulses are seldom palpable at this stage, and if doubt exists an operative arteriogram may be done to show any morphological abnormality (*Fig. 1.20*). Haemodynamic information can be obtained by insonating the vessels with a sterile Doppler probe or by applying an electromagnetic flowmeter. It is helpful to repeat the measurements after 15–20 minutes to allow conditions to stabilize fully following clamp release. The pulse volume recorder (PVR) has helped to provide immediate confirmation of a successful limb reconstruction. The PVR is a segmental air plethysmograph which is linked to the patient by an air-filled sphygmomanometer cuff applied to the extremity to be revascularized. The PVR recording corresponds to the arterial pressure pulse and typically is damped and of low amplitude prior to reconstruction; at 5 minutes after removal of the clamps, the PVR waveform shows increased pulsatility and/or amplitude. The recordings are repeated at 20 minutes and checked in the recovery room. The technique is simple and will confirm a good result in the majority of cases as well as drawing immediate attention to less-than-ideal distal perfusion so that the cause is actively sought and dealt with before the operative wound is closed.

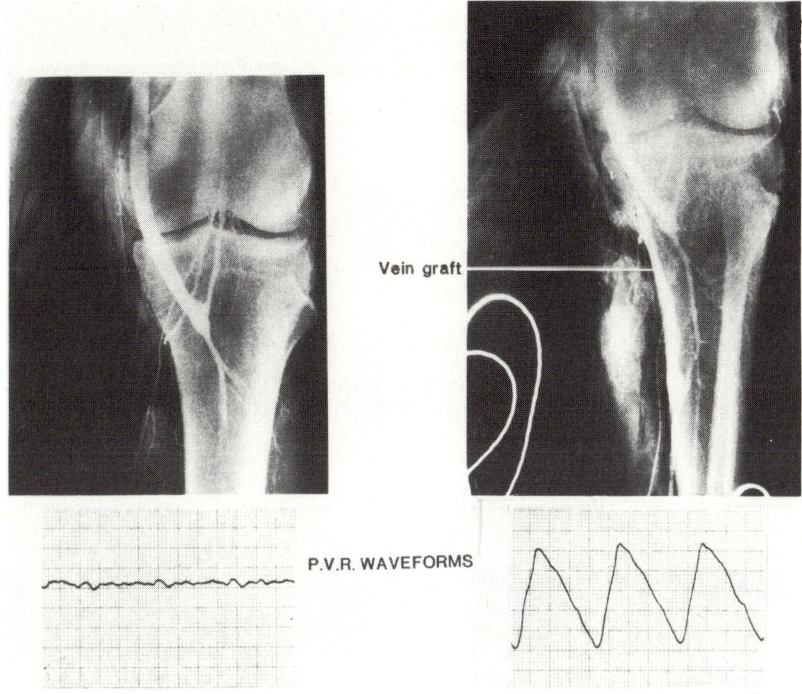

Fig. 1.20. Operative arteriogram (*left*) of a femoropopliteal graft that failed to result in pulsatile flow in calf pulse volume recordings (PVR). Repeat operative arteriogram after a graft extension to the peroneal artery (*right*) shows a pulsatile PVR.

CONCLUSION

The ultrasound, plethysmographic and related techniques described in this chapter provide a better understanding of the pathophysiology of arterial disease. These measurements are complementary to clinical evaluation and arteriography, and their use has resulted in a more precise assessment of the extent and haemodynamic effects of arterial diseases, as well as monitoring the results of treatment.

BIBLIOGRAPHY

General Reading

Baird R. N. and Woodcock J. P. (ed.) (1980) *Diagnosis and Monitoring in Arterial Surgery*. Bristol, Wright.

Dawber T. R. (1980) *The Framingham Study. The Epidemiology of Atherosclerotic Disease*. Cambridge, Mass., Harvard University Press.

Rutherford R. B. (ed.) (1977) *Vascular Surgery*. Philadelphia, Saunders.
da Silva A. and Widmer L. K. (1980) *Occlusive Peripheral Artery Disease: Early Diagnosis, Incidence, Course, Significance*. Berne, Huber.
Woodcock J. P. (1981) Special ultrasonic methods for the assessment and imaging of systemic arterial disease. *Br. J. Anaesth.* **53**, 719–30.

Lower Limb Ischaemia

Angelides N. S. and Nicolaides A. N. (1980) Simultaneous isotope clearance from the muscles of the calf and thigh. *Br. J. Surg.* **67**, 220–4.
Baird R. N., Bird D. R., Clifford P. C. et al. (1980) Upstream stenosis. Its diagnosis by Doppler signals from the femoral artery. *Arch. Surg.* **115**, 1316–22.
Baird R. N., Lusby R. J., Bird D. R. et al. (1979) Pulsed Doppler angiography in lower limb ischaemia. *Surgery* **86**, 818–25.
Charlesworth D., Harris P. L. and Cave F. D. (1975) Undetected aorto-iliac insufficiency: a reason for early failure of saphenous vein bypass grafts for obstruction of the superficial femoral artery. *Br. J. Surg.* **62**, 567–70.
Evans D. H., Quin R. O. and Bell P. R. F. (1980) The significance of blood pressure measurements in patients with peripheral vascular disease. *Br. J. Surg.* **67**, 238–41.
Hurlow R. A., Chandler S. T., Hardman J. et al. (1978) The non-invasive assessment of aorto-iliac disease; a comparison of dynamic isotope angiology with thigh/brachial pressure index. *Surgery* **84**, 278–82.
Johnston K. W. (1978) Role of Doppler ultrasonography in determining the haemodynamic significance of aorto-iliac disease. *Can. J. Surg.* **21**, 319–25.
Laing S. P. and Greenhalgh R. M. (1980) Standard exercise test to assess peripheral arterial disease. *Br. Med. J.* **1**, 13–15.
Robinson K. (1980) Amputation in vascular disease. *Ann. R. Coll. Surg. Engl.* **62**, 87–91.
Yates C. J., Berent A., Andrews V. et al. (1979) Increase in leg blood flow by normovolaemic haemodilution in intermittent claudication. *Lancet* **2**, 166–8.

Cerebrovascular Disease

Blackshear W. M., Phillips D. J., Thiele B. L. et al. (1979) Detection of carotid occlusive disease by ultrasonic imaging and pulsed Doppler spectral analysis. *Surgery* **86**, 698–706.
Busuttil R. W., Baker J. D., Davidson R. K. and Machleder H. I. (1981) Carotid artery stenosis—haemodynamic significance and clinical course. *JAMA* **245**, 1438–41.
Kistler J. P., Lees R. S., Miller A., Cromwell R. M. and Roberson G. (1981) Correlation of spectral phono-angiography and carotid angiography with gross pathology in carotid stenosis. *N. Engl. J. Med.* **305**, 417–19.
Lusby R. J., Machleder H. I., Jeans W. D. et al. (1981) Vessel wall and blood flow dynamics in arterial disease. *Phil. Trans. R. Soc. Lond. B* **294**, 231–9.
Padayachee T. S., Lewis R. R. and Gosling R. G. (1982) Detection of carotid bifurcation disease: comparison of ultrasound tests with angiography. *Br. J. Surg.* **69**, 218–22.

Intraoperative Monitoring

Baird R. N., Davies P. W. and Bird D. R. (1979) Segmental air plethysmography during arterial reconstruction. *Br. J. Surg.* **66**, 718–22.
Cotton L. T., Hamilton W. A. P., Horrocks M. et al. (1980) The detection and measurement of blood flow in arterial surgery. In: Taylor S. (ed.) *Recent Advances in Surgery, 10*. Edinburgh, Churchill Livingstone, pp. 65–91.
Courbier R., Jausseran J. M. and Reggi M. (1977) Detecting complications of direct arterial surgery—the role of intraoperative arteriography. *Arch. Surg.* **112**, 1115–19.
Prys-Roberts C. (1981) Cardiovascular monitoring in patients with vascular disease. *Br. J. Anaesth.* **53**, 767–76.

G. D. O. Lowe and C. R. M. Prentice

2 Haemostatic and Haemorheological Factors in Peripheral Vascular Disease

A review of haemostatic and rheological factors in peripheral arterial disease is timely, for in recent years there has been increasing interest in their relationship to atherosclerosis, thrombosis and vasospasm. The treatment or prevention of these disorders by modifying such factors in the blood or vessel wall has also attracted attention. In this chapter we shall review the relationships of haemostasis and blood rheology to arterial disease. Therapeutic aspects are considered in Chapter 9.

HAEMOSTASIS

Factors involved in prevention of bleeding or cessation of bleeding may be grouped as follows:

1. Vessel wall factors.
2. Platelet factors.
3. Coagulation factors.
4. Fibrinolytic factors.

Vessel Wall

Vessel wall injury may stimulate constriction of the vessel, which may allow temporary arrest of bleeding. However, the major mechanism securing permanent haemostasis is the formation of a platelet-fibrin plug—the haemostatic plug. There appear to be several mechanisms by which vessel wall injury could initiate activation of platelets and blood coagulation. In recent years much attention has focused on prostacyclin (PGI_2), a product of arachidonic acid and prostaglandin metabolism in the wall of both arteries and veins. Prostacyclin is a potent vasodilator, and is also the most potent inhibitor of platelet aggregation known. Prostacyclin is an unstable compound (half-life 3 minutes) which breaks down to the stable, inactive compound 6-keto-$PGF_{1\alpha}$. The concentrations of prostacyclin and the enzyme responsible for its formation (prostacyclin synthetase) are highest in the intima and decrease progressively across the vascular wall to the adventitia [1]. Conversely, collagen and other elements of the vascular wall which promote platelet activation increase in concentration towards the adventitia. Thus, vessel wall injury removes the 'protective' anti-platelet influence of prostacyclin and exposes blood to subendothelial substances that promote platelet activation and adhesion [1]. Vessel wall damage also initiates activation of blood coagulation. Exposed collagen activates the intrinsic pathway of coagulation, and release of tissue thromboplastin from damaged tissues activates the extrinsic coagulation pathway. The interaction of blood and vessel wall is summarized in *Fig. 2.1.*

Platelets

The first visible components of the haemostatic plug are platelets, which rapidly adhere to exposed subendothelial collagen: further platelets then aggregate to form an initial, friable platelet plug. The shearing action of blood flow may initially fragment this continually forming platelet-aggregate, but after some minutes fibrin strands can be demonstrated among the platelets, and this fibrin reinforces and stabilizes the plug. The platelets undergo autolysis and the plug is eventually composed of fibrin only. Platelet activation involves several stages—adhesion, shape change, aggregation, secretion, arachidonic acid metabolism and coagulant activity.

Adhesion

Adhesion of platelets to exposed vessel wall collagen and other subendothelial structures has already been mentioned: platelets adhere also to fibrin and to artificial surfaces in contact with blood (grafts, heart valves, shunts, heart/lung bypass and haemodialysis equipment)—such artificial surfaces, of course, lack platelet-inhibitory prostacyclin. Collagen appears to be the most important component of subendothelium in platelet–vessel wall interaction. Anticoagulants such as heparin and coumarin derivatives have little effect on platelet adhesion: on the other hand, prostacyclin release from the vessel wall inhibits adhesion [2]. The molecule which is related to coagulation Factor VIII (anti-haemophilic factor) is required for normal platelet adhesion. This Factor VIII molecule, which can be detected immunologically, is synthesized by endothelial cells and released into plasma. Haemophiliacs have normal plasma levels of the Factor VIII molecule, but the molecule lacks coagulant activity. On the other hand, patients with von Willebrand's disease lack the whole Factor VIII molecule, including that part required for platelet adhesion (Willebrand factor), and hence not only have defective coagulant activity but also defective platelet adhesion [2].

Platelet adhesion is also related to physical factors [2]. Shear rate at the vessel wall (ratio of flow rate to vessel diameter) appears to be more

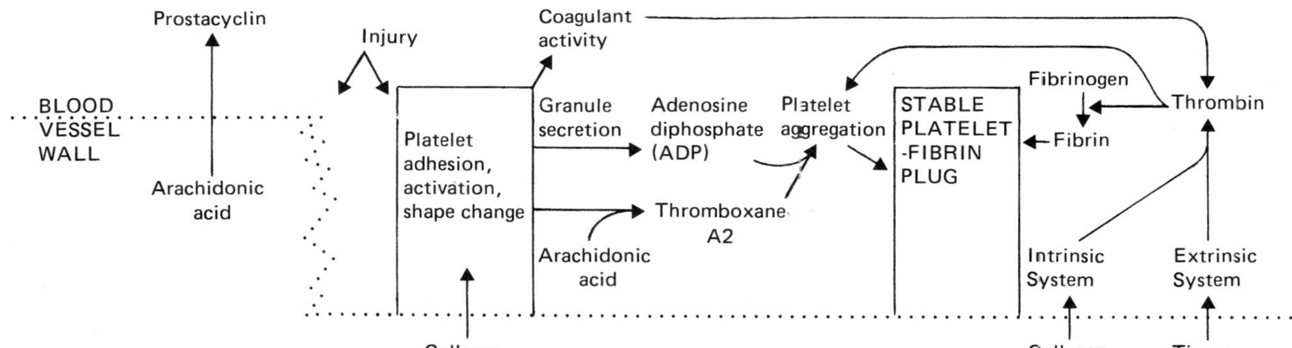

Fig. 2.1. Interaction of blood and vessel wall to form haemostatic plug. Vessel wall injury removes the inhibiting effects of prostacyclin on platelet adhesion and aggregation, and exposes flowing blood to collagen, which promotes platelet adhesion and aggregation. Exposed collagen activates the intrinsic pathway of coagulation and release of tissue thromboplastin from damaged tissues activates the extrinsic coagulation pathway.

important than flow rate. High shear rates increase the rate of platelet adhesion and are found in stenosed arteries, at bifurcations, and in arterioles and capillaries; whereas low shear rates occur in large arteries and veins. Red cells markedly enhance platelet adhesion, which therefore increases strongly with the haematocrit. This effect is partly due to physical factors (enhanced diffusion of platelets towards the vessel wall), but may also involve chemical factors (platelet-active factors released from red cells, or binding of prostacyclin by red cells).

Shape Change

Activation of platelets is accompanied by their changing shape, from a disc to a sphere with long pseudopodia. This shape change is due to contraction of a submembranous net of actomyosin filaments. While this shape change would be expected to facilitate adhesion of platelets to the vessel wall and to each other (aggregation), it may not be essential for these phenomena to occur [3].

Platelet Aggregation

Aggregation of platelets is essential for the formation of the haemostatic plug, as well as for platelet thrombus formation. Primary aggregation is not associated with arachidonic acid metabolism or platelet secretion (*see below*) and can be induced by ADP (released from red cells) or by thrombin (formed after activation of blood coagulation). Secondary aggregation follows platelet activation, arachidonic acid liberation and formation of thromboxane A2, and platelet secretion of ADP; collagen-induced aggregation is an example of secondary aggregation. Fibrinogen and calcium ions are required for platelet aggregation, and ADP-induced aggregation is associated with binding of fibrinogen to platelets.

Secretion

Activated platelets specifically release several compounds from their intracellular storage granules. Three types of storage granules have been identified [4]. Dense granules contain simple compounds, including adenosine diphosphate (ADP), adenosine triphosphate (ATP), catecholamines, pyrophosphate, serotonin (5-hydroxytryptamine or 5HT) and divalent cations. Alpha-granules contain proteins, including the platelet-specific protein beta-thromboglobulin and its precursor, platelet Factor 4 (which has anti-heparin properties); proteins which are also present in plasma and which may have entered platelets from the plasma by endocytosis—albumin, fibrinogen, fibronectin, coagulation Factor V; and other proteins with activities related to cell growth, vascular permeability, chemotaxis and killing of bacteria. Thirdly, vesicles which contain acid hydrolases have been defined. Of the released compounds, ADP, catecholamines and serotonin promote further platelet activation and aggregation.

Platelet Arachidonic Acid Metabolism

Upon activation of platelets, arachidonic acid is cleaved from membrane phospholipids by the enzyme phospholipase A2. Arachidonic acid is converted by the enzyme cyclo-oxygenase to cyclic endoperoxides, which are then converted by the enzyme thromboxane synthetase to thromboxane A2 (TXA2), a potent vasoconstrictor and inducer of platelet aggregation. Thromboxane A2 is an unstable compound (half-life 30 seconds), which breaks down to the stable inactive compound thromboxane B2 (TXB2). This platelet metabolism of arachidonic acid to thromboxane A2, a vasoconstrictor and platelet aggregator, can be contrasted with vessel wall metabolism of arachidonic acid to prostacyclin (*see above*), a vasodilator and inhibitor of platelet adhesion and aggregation. A balance between vascular prostacyclin formation and platelet thromboxane A2 formation may be important in platelet–vessel wall interaction and thrombus formation [1]. Arachidonic acid and thromboxane A2 stimulate platelet activation; however, platelet activation by other agents, such as thrombin, is not dependent on generation of cyclic endoperoxides and thromboxanes [5].

Coagulant Activity

Platelets promote blood coagulation in several ways [6]. The platelet surface may protect activated clotting factors from inactivation by inhibitors. Platelets appear able to initiate coagulation by the intrinsic pathway, and to facilitate coagulation by exposure of membrane phospholipid (platelet Factor 3). Finally, platelet Factor 4, released from platelet granules, has anti-heparin activity.

Coagulation

Fibrin is required to stabilize the initial platelet plug, and the conversion of circulating fibrinogen to fibrin requires the formation of the active enzyme, thrombin, from its inert precursor, prothrombin. Activation of prothrombin to thrombin may occur by two pathways. The intrinsic system is initiated by contact of blood with a non-endothelial surface (such as collagen): all factors in this pathway are contained within the blood (that is, intrinsic). Blood or plasma takes several minutes to clot by this pathway. Addition of tissue extracts to blood shortens the clotting time to several seconds: the tissue extract contains a lipoprotein clot-promoting factor (tissue thromboplastin) and this shorter pathway is the extrinsic system (*Fig. 2.1*).

The coagulation factors involved in these pathways are shown in *Fig. 2.2*: they are identified by Roman numerals from I to XIII. Tissue thromboplastin was formerly known as Factor III. Calcium ions were known as Factor IV: they are required at several stages, and blood samples are anticoagulated by adding sodium or potassium citrate, oxalate or edetate, which remove calcium ions. Factor VI does not exist. All other coagulation factors are plasma proteins. Fibrinogen is Factor I: prothrombin is Factor II. Factors I, II, V, VII, IX, X and XIII are synthesized in the liver: vitamin K is required for hepatic synthesis of Factors II, VII, IX and X.

Intrinsic System

Contact with a non-endothelial surface activates Factor XII to Factor XIIa, which then converts plasma prekallikrein to kallikrein. Kallikrein converts high molecular weight kininogen to kinins, peptides which mediate inflammatory reactions. High molecular weight kininogen and kallikrein are also involved in further activation of Factor XIIa to Factor XIIa′, which not only initiates blood coagulation, but also fibrinolysis (*see below*). Thus, Factor XII links three important biological systems: coagulation, fibrinolysis and the kinin system [7].

Formation of Factor XIIa′ results in sequential activation of four further coagulation factors (XI, IX, X and II). These four activated factors are enzymes with a similar biochemical active site (serine proteases). This chain reaction is a biological amplification system, trace amounts of Factor XIIa′ being capable of producing large quantities of thrombin. Naturally *coagulation inhibitors* have evolved to prevent excessive thrombin formation: the major inhibitor, antithrombin III, inhibits not only thrombin (IIa) but also the other three serine proteases (XIa, IXa and Xa). Heparin catalyses all these inhibitory actions of antithrombin III and hence interferes with blood coagulation at several stages, which may explain its potent anticoagulant effect [8].

The activation of Factor X by Factor IXa, and the activation of prothrombin by Factor Xa both require calcium ions and phospholipid (the latter derived from platelets). Factor VIII and Factor V respectively are also required as cofactors for these reactions. Thrombin converts fibrinogen to fibrin monomer, which polymerizes to insoluble fibrin. The fibrin clot is stabilized by Factor XIII, which is activated by thrombin and which again requires calcium ions.

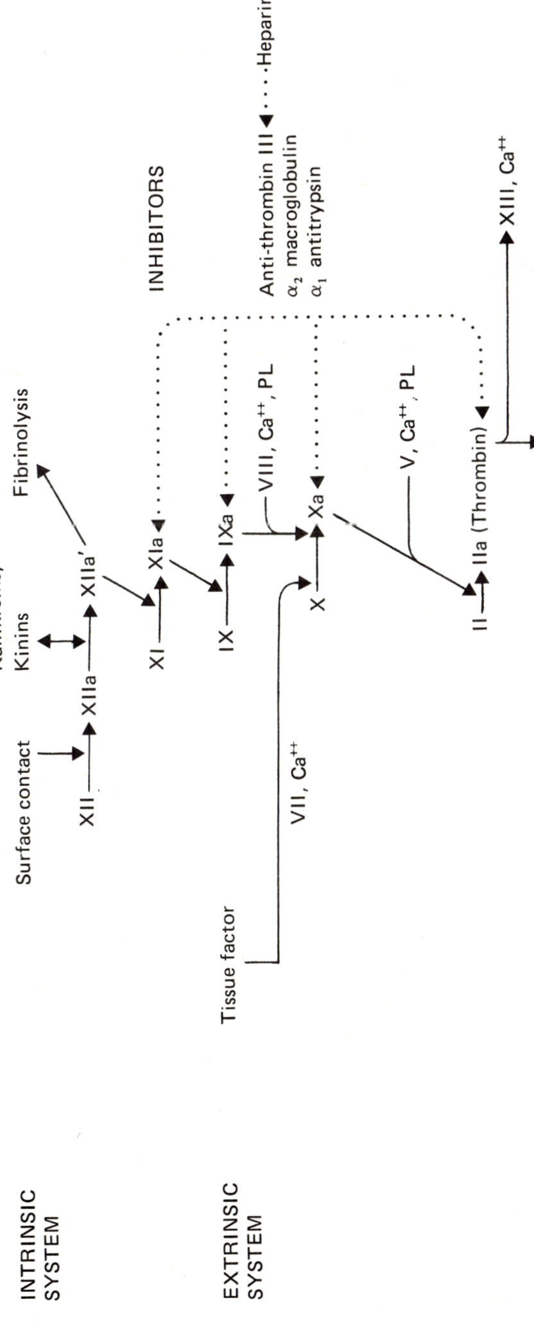

Fig. 2.2. The blood coagulation system. For explanation *see* text. (PL = platelet phospholipid.)

Extrinsic System

Tissue thromboplastin, Factor VII and calcium ions are able to activate Factor X without involvement of prior stages of the intrinsic pathway.

Fibrinolysis

The fibrin plug is eventually broken down by the specific fibrinolytic enzyme, plasmin, as well as by non-specific proteases from leucocytes and macrophages. Plasmin is generated from its inactive plasma precursor, plasminogen, by activators which can be demonstrated in tissues, plasma and urine. Characterization of these activators is limited compared with the coagulation factors. Tissue activators are found especially in the vascular endothelium of small veins. Plasma activators are derived mainly from release of endothelial activator, following stimuli including catecholamine release, exposure to other vasoactive agents and endothelial damage. Urine activator (urokinase) is synthesized in the kidney: it can now be produced commercially from tissue cultures as an alternative therapeutic fibrinolytic agent to streptokinase, which is obtained from streptococcal extracts.

Plasmin digests not only fibrin but also circulating fibrinogen and other coagulation factors (V and VIII). Fibrin and fibrinogen are degraded into small proteins and peptides (fibrinogen/fibrin degradation products or FDP). As with the coagulation system, potent inhibitors of plasmin and plasminogen activators have developed to prevent excessive plasmin activity: a recently discovered α_2-globulin, α_2-antiplasmin, is the major inhibitor.

An outline of the fibrinolytic system is shown in *Fig. 2.3*.

Haemostatic Defects

Vessel wall and platelet defects

Abnormal bleeding from vessel wall or platelet dysfunction is commonly manifest as purpura, bleeding from mucous membranes and excessive bleeding after trauma. Post-traumatic bleeding usually arises immediately after trauma, and may be controlled by pressure. The most helpful initial investigations are the platelet count and the bleeding time. Thrombocytopenia (platelet count less than 150×10^9/l) may be associated with post-traumatic bleeding when the platelet count is less than 100×10^9/l, and with spontaneous bleeding when less than 50×10^9/l. Bone-marrow biopsy is usually indicated and will reveal causes of decreased platelet production, which include aplasia (e.g. from radiation, chemicals or drugs), neoplasia (e.g. leukaemia, lymphoma, metastatic carcinoma) and megaloblastic anaemia (due to deficiency of vitamin B12 or folic acid). Thrombocytopenia may also be due to increased platelet destruction, which occurs in the defibrination

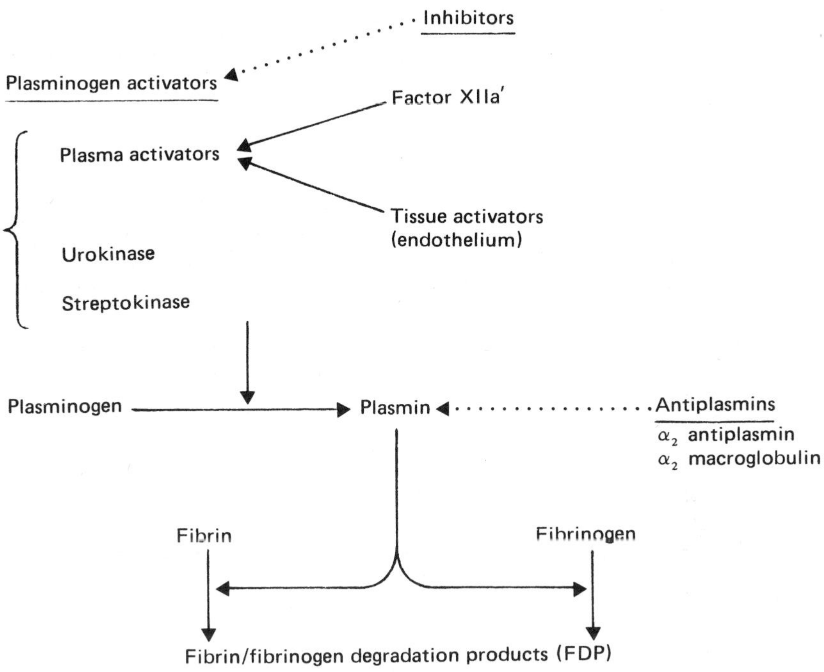

Fig. 2.3. The fibrinolytic system. For explanation *see* text.

syndrome (*see below*) or as a result of immunological abnormalities—idiopathic thrombocytopenic purpura (ITP) probably falls into this group. Splenic pooling of platelets causes thrombocytopenia in patients with splenomegaly from several causes (hypersplenism).

Prolongation of the bleeding time with a normal platelet count suggests either a defect in platelet function or a vessel wall defect. Platelet function defects are revealed by testing platelet aggregation in response to agents such as ADP, adrenaline, collagen and thrombin in a photometric aggregometer, and sometimes by other platelet function tests. There are several uncommon congenital disorders of platelet function; acquired defects are common and include drug effects (aspirin and other non-steroidal anti-inflammatory agents, dextrans, high-dose penicillins), renal failure and myeloproliferative disorders [9]. As discussed above, the congenital disorder, von Willebrand's disease, is associated with defective platelet adhesion to glass and collagen: platelets also fail to aggregate in response to the antibiotic ristocetin. These abnormalities of platelet function are due to deficiency of the Factor VIII molecule, and are reversed by therapeutic infusion of Factor VIII concentrates. Vessel wall defects include rare congenital connective tissue disorders, senile purpura due to collagen atrophy with age, deficiency of vitamin C which is required for connective tissue synthesis, corticosteroid excess which causes catabolism of connective tissue, and vasculitis due to septicaemia (e.g. meningococcal infection), allergy (e.g. Henoch–Schönlein purpura) or connective tissue disorders.

Coagulation factor deficiencies

Coagulation factor deficiencies manifest as extensive skin bruising, muscle haematomas, haemarthrosis, bleeding from mucous membranes and post-traumatic bleeding which may be delayed for hours or days and which is not controlled by pressure. Three clotting time tests commonly performed as a 'coagulation screen' are the activated partial thromboplastin time, which tests the intrinsic pathway, the prothrombin time, which tests the extrinsic pathway, and the thrombin time, which tests the conversion of fibrinogen to fibrin. Congenital deficiencies are rare with the exception of haemophilia A (Factor VIII deficiency) and haemophilia B (Factor IX deficiency), which are both sex-linked recessive disorders and hence manifest in males but are transmitted by female 'carriers' who are usually asymptomatic. The activated partial thromboplastin time is prolonged in the haemophilias, and specific coagulation factor assays establish which factor is deficient. Common causes of extrinsic coagulation defects (prolonged prothrombin time) include liver disease (defective hepatic synthesis of clotting factors), vitamin K deficiency due to biliary obstruction or malabsorption and oral anticoagulant drugs which antagonize vitamin K. Heparin increases the ability of antithrombin III to inactivate several coagulation factors (*see above*), resulting in prolongation of all clotting times.

In the absence of heparin, a prolonged thrombin time suggests the defibrination syndrome, which may complicate surgery and a wide variety of conditions, including obstetric accidents, malignant disease, septicaemia, burns and transfusion of incompatible blood. In such illnesses there is massive activation of blood coagulation, due to widespread endothelial damage and/or release of tissue thromboplastin into the circulation. Consequently, small platelet-fibrin thrombi are deposited diffusely in small blood vessels (disseminated intravascular coagulation or DIC), damaging vital organs such as the lungs (hypoxia, oedema, infiltrates, 'shock lung'), brain (confusion, coma), heart (hypotension, dysrhythmias), kidney (renal failure) and red blood cells (fragmentation of red cells by fibrin strands in small blood vessels—these 'chopped cells' may be seen on the blood film and result in microangiopathic haemolytic anaemia). These abnormalities may be overlooked in sick patients and disseminated intravascular coagulation diagnosed only when the patient starts to bleed due to defibrination. Following widespread thrombosis there is secondary activation of the fibrinolytic system, resulting in plasmin digestion of fibrin and fibrinogen and the formation of high concentrations of circulating fibrin/fibrinogen degradation products (FDP), which inhibit thrombin activity as well as fibrin polymerization. Plasmin also digests other coagulation factors (VIII, V), and platelets are consumed in the thrombotic process. Bleeding results from these multiple haemostatic defects. Laboratory tests show a prolonged thrombin time (due to low plasma fibrinogen levels and the effects of increased FDP), high levels of circulating FDP and thrombocytopenia. Management includes treatment of the underlying illness and replacement infusions of blood, plasma, clotting factor concentrates and platelet concentrates.

Haemostatic Factors in Peripheral Arterial Disease

From the previous section it is apparent that bleeding may arise from deficient vessel walls, platelets or coagulation factors; or from increased fibrinolytic activity. In developed countries life and limb are now threatened more commonly by ischaemia than by bleeding, and many workers have investigated the possibility that processes contributing to ischaemia (atherosclerosis, thrombosis, embolism, spasm) may be related to excessive haemostatic activities (whether of vessel walls, platelets or coagulation), or to decreased fibrinolytic activity. The literature on these relationships is vast, and their interpretation is difficult [10]. Nevertheless, it is quite plausible that such investigations will progressively increase our understanding of the pathogenesis of ischaemia and open up new therapeutic possibilities.

Haemostatic Factors, Thrombosis and Atherosclerosis

Non-traumatic arterial thrombosis usually occurs on atherosclerotic plaques, especially ulcerated or fissured plaques. In addition, most workers now recognize that thrombosis may contribute to the growth of atherosclerotic plaques [11]. Since arterial thrombi and atherosclerotic plaques contain material derived from platelets, as well as fibrin, it is conceivable that haemostatic abnormalities could promote not only thrombosis, but also atherosclerosis following incorporation of mural thrombi into atherosclerotic plaques.

Recent work raises the possibility that platelets and clotting factors may also contribute to atherosclerotic plaques independently of thrombosis. Ross and Glomset [12] have identified a factor released by platelets during secretion (*see above*) which promotes proliferation of arterial wall smooth muscle cells. It is therefore possible that platelets that adhere to exposed subendothelial connective tissue could release such substances, which might then diffuse into the artery wall and promote proliferation of smooth muscle cells from the arterial wall media into the intima, forming arterial lesions. As regards coagulation factors, Smith et al. [13] have shown that not only lipoproteins, but also other plasma proteins including clotting factors such as fibrinogen, are present in arterial intima. It appears that clotting factors infiltrate the arterial wall from the plasma, as well as being incorporated into the arterial wall as components of mural thrombi. Developing arterial lesions accumulate fibrinogen more than lipoprotein [13].

Atheromatous lesions also contain fibrin, which appears to bind not only lipoprotein but also clotting factors. The ratio of bound clotting factors to bound coagulation inhibitors is increased, favouring further fibrin formation: thus a self-amplifying system appears to exist in the arterial wall [14].

There appears to be a reasonable pathological basis for the involvement of haemostatic factors in atherosclerosis and arterial thrombosis. What is the evidence that these haemostatic factors are related to peripheral occlusive arterial disease?

Vessel Wall

The role of prostacyclin in preventing platelet adhesion and aggregation on the vessel wall has been previously mentioned. Prostacyclin synthetase—the enzyme generating prostacyclin—is inhibited by lipid peroxides, and Szczeklik [15] has summarized evidence that increased lipid peroxides promote atherosclerosis by inhibiting arterial prostacyclin formation. Prostacyclin deficiency has been reported in atherosclerotic lesions [16] and in diabetes [17]; studies of prostacyclin production in peripheral arterial disease are awaited.

Platelets

Platelet behaviour can be assessed in several ways: the relationships between the various tests have yet to be clearly defined. Methodologies are also diverse, and many illnesses and commonly used drugs alter platelet behaviour. Therefore it is not surprising that reports of platelet behaviour in atherosclerosis are often conflicting. Reported abnormalities include a shortened bleeding time [18], increased platelet turnover [19, 20], decreased platelet count and increased mean platelet volume [18] and increased platelet adhesiveness [21]. Platelet aggregation *in vitro* is usually measured photometrically after exposure to aggregating agents such as ADP, adrenaline, collagen or thrombin: patients with peripheral arterial disease have been reported to have increased aggregation [22], normal aggregation [20] or decreased aggregation [18, 23]. Wu and Hoak [24] reported an increased frequency of 'spontaneous' aggregation in the photometer, that is, aggregation without addition of aggregating agents. Lowe et al. [25] described increased 'circulating' platelet aggregates in patients with ischaemic rest pain, measured by formalin fixation in freshly drawn blood. Platelet secretion *in vivo* can be assessed by plasma levels of beta-thromboglobulin or platelet Factor 4, proteins which are secreted from platelet alpha-granules and which are measured by radioimmunoassay. Cella et al. [20] reported increased plasma beta-thromboglobulin levels in peripheral arterial disease.

Coagulation

Blood coagulation may also be assessed in several ways. Patients with peripheral arterial disease have been reported to have shortened clotting times [26] and increased levels of clotting factors such as fibrinogen [26–28] and Factor VIII [26]. Banerjee et al. [29] reported decreased levels of the coagulation inhibitor, antithrombin III, but other groups have not confirmed this (26). There is little evidence for increased intravascular fibrin formation in peripheral arterial disease, as measured by increased levels of circulating soluble fibrin or fibrin degradation products.

Fibrinolysis

Decreased blood fibrinolytic activity in peripheral arterial disease has been reported [26, 30–32]; Browse et al. [33] also reported decreased fibrinolytic activity of vein walls, but the relevance of *venous* fibrinolysis to arterial disease is not known. Decreased levels of the fibrinolytic inhibitor, α_2-antiplasmin, have been recently reported [34].

Interpretation of these associations of peripheral arterial disease with blood tests is difficult. The relationship may be cause, consequence or coincidence. While increased platelet or coagulation activities or decreased fibrinolytic activity may promote thrombosis or atherosclerosis, it is also possible that these blood abnormalities may *result* from extensive arterial disease and endothelial damage [26]. Alternatively, they may be related to 'risk factors' for arterial disease such as age, cigarette smoking, hypertension, hyperlipidaemia and diabetes [10]. Larger studies with multivariate analysis are required to resolve this problem.

Dormandy et al. [35] associated high fibrinogen levels with poor prognosis in patients with peripheral arterial disease. However this association could be due to correlations with other factors such as smoking, which is associated with adverse prognosis [28].

Haemostatic Factors and Arterial Grafts

Platelets and fibrin are deposited from the blood on to prosthetic arterial grafts. Eventually a pseudo-intima develops, but despite newer, less thrombogenic materials there remains a risk of graft occlusion by platelet–fibrin thrombus, especially in the first year. Kinetic studies using radio-labelled platelets and fibrinogen have shown increased platelet turnover for 9 months, and increased fibrinogen consumption for 6 months, after Dacron aortofemoral grafting [36]. Hamer et al. [37] associated increased platelet adhesiveness and plasma fibrinogen, and decreased fibrinolysis, with the prognosis for graft occlusion. Postlethwaite [38] and Harris et al. [39] also associated raised fibrinogen levels with subsequent graft occlusion. However, once again these associations may reflect correlations with other factors such as smoking, which increases the risk of graft occlusion [40].

Haemostatic Factors and Cardiac Embolism

Patients with diseased or prosthetic heart valves have been reported to have increased platelet turnover, especially in patients with embolism [41, 42] and increased platelet secretion as measured by plasma levels of platelet Factor 4 or β-thromboglobulin [43]. These abnormalities are presumably related to interaction of platelets with the abnormal valves.

Haemostatic Factors and Raynaud's Syndrome

While the cause of Raynaud's syndrome remains obscure, there have been several recent reports of abnormal haemostasis. Blunt et al. [26] observed increased platelet aggregation to ADP and increased Factor VIII in females with Raynaud's syndrome, and shortened clotting time and decreased fibrinolytic activity in males with vibration-induced Raynaud's syndrome. Zahavi et al. [44] reported increased platelet secretion (plasma β-thromboglobulin level) and increased platelet aggregation to ADP. These abnormalities were reversed by plasma exchange, which also appeared to induce clinical improvement. It is not known whether these haemostatic changes reflect ischaemic endothelial damage secondary to vascular spasm, or whether haemostatic factors are involved in production of the vasoconstriction. With regard to the latter possibility, it has been mentioned that activated platelets produce thromboxane A_2, which is a potent vasoconstrictor.

Platelets and Microvascular Ischaemia

Patients with recurrent attacks of pain and cyanosis in the fingers and toes, with normal pulses, have been reported to have various platelet abnormalities. These include high platelet counts (e.g. in myeloproliferative diseases), 'spontaneous' aggregation *in vitro* and increased 'circulating' platelet aggregates. The symptoms respond to aspirin, which inhibits platelet aggregation [45–47].

HAEMORHEOLOGY

In contrast to the obvious anatomical obstructions to blood flow (atherosclerosis, thromboembolism, spasm), the intrinsic flow-resisting properties of blood have received relatively little attention as possible causes of ischaemia. However, in recent years there has been increasing clinical interest in blood rheology [48, 49] not least because 'if you can't change the vessel, you can at least change the blood'. As regards tissue perfusion, improvement in the flow properties of blood is a logical and feasible therapeutic alternative to improvement of vessel calibre.

Rheology is the study of deformation and flow of matter, and haemorheology is the study of the flow properties of blood. Blood viscosity is the property which has received most attention: viscosity describes the resistance of a liquid to flow, and is the reciprocal of fluidity. Resistance within a flowing liquid arises from internal friction between adjacent 'streamlines', which move parallel to each other (shearing). The applied force which produces shearing is termed the 'shear stress', and the resulting gradient of velocity across the sheared fluid is termed the 'shear rate'. Viscosity is defined as the ratio of shear stress to shear rate:

$$\text{Viscosity (mPa.s)} = \frac{\text{shear stress (mPa)}}{\text{shear rate } (\text{s}^{-1})}.$$

The SI (Système Internationale) unit of viscosity is the millipascal-second (mPa.s), which is equal to the old unit, the centipoise (cP). From the equation it can be seen that the higher the viscosity of the liquid, the greater the shear stress (or force) which must be applied to produce the same shear rate (or flow rate).

Determinants of Blood Viscosity

The major determinants of blood viscosity are: temperature, shear rate, haematocrit, plasma proteins (which affect plasma viscosity and red cell aggregation) and red cell deformation (*Fig. 2.4*). These factors have been reviewed in detail by Chien [50] and Schmid-Schönbein [51].

Temperature

As with any other liquid, a decrease in temperature results in an increase in blood viscosity. This may be of clinical relevance in the cold extremities of patients with peripheral arterial disease.

Shear rate

At the high shear rates which have been calculated to exist in the majority of blood vessels in the normal circulation (100–200 s^{-1}),

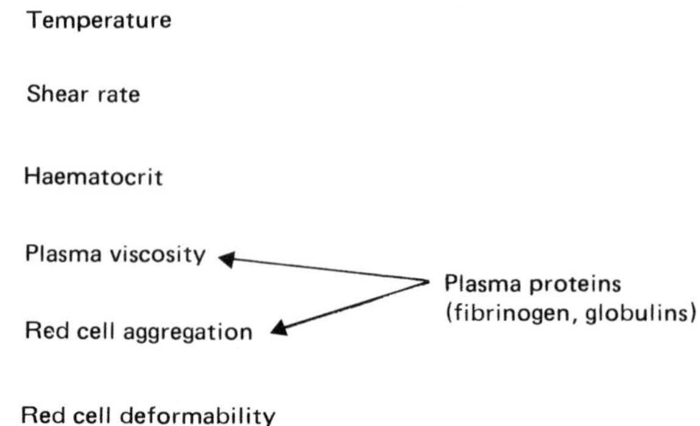

Fig. 2.4. Determinants of blood viscosity.

blood viscosity is low (normal range at 37 °C, 3·5–6·5 mPa.s). For comparison, the viscosity of water at 37 °C is about 0·7 mPa.s, hence blood at high shear and normal temperature is 5–9 times thicker than water, and presents relatively little hindrance to blood flow. With decrease in shear rate, blood viscosity rises exponentially. At the shear rate of $1\ s^{-1}$, normal blood viscosity ranges from 10 to 25 mPa.s (15–35 times thicker than water), and at lower shear rates blood viscosity may exceed the viscosity of water by several hundredfold. Under such low shear conditions, therefore, the resistance of blood to flow is considerably increased. Again this may be clinically relevant in the diseased peripheral circulation with low flow rates.

This change in blood viscosity with shear rate is due both to red cell deformation at high shear rates and also to red cell aggregation at low shear rates [52]. At high shear rates, all aggregates of red cells are dispersed, and red cells are deformed into ellipsoids in parallel with the flow streamlines. The red cell membrane rotates around its haemoglobin contents like the caterpillar tread of a military tank, and the liquid haemoglobin also participates in flow. At low shear rates, red cells are no longer deformed, and are aggregated into rouleaux by large plasma globulins which form bridges between the cells. This rouleaux network is responsible for the great increase in viscosity of slowly flowing blood. It also gives rise to a yield stress in blood—the minimum force or shear stress which must be applied to resting blood to start it flowing.

The alteration of blood viscosity with shear rate also makes it necessary to measure viscosity at a range of defined shear rates. This is accomplished in rotational viscometers, in which various defined shear rates can be established throughout the blood sample. It is common practice to measure blood viscosity at a high shear rate ($100–200\ s^{-1}$) and at a low shear rate ($0{\cdot}1–1\ s^{-1}$).

Haematocrit

The ratio of red cells to plasma (packed cell volume or haematocrit) has major effects on viscosity, even within the normal range of haematocrit (0·35–0·55). Linear increase in haematocrit produces a logarithmic increase in viscosity, and the increase in viscosity is greater at low shear rates than at high shear rates. An increase in haematocrit from 0·35 to 0·55 doubles blood viscosity at shear rate $100\,s^{-1}$, trebles viscosity at shear rate $1\,s^{-1}$ and quadruples viscosity at shear rate $0{\cdot}1\,s^{-1}$.

Plasma Proteins

Large plasma globulins also have important effects on blood viscosity. Increases in plasma levels of fibrinogen, α_2-macroglobulin and immunoglobulins result in increased blood viscosity at high shear rates, due to increased plasma viscosity. At low shear rates a greater rise in blood viscosity is observed, as these large globulins markedly enhance red cell aggregation.

Red Cell Deformation

Normal red cells are highly deformable, and as previously mentioned this ensures low blood viscosity at the high shear rates encountered in the normal circulation. Furthermore, red cell deformability is essential to allow a cell whose mean resting diameter is about 7·5 μm to spend most of its life traversing capillaries with diameters of between 3 and 5 μm. The deformability of normal red cells is due to several factors—excess ratio of surface area to volume, cell shape, membrane flexibility and intracellular viscosity. Red cell deformability is usually measured by filterability of red cell suspensions through filters with pore diameter 3–5 μm.

Other Cells

Platelets have minimal effect on blood viscosity, but white cells may have important effects in leukaemic patients with a high circulating white cell mass.

Blood Viscosity and Blood Flow

According to Poiseuille's Law, the volume rate of steady flow of a simple liquid in a straight, rigid tube depends on the pressure gradient, the length and diameter of the tube and the viscosity of the fluid. An increase in fluid viscosity should produce a decrease in flow rate, unless compensated by increased vessel diameter or increased driving pressure. Although Poiseuille's Law cannot be applied directly to the complex human circulation, it seems reasonable to expect that changes in blood viscosity are associated with changes in blood flow.

There are, however, at least two factors that complicate the simple inverse relationship of blood viscosity and blood flow. First, an increase in blood viscosity not only tends to reduce blood flow, it also tends to reduce the likelihood of turbulence in large arteries, and hence tends to reduce energy loss as blood is transported through these vessels [53]. Whether or not increased blood viscosity reduces blood flow will therefore depend on a balance of these two opposing effects.

Secondly, although blood viscosity measured *in vitro* rises steeply with increase in haematocrit, the reduction in blood flow *in vivo* appears to be less than predicted by *in vitro* viscometry [54–56]. This is because haematocrit and viscosity fall below venous haematocrit and viscosity in the major resistance vessels—the arterioles and capillaries. This phenomenon is known as the Fahraeus–Lindqvist effect [57]. There are several possible mechanisms by which this reduction in microcirculatory haematocrit could occur. The most important appears to be axial migration of red cells in narrow vessels. This leads to more rapid transit of red cells in the central rapidly flowing zone of the parabolic velocity profile, compared to the peripheral plasma. Because of this low microcirculatory haematocrit, most workers record blood viscosity not only at native venous haematocrit, but also after correction to a standard haematocrit (usually 0·45).

Despite these reservations, experimental animal studies have indeed confirmed that increased blood viscosity is associated with decreased blood flow [54–56, 58]. Of particular interest is the study of Fischer and Ames [59]. Following temporary arterial ligation, blood flow may not recommence immediately the obstruction is relieved—the 'no-reflow' phenomenon. Such failure of reflow could be due in part to the intrinsic flow resistance of aggregated, static blood. Prior haemodilution of the animal, which lowers blood viscosity and yield stress, eliminated the 'no-reflow' phenomenon [59].

In man, there is now reasonable evidence that increased blood viscosity is related to impaired cerebral blood flow and retinal blood flow, and that therapeutic blood viscosity reduction increases flow and improves cerebral and retinal function (*see* review by Lowe and Forbes [60]). Whether or not blood viscosity is related to limb blood flow in man is more controversial. Valnes et al. [61] found normal leg flow patterns in 5 patients with high blood viscosity due to paraproteinaemias. Dormandy [62] observed increased limb blood flow following acute haemodilution with intravenous fluids. However Humphreys et al. [63] concluded that such flow changes were related to changes in vascular tone consequent upon increased blood volume, rather than to decreased blood viscosity. In patients with peripheral arterial disease, increased leg blood flow has been reported after viscosity reduction by normovolaemic haemodilution [64, 65] or defibrination [66, 67]. In Raynaud's syndrome, increased digital blood flow has been reported after viscosity reduction by plasma exchange [68]. These flow increases cannot be explained by changes in blood volume, nor by compensation for reduced oxygen carriage after haemodilution. While one may tentatively accept that these flow increases were consequent upon decreased blood viscosity, further studies of the relationship between blood rheology and limb blood flow in man are desirable.

Blood Rheology Factors in Peripheral Arterial Disease

Overt blood hyperviscosity syndrome is found in three groups of patients—polycythaemics (due to a raised haematocrit), leukaemics (due to high circulating white cell mass) and paraproteinaemics (due to high levels of immunoglobulins in macroglobulinaemia, myeloma or rheumatoid arthritis). Clinical features are largely due to hypoperfusion of the brain and retina: symptoms and abnormal retinal appearances respond rapidly to blood viscosity reduction. Urgent reduction of viscosity is indicated for cerebral or retinal symptoms, and is achieved by venesection in polycythaemia, leucopheresis in leukaemia and plasma exchange in paraproteinaemia. Long term prevention of hyperviscosity is accomplished by ^{32}P therapy in polycythaemia vera, and by cytotoxic therapy in leukaemia and paraproteinaemia (for references *see* Lowe and Forbes [60]. Peripheral arterial occlusion appears rare in paraproteinaemia or leukaemia (apart from priapism), but is well recognized in polycythaemia vera.

Increased blood viscosity in chronic peripheral occlusive arterial disease, associated with high plasma fibrinogen levels, has been reported [26, 27, 48, 69]. Increased haemoglobin levels may also contribute to hyperviscosity [70]. Similar changes have been described in chronic coronary artery disease [71–73]. Decreased red cell deformability has also been reported in peripheral arterial disease, as measured by reduced filterability of whole blood [74, 75]. However, this may reflect leucocytosis [76] or hyperfibrinogenaemia [77] rather than red cell abnormalities.

The cause of the rheological disturbance in peripheral arterial disease is uncertain; but is probably partly due to cigarette smoking. Smokers have higher levels of blood and plasma viscosity than non-smokers, due to increased levels of haematocrit and fibrinogen [78, 79]. The increased levels of haematocrit and haemoglobin appear to be related to the higher level of carboxyhaemoglobin from inhaled carbon monoxide. This reduces blood oxygen-carrying capacity and increases blood-oxygen affinity: the resulting tissue hypoxia leads to increased synthesis of haemoglobin and red cells [80]. The circulating level of functioning haemoglobin is therefore maintained, but at the rheological cost of increased blood viscosity, which rises logarithmically with linear increase in haematocrit. Smoking is increasingly recognized as a potentially reversible cause of polycythaemia, and we have observed dramatic falls in haematocrit in patients with peripheral arterial disease who can be persuaded to stop smoking. The mechanisms by which fibrinogen is elevated in smokers are not understood: hyperfibrinogenaemia does not appear to be related to bronchitis and reduced lung function [81]. Smoking has also been shown to decrease red cell filterability [82, 83], and this does not appear to be related to carboxyhaemoglobin [83].

There is some evidence that blood rheology factors are related to adverse prognosis in peripheral arterial disease and vascular surgery. Dormandy et al. [35] related increased blood viscosity and fibrinogen levels to adverse prognosis in claudication. Bouhoutsos et al. [70] associated high preoperative haemoglobin levels with complications following arterial surgery. Reference has already been made to the relationship between high plasma fibrinogen levels and graft occlusion [37, 39]. As previously discussed, these associations may reflect correlations of fibrinogen and haemoglobin with other factors such as smoking, which worsens the prognosis of the disease [84] and of the graft [40].

Bailey et al. [85] found that failure of limited amputations in diabetics was associated with higher haemoglobin levels than successful operations, regardless of smoking habit. Increased blood viscosity in diabetics is now well recognized [86, 87].

Increased blood viscosity in Raynaud's syndrome has been described by several groups [26, 88–90], but not by all [91]. Vasoconstriction reduces flow rates and temperature in the digits, hence a further rise in blood viscosity could occur peripherally due to decreased shear rate and decreased temperature. Goyle and Dormandy [90] reported an abnormal increase in viscosity at low temperature in Raynaud's syndrome, but this was not confirmed by Blunt et al. [26]. The increase in viscosity is similar in idiopathic Raynaud's disease, connective tissue disorders and vibration-induced Raynaud's syndrome [25]. Decreased red cell deformability has also been reported [68, 92].

REFERENCES

1. Moncada S. and Vane J. R. (1978) Unstable metabolites of arachidonic acid. *Br. Med. Bull.* **34**, 129–35.
2. Baumgartner H., Muggli R. and Tschopp T. B. (1980) Interaction of platelets with subendothelium in flowing blood. In: Rotman A., Meyer F. A., Gitler C. et al. (ed.) *Platelets—Cellular Response Mechanisms and their Biological Significance.* Chichester, Wiley, pp. 17–28.
3. Born G. V. R. (1977) Fluid-mechanical and biochemical interactions in haemostasis. *Br. Med. Bull.* **33**, 193–7.

4. Holmsen H. (1980) Mechanisms of platelet secretion. In: Rotman A., Meyer F. A., Gitler C. et al. (ed.) *Platelets—Cellular Response Mechanisms and their Biological Significance*. Chichester, Wiley, pp. 249–63.
5. White J. G., Rao G. H. R. and Gerrard J. M. (1980) Prostaglandins in platelet activation. In: Rotman A., Meyer F. A., Gitler C. et al. (ed.) *Platelets—Cellular Response Mechanisms and their Biological Significance*. Chichester, Wiley, pp. 201–11.
6. Walsh P. N. (1978) The significance of platelet coagulant activities in hemostasis and thrombosis. In: Day H. J., Holmsen H. and Zucker M. B. (ed.) *Platelet Function Testing*. Washington, DC, US Dept of Health, Education and Welfare, pp. 436–60.
7. Ogston D. and Bennett B. (1978) Surface mediated reactions in the formation of thrombin, plasmin and kallikrein. *Br. Med. Bull.* **34**, 107–12.
8. Rosenberg R. D. (1975) Actions and interactions of antithrombin and heparin. *N. Engl. J. Med.* **292**, 146–51.
9. Hardisty R. M. (1977) Disorders of platelet function. *Br. Med. Bull.* **33**, 207–12.
10. Lowe G. D. O. (1981) Laboratory evaluation of hypercoagulability. *Clin. Haematol.* **10**, 407–42.
11. Woolf N. (1978) Thrombosis and atherosclerosis. *Br. Med. Bull.* **34**, 137–42.
12. Ross R. and Glomset J. A. (1976) The pathogenesis of atherosclerosis (Part 1). *N. Engl. J. Med.* **295**, 369–77.
13. Smith E. B., Alexander K. M. and Massie I. B. (1976) Insoluble 'fibrin' in human aortic intima. Quantitative studies on the relationship between insoluble 'fibrin', soluble fibrinogen and low density lipoprotein. *Atherosclerosis* **23**, 19–26.
14. Smith E. and Staples E. (1981) Haemostatic factors in human aortic intima. *Lancet* **1**, 1171–4.
15. Szczeklik A. (1980) Prostacyclin and atherosclerosis. *Triangle* **19**, 61–7.
16. Sinzinger H., Feigl W. and Silberbauer K. (1979) Prostacyclin generation in atherosclerotic arteries. *Lancet* **2**, 469.
17. Dollery C. T., Friedman L. A., Hensby C. N. et al. (1979) Circulating prostacyclin may be reduced in diabetes. *Lancet* **2**, 1365.
18. O'Brien J. R., Etherington M. D., Jamieson S. et al. (1975) Blood changes in atherosclerosis and long after myocardial infarction and venous thrombosis. *Thromb. Diath. Haem.* **34**, 483–97.
19. Murphy E. A. and Mustard J. F. (1962) Coagulation tests and platelet economy in atherosclerotic and control subjects. *Circulation* **25**, 124–5
20. Cella G., Zahavi J., de Haas H. A. et al. (1979) Beta-thromboglobulin, platelet production time and platelet function in vascular disease. *Br. J. Haematol.* **43**, 127–36.
21. Evans G. and Irvine W. T. (1966) Long-term arterial-graft patency in relation to platelet adhesiveness, biochemical factors and anticoagulant therapy. *Lancet* **2**, 353–5.
22. Ward A. S., Porter N., Preston F. E. et al. (1978) Platelet aggregation in patients with peripheral vascular disease. *Atherosclerosis* **29**, 63–8.
23. Kobayashi H. and Mishima Y. (1980) Platelet aggregability in chronic arterial occlusive diseases of the extremities. *Thromb. Res.* **20**, 363–73.
24. Wu K. K. and Hoak J. C. (1976) Spontaneous platelet aggregation in arterial insufficiency: mechanisms and implications. *Thromb. Haem.* **35**, 702–11.
25. Lowe G. D. O., Reavey M. M., Johnston R. V. et al. (1979) Increased platelet aggregates in vascular and non-vascular illness: correlation with fibrinogen and effect of ancrod. *Thromb. Res.* **14**, 377–86.
26. Blunt R. J., George A. J., Hurlow R. A. et al. (1980) Hyperviscosity and thrombotic changes in idiopathic and secondary Raynaud's syndrome. *Br. J. Haematol.* **45**, 651–8.

27. Dormandy J. A., Hoare E., Colley J. et al. (1973) Clinical, haemodynamic, rheological and biochemical findings in 126 patients with intermittent claudication. *Br. Med. J.* **4**, 576–81.
28. Hughson W. G., Mann J. I., Tibbs D. J. et al. (1978) Intermittent claudication: factors determining outcome. *Br. Med. J.* **1**, 1377–9.
29. Banerjee R. N., Sahni A. L., Kumar V. et al. (1974) Antithrombin III deficiency in maturity onset diabetes mellitus and atherosclerosis. *Thromb. Diath. Haem.* **31**, 339–45.
30. Nestel P. J. (1959) Fibrinolytic activity of blood in intermittent claudication. *Lancet* **2**, 373–4.
31. Naimi S., Goldstein R. and Proger S. (1963) Studies on the coagulation and fibrinolysis of the arterial and venous blood in normal subjects and patients with atherosclerosis. *Circulation* **27**, 904–18.
32. Turpie A. G. G., Forbes C. D. and McNicol G. P. (1967) Idiopathic gangrene in African children. *Br. Med. J.* **2**, 646–8.
33. Browse N. J., Gray L., Jarrett P. E. M. et al. (1977) Blood and vein-wall fibrinolytic activity in health and vascular disease. *Br. Med. J.* **1**, 478–81.
34. Frisch E. P. (1980) Decreased α2-antiplasmin levels in patients suffering from obstructive peripheral arterial disease. *Thromb. Res.* **19**, 701–3.
35. Dormandy J. A., Hoare E., Khattab A. M. et al. (1973) Prognostic significance of rheological and biochemical findings in patients with intermittent claudication. *Br. Med. J.* **4**, 581–3.
36. McCollum C. N., Kester R. C., Rajah S. M. et al. (1981) Arterial graft maturation: the duration of thrombotic activity in Dacron aortobifemoral grafts measured by platelet and fibrinogen kinetics. *Br. J. Surg.* **68**, 61–4.
37. Hamer J. D., Ashton F. and Meynell M. J. (1973) Factors influencing prognosis in the surgery of peripheral vascular disease: platelet adhesiveness, plasma fibrinogen and fibrinolysis. *Br. J. Surg.* **60**, 386–9.
38. Postlethwaite J. C. (1976) The importance of plasma fibrinogen in vascular surgery. *Ann. R. Coll. Surg. Engl.* **58**, 457–64.
39. Harris P. L., Harvey D. R. and Bliss B. P. (1978) The importance of plasma lipids, glucose, insulin and fibrinogen in femoropopliteal surgery. *Br. J. Surg.* **65**, 197–200.
40. Myers K. A., King R. B., Scott D. F. et al. (1978) The effect of smoking on the late patency of arterial reconstructions in the legs. *Br. J. Surg.* **65**, 267–71.
41. Steele P. P., Weilly H. S., Davies H. (1974) Platelet survival in patients with rheumatic heart disease. *N. Engl. J. Med.* **290**, 537–9.
42. Weily H. S., Steele P. P., Davies H. et al. (1974) Platelet survival in patients with substitute heart valves. *N. Engl. J. Med.* **290**, 534–7.
43. Cella G., Schivarazappa L., Casonato A. et al. (1980) *In vivo* platelet release reaction in patients with heart valve prosthesis. *Haemostasis* **9**, 263–275.
44. Zahavi J., Hamilton W. A. P., O'Reilly M. J. G. et al. (1980) Plasma exchange and platelet function in Raynaud's phenomenon. *Thromb. Res.* **19**, 85–93.
45. Vreeken J. and van Aken W. G. (1971) Spontaneous aggregation of blood platelets as a cause of idiopathic thrombosis and recurrent painful toes and fingers. *Lancet* **2**, 1394–7.
46. Preston F. E., Emmanuel I. G., Winfield D. A. et al. (1974) Essential thrombocythemia and peripheral gangrene. *Br. Med. J.* **3**, 548–52.
47. Morris-Jones W. and Preston F. E. (1979) The 'dead digit, palpable pulse' syndrome: a preliminary study of the value of antiplatelet drugs in this disorder. *Thromb. Haem.* **42**, 62.
48. Dormandy J. A. (1975) Blood: its viscosity and circulation. In: Harcus A. W. and Adamson L. (ed.) *Arteries and Veins*. Edinburgh, Churchill Livingstone, pp. 99–134.

49. Lowe G. D. O., Barbenel J. C. and Forbes C. D. (ed.) (1981) *Clinical Aspects of Blood Viscosity and Cell Deformability*. Berlin, Springer-Verlag.
50. Chien S. (1975) Biophysical behaviour of red cells in suspensions. In: Surgenor D. M. (ed.) *The Red Blood Cell*, volume 2, 2nd ed. New York, Academic Press, pp. 1031–1133.
51. Schmid-Schönbein H. (1976) Microrheology of erythrocytes, blood viscosity, and the distribution of blood flow in the microcirculation. *Int. Rev. Physiol.* **9**, 1–62.
52. Chien S. (1970) Shear dependence of effective cell volume as a determinant of blood viscosity. *Science* **168**, 977–8.
53. Charlesworth D. (1981) Relationship of blood rheology to blood flow. In: Lowe G. D. O., Barbenel J. C. and Forbes C. D. (ed.) *Clinical Aspects of Blood Viscosity and Cell Deformability*. Berlin, Springer-Verlag, pp. 91–6.
54. Whittaker S. R. F. and Winton F. R. (1933) The apparent viscosity of blood flowing in the isolated hindlimb of the dog and its variations with corpuscular concentration. *J. Physiol.* **78**, 339–69.
55. Skovborg F., Nielsen A. V. and Schlichtkrull J. (1968) Blood viscosity and vascular flow rate. *Scand. J. Clin. Lab. Invest.* **21**, 83–8.
56. Barrie W. W. (1980) MD Thesis, University of Glasgow.
57. Fahraeus R. and Lindqvist T. (1931) The viscosity of the blood in narrow capillary tubes. *Am. J. Physiol.* **96**, 562–8.
58. Driessen G. K., Heidtmann H. and Schmid-Schönbein H. (1979) Effects of hemodilution and hemoconcentration on red cell flow velocity in the capillaries of the rat mesentery. *Pflugers Arch. Eur. J. Physiol.* **380**, 1–6.
59. Fischer E. G. and Ames A. (1972) Studies on mechanisms of impairment of cerebral circulation following ischaemia: effect of hemodilution and perfusion pressure. *Stroke* **3**, 538–42.
60. Lowe G. D. O. and Forbes C. D. (1981) Blood rheology and thrombosis. *Clin. Haematol.* **10**, 343–67.
61. Valnes K., Lorentsen E. and Holter B. (1979) Calf blood flow and systolic blood pressure in patients with hyperviscosity of the blood. *Angiology* **30**, 313–16.
62. Dormandy J. A. (1971) Influence of blood viscosity on blood flow and the effect of low molecular weight dextran. *Br. Med. J.* **2**, 716–19.
63. Humphreys W. V., Walker A., Cave F. D. et al. (1976) The effect of an infusion of low molecular weight dextran on peripheral resistance in patients with arteriosclerosis. *Br. J. Surg.* **63**, 691–3.
64. Reiger H., Kohler M., Schoop W. et al. (1979) Hemodilution (HD) in patients with ischemic skin ulcers. *Klin. Wochenschr.* **57**, 1153–61.
65. Yates C. J. P., Andrews V., Berent A. et al. (1979) Increase in leg blood-flow by normovolaemic haemodilution in intermittent claudication. *Lancet* **2**, 166–8.
66. Ehringer H., Dudczak R. and Lechner K. (1974) A new approach in the treatment of peripheral arterial occlusions: defibrination with arvin. *Angiology* **25**, 279–89.
67. Lowe G. D. O., Morrice J. J., Forbes C. D. et al. (1979) Subcutaneous ancrod therapy in peripheral arterial disease: improvement in blood viscosity and nutritional blood flow. *Angiology* **30**, 594–9.
68. Dodds A. J., O'Reilly M. J. G., Yates C. J. P. et al. (1979) Haemorheological response to plasma exchange in Raynaud's syndrome. *Br. Med. J.* **4**, 1186–7.
69. Stormer B., Horsch R., Kleinschmidt F. et al. (1974) Blood viscosity in patients with peripheral vascular diseases in the areas of low shear rates. *J. Cardiovasc. Surg.* **15**, 577–84.
70. Bouhoutsos J., Morris T., Chavatzas D. et al. (1974) The influence of haemoglobin and platelet levels on the results of arterial surgery. *Br. J. Surg.* **51**, 984–6.
71. Mayer G. A. (1964) Blood viscosity in healthy subjects and patients with coronary heart disease. *Can. Med. Assoc. J.* **91**, 951–4.

72. Nicolaides A. N., Bowers R., Horbourne T. et al. (1977) Blood viscosity, red-cell flexibility, haematocrit and plasma fibrinogen in patients with angina. *Lancet* **2**, 943–5.
73. Lowe G. D. O., Drummond M. M., Lorimer A. R. et al. (1980) Relation between extent of coronary artery disease and blood viscosity. *Br. Med. J.* **1**, 673–4.
74. Reid H. L., Dormandy J. A., Barnes A. J. et al. (1976) Impaired red cell deformability in peripheral vascular disease. *Lancet* **1**, 666–8.
75. Drummond M. M., Lowe G. D. O., Belch J. J. F. et al. (1980) An assessment of red cell deformability using a simple filtration method. *J. Clin. Pathol.* **33**, 373–6.
76. Alderman M. J., Ridge A., Morley A. A. et al. (1981) The effect of total leucocyte count on whole blood filterability in patients with peripheral vascular disease. *J. Clin. Pathol.* **34**, 163–6.
77. Kenny M. W., Meakin M. J. and Stuart J. (1981) Measurement of erythrocyte filterability using washed-erythrocyte and whole-blood methods. *Clin.. Hemorheol.* **1**, 135–46.
78. Dintenfass L. (1975) Elevation of blood viscosity, aggregation of red cells, haematocrit values and fibrinogen levels in cigarette smokers. *Med. J. Aust.* **1**, 617–20.
79. Lowe G. D. O., Drummond M. M., Forbes C. D. et al. (1980) The effects of age and cigarette-smoking on blood and plasma viscosity in men. *Scott. Med. J.* **25**, 13–17.
80. Sagone A. L., Lawrence T. and Balcerzak S. P. (1971) Smoking—a cause of 'spurious' polycythaemia. *Blood* **38**, 826.
81. Korsan-Bengtsen K., Wilhelmsen L. and Tibblin G. (1972) Blood coagulation and fibrinolysis in a random sample of 788 men 54-years-old. II. Relations of the variables to 'risk factors' for myocardial infarction. *Thromb. Diath. Haem.* **28**, 99–108.
82. Lowe G. D. O., Drummond M. M., Forbes C. D. et al. (1981) Effects of cigarette-smoking on blood rheology. In: Stolz J. F. and Drovin P. (ed.) *Proceedings of European Symposium on Hemorheology and Diseases, Nancy, 1979*. Paris, Doin Ed., pp. 349–52.
83. Norton J. M. and Rand P. W. (1981) Decreased deformability of erythrocytes from smokers. *Blood* **57**, 671–4.
84. Hughson W. G., Mann J. I. and Garrod I. (1978) Intermittent claudication: prevalence and risk factors. *Br. Med. J.* **1**, 1379–81.
85. Bailey M. J., Yates C. J. P., Johnston C. L. W. et al. (1979) Preoperative haemoglobin as predictor of outcome of diabetic amputation. *Lancet* **2**, 168–70.
86. Barnes A. J., Locke P., Scudder P. R. et al. (1977) Is hyperviscosity a treatable component of diabetic microcirculatory disease? *Lancet* **2**, 789–91.
87. Lowe G. D. O., Lowe J. M., Drummond M. M. et al. (1980) Blood viscosity in young male diabetics with and without retinopathy. *Diabetol.* **18**, 359–63.
88. Pringle R., Walder D. N. and Weaver J. P. A. (1965) Blood viscosity and Raynaud's disease. *Lancet* **1**, 1086–9.
89. Walder D. N. (1973) Blood viscosity and Raynaud's disease. *J. R. Coll. Surg. Edinb.* **18**, 277–80.
90. Goyle K. B. and Dormandy J. A. (1976) Abnormal blood viscosity in Raynaud's phenomenon. *Lancet* **1**, 1317–18.
91. Jahnsen T., Neilsen S. L. and Skovborg F. (1977) Blood viscosity and local response to cold in primary Raynaud's phenomenon. *Lancet* **2**, 1001–2.
92. Dintenfass L. (1977) Haemorheological factors in Raynaud's phenomenon. *Angiology* **28**, 472–81.

J. G. Pollock and A. J. McKay
Frank J. Veith and Sushil K. Gupta
Herbert Dardik
D. Annis and R. M. Clarke

3 Modern Vascular Prosthetic Materials

I. Dacron

J. G. Pollock and A. J. McKay

INTRODUCTION

For large-vessel reconstruction in the aorto-iliac or aortofemoral segment, the challenge to provide an acceptable arterial substitute has largely been met. Knitted or woven Dacron prostheses are biocompatible, have satisfactory handling characteristics, are readily conformable and can be produced in many configurations. Consequently, this material has found widespread acceptance for use in large-vessel, high-flow reconstructive surgery, although further refinements are continually being made.

Such a satisfactory situation does not exist for femoropopliteal or femorotibial reconstruction, where autologous saphenous vein remains the conduit of choice. Apart from its almost ideal handling characteristics and conformability, the flow surface of the vein is non-thrombogenic owing to the presence of an intact endothelium which, amongst other things, produces the prostaglandin PG12 (prostacyclin) which prevents platelet aggregation. No other vascular conduit has these properties and thus saphenous vein remains the first choice.

None the less, using the saphenous vein is not without problems. Occasionally the vein will have been previously removed or will be found to be unsuitable, usually because of varicosity. More commonly, the vein will be present but of inadequate size. Even when a suitable vein is present, harvesting it is time-consuming and the incision required for its exposure contributes to postoperative morbidity. In the severely ill patient or in the patient who has already undergone aortofemoral bypass and requires femoro-distal reconstruction, the time taken for retrieval and preparation of the vein may be considered unacceptable. Finally, patients with peripheral vascular disease inevitably have a higher incidence of coronary artery disease than the normal population and since the saphenous vein remains virtually the only suitable conduit for aorto-coronary bypass, any acceptable alternative conduit for distal arterial reconstruction would clearly merit consideration.

For these reasons alternatives to saphenous vein have been developed for use in small-vessel, low-flow situations and tested over the past 30 years. Following the observation by Voorhees and his colleagues that Vinyon-N could be constructed to function as an arterial conduit [1], extensive animal research led to the development of Dacron for use in the human situation [2]. However, other potential arterial substitutes were tried. Chemically modified bovine arterial substitutes were used for below-knee reconstruction but later abandoned because of early thrombosis and aneurysm formation as well as limited size range and cost [3]. The Sparks Mandril graft was an autogenous fibrous tissue tube supported by a Dacron mesh but again, although early results were encouraging, it is no longer used due to thrombosis, aneurysm formation and haemorrhage, which occurred all too frequently [4].

Apart from Dacron, there are only two alternative grafts presently being used in any numbers. These are expanded polytetrafluoroethylene (PTFE) (Gore-Tex) and Biograft (Dardik) both of which are dealt with in detail later in this chapter. Gore-Tex is composed of expanded Teflon arranged as nodules and connected by thin fibrils. The microporous structure of this material means that although tissue ingrowth does occur, the graft does not leak and has the considerable advantage that it requires no pre-clotting. Furthermore, it has been suggested that Gore-Tex has a lower thrombogenic potential than Dacron [5]. Among its potential disadvantages are the cost of the material, which is currently significantly more expensive than Dacron. Late thrombosis in the material has been attributed in part to neo-intimal hyperplasia and some workers have suggested that aspirin and dipyridamole should be used to prevent this complication [6].

Technical precision is required when inserting Gore-Tex grafts, most workers favouring the use of a 6/0 or smaller monofilament suture. It is recommended that an interrupted suture is placed at the heel and toe of any anastomosis with continuous suturing in between. The tension of the graft must be precise and, for example, in the femoropopliteal segment, a gentle loop must be left below the knee to allow for extension of the joint. The graft must be kept absolutely dry before flow is established.

There are, of course, many areas apart from peripheral vascular disease where a suitable vascular prothesis can find application, and the use of Gore-Tex grafts has met with several favourable reports in many situations. In most patients who require long term haemodialysis vascular access is afforded by the formation of an arteriovenous fistula in an appropriate site, usually the forearm. When such a fistula fails (for example due to thrombosis, infection or aneurysm formation) it is often necessary to fashion an arteriovenous shunt. Many materials have been used for such a shunt, including saphenous vein, modified bovine heterografts, Sparks Mandril and vein homografts [7–9]. Gore-Tex has been widely used in this context and appears particularly suitable since it does not fray on cutting and its pliable construction allows very fine placement of sutures and thus a precise anastomosis can be performed to these small vessels.

Following early experimental work on large vein replacement in animals [10–12], there have been an increasing number of reports commenting on the use of the Gore-Tex graft as a venous substitute both to bypass large vein thrombosis [13] and also in portal hypertension either as distal splenorenal shunts or as side-to-side mesocaval shunts [14].

Paediatric cardiac surgeons have also made use of Gore-Tex in the treatment of systemic pulmonary shunts and other forms of cyanotic congenital heart disease [15, 16]. While the saphenous vein remains by far the conduit of choice for aorto-coronary bypass surgery, in those patients who do not have a suitable vein, Gore-Tex has been used with promising early results [17, 18]. General surgeons have also made use of Gore-Tex to allow replacement of the portal vein, permitting more aggressive surgery in the treatment of pancreatic carcinoma [19].

This chapter reviews the use of Dacron, Gore-Tex and Biograft, and concludes with a discussion on the inherent problems derived from the insertion of an essentially rigid tube in a pulsatile flow system. A possible solution to this problem—the 'Liverpool' graft—will be discussed and early results presented. Each of the contributors to this chapter emphasizes the importance of careful patient selection, correct choice of procedure and rigid application of precise surgical technique. Without these the best prosthesis available is doomed to failure. Lastly, it is worth noting that while it is agreed that the ideal conduit should be lightweight yet strong, easily sutured, conformable, non-thrombogenic, biocompatible and readily available, it should also be cheap. In the choice of which material to use, this last factor may assume increasing importance, with the most expensive of these materials presently costing £6·00 per centimetre in the United Kingdom.

DACRON

Having assessed several fabrics (e.g. Nylon, Orlon, Teflon and Ivalon) as possible arterial substitutes, DeBakey showed in the early 1950s that

Dacron could be knitted into a suitable tube for use as an arterial prosthesis [20]. Dacron is a polyester (chemical name polyethylene terephthalate) that is highly resistant to most organic and inorganic compounds such as oils, fats, chlorinated hydrocarbons and acids.

Although the earliest grafts were hand-knitted, the application of established textile industry techniques quickly led to the development of a knitting machine that allowed grafts of varying size and porosity to be made available. Since that time, the further development of this material has centred around modification of the pore size and the addition of a velour or filamentous surface either on the outside of the tube alone or on both the outer and flow surfaces. The porosity in a knitted graft must be low enough to allow pre-clotting but high enough not to delay healing. With these developments the handling characteristics of the material have greatly improved, as has the suturability. Modern knitting techniques produce a warp lock knit structure which is highly stable, consistent, conformable and strong even at the cut edge. The pile height can be varied either by increasing the amount of thread used in the knitting process or by raising a series of loops. The filamentous height ranges from zero in the knitted graft to 250 microns in the knitted graft with velour surface. Currently these grafts are available with variable porosity and all require pre-clotting.

In man complete healing of a Dacron graft (that is, the development of a continuous endothelium) probably never occurs and initially the Dacron merely provides a support which acts as a conduit. Healing of the graft then occurs with ingrowth of perigraft fibrous tissue and the final inner flow surface is compacted fibrin. True endothelium has been reported in up to 32 per cent of the flow surface but the healing at best is patchy [21]. The velour surface which is now added to most knitted Dacron prostheses has been shown to improve anchorage of the graft to the surrounding tissues and to promote rapid tissue ingrowth.

The alternative to a porous knitted graft which requires pre-clotting is the woven Dacron graft. This structure is not as stable as the knit, particularly at the edges, where fraying occurs. For this reason it has been suggested that it be cut with a hot wire. It is possible to produce a velour surface on a woven graft by brushing the surface to raise a pile. The major advantage of this material is that no pre-clotting is required and blood loss through the graft is minimal. Where blood loss is critical (ruptured abdominal aneurysm) this advantage makes it the graft of choice. The major disadvantage of the woven material is that it is more rigid than its knitted counterpart and therefore handles and sutures less well. Although the healing process cannot occur to the same extent, there is no published evidence that long term patency rates in the aorto-iliac segment are lower than for knitted Dacron. Woven Dacron is significantly cheaper.

USES OF DACRON

Aorto-iliac/Aortofemoral Reconstruction

A Gore-Tex aortic bifurcation graft is now available and the nature of this material allows the formation of a precisely sculptured bifurcation. None the less, the cost of such a graft and the excellent results that are possible using knitted Dacron have meant that in the aorto-iliac/femoral segment, knitted Dacron is used almost exclusively. Crimping of the Dacron tube means that the graft can be taken to the femoral vessels and yet it will resist kinking during flexion of the groin. Single or double velour knitted grafts give excellent long term patency rates in this high-flow, large-vessel replacement, although long term patency rates vary widely in the literature. Some authors have claimed a 10-year patency of around 80 per cent [22–24] but if success is measured in terms of functional improvement, a more realistic figure for long term success is around 50–60 per cent [25]. Considering the type of patient undergoing this surgery, these results are encouraging.

The surgical approach to the abdominal aorta and femoral vessels has become standardized, as has the technique for insertion of the graft material. Inevitably personal preferences are apparent in different centres with, for example, many surgeons favouring an end-to-side construction of the aortic anastomosis. For many years we have favoured resection of the abdominal aorta and bifurcation with subsequent end-to-end anastomosis. Rheologically, this is the favoured technique, although it is more time-consuming and technically more demanding. While it is our procedure of choice if the aortic bifurcation is heavily calcified or densely adherent to the iliac veins, in the interest of safety we occasionally make use of the end-to-side method. Although this is both faster and easier to perform, the final position of the graft is not anatomically ideal and separation of the graft from the peritoneal contents can be more difficult. However, if this onlay technique is used, the presacral neural plexus is not distributed and in male patients this may be an important consideration in preventing postoperative impotence. Furthermore, where severe occlusive aorto-iliac disease is present and distal flow is largely maintained through collateral circulation, we would be reluctant to sacrifice this collateral flow by excising the aorta and would therefore favour the end-to-side technique. Whichever technique is used, haematoma formation must be prevented since this not only leads to infection but also delays graft healing. Although initially silk sutures were used for the anastomoses [26], this material has now been almost universally abandoned in vascular surgery. Our preference is for a siliconized braided Terylene used as a continuous suture, but others successfully use monofilament polypropylene sutures.

Whichever technique is used most surgeons are agreed that Dacron is the graft of choice in the aorto-iliac segment. Long term patency rates are good and complications relatively infrequent. The future development of the Dacron prosthesis will centre on the production of ultra low porosity knitted grafts perhaps with the incorporation of elastic fibres to allow for a degree of compliance. In addition, various chemicals may be leeched to the structure lessening thrombogenicity. This modification has already been attempted with carbon and heparin but other substances seem sure to follow. Even in current grafts of woven construction porosity can be further lowered by pre-clotting with autologous platelet-rich plasma.

Femoropopliteal Reconstruction

Two major factors influence the success of arterial reconstruction in this segment. First, whether the distal anastomosis is above or below the knee joint, and secondly, if the distal anastomosis is below the knee, the number and quality of the distal run-off vessels. If the reconstruction is performed entirely above the knee, patency rates of up to 90 per cent at 1 year [27] and 60–70 per cent at 5 years [28, 29] using a Dacron tube graft of 8–10 mm diameter have been reported.

However, it is when the graft needs to cross the knee joint or be implanted into a small vessel in a limb with poor run-off that the deficiencies of Dacron have emerged with reported patencies at 1 year of 11 per cent [27]. It is clear that when an adequate saphenous vein is not available, Dacron has not proved satisfactory for below-knee reconstruction. Claims have been advanced for a non-crimped externally supported Dacron graft but it is too early to state with any confidence whether long term patency rates are appreciably better with this material [30].

Axillofemoral and Femorofemoral Bypass

This so-called extra-anatomically formed arterial bypass was first described less than 20 years ago [31]. Specific indications for its use vary from centre to centre [32, 33] and although both Gore-Tex and Dacron have been successfully used at the present time, the most popular choice of graft material for such reconstructions appears to be 8 mm or 10 mm knitted Dacron. Essentially, this means of reconstruction is chosen in the high-risk patient who has a threat to limb viability, in the patient with infection of an aortofemoral prosthesis or an aortoenteric fistula and in patients in whom access to aortic or iliac occlusion is deemed to be unduly hazardous. Since the technique is relatively straightforward and involves minimal dissection it can be used in the severely ill patient who would not tolerate major abdominal surgery. If at all possible, a crossover femorofemoral graft should be performed at the same time as the axillofemoral bypass since it has been shown that this reduces the distal run-off resistance thereby increasing long term patency rates. The graft itself lies in a gentle curve from the axillary artery to the femoral artery and lies in a subcutaneous position. If thrombosis does occur thrombectomy can be successfully performed relatively simply due to the easy access to the graft. Details of graft insertion appear in standard texts.

Other Uses

Dacron, PTFE (Gore-Tex) and vein are frequently used for vessel patching either after injury or following open endarterectomy. Cardiac surgeons make use of Dacron patches both to buttress stitches in soft endocardial tissues and also to repair defects following the excision of ventricular aneurysms. The use of Dacron for aortic arch, subclavian and carotid artery reconstruction is thoroughly discussed elsewhere (*see* Chapter 4).

REFERENCES

1. Voorhees A. B., Jaretzki A. and Blakemore A. H. (1952) The use of tubes constructed from Vinyon-N cloth in bridging arterial defects. *Ann. Surg.* **135**, 332.
2. DeBakey M. E., Cooley D. A., Crawford E. S. et al. (1958) Clinical application of a new flexible knitted Dacron arterial substitute. *Am. J. Surg.* **24**, 862.
3. Dale W. A. and Lewis M. R. (1976) Further experiences with bovine arterial grafts. *Surgery* **80**, 711.
4. Hallin R. W. and Sweetman W. R. (1976) The Sparks Mandril graft. *Am. J. Surg.* **132**, 221.
5. Hamlin G. W., Rajah S. M., Crow M. J. et al. (1978) Evaluation of the thrombogenic potential of three types of arterial graft studied in an artificial circulation. *Br. J. Surg.* **65**, 272.
6. Oblath R. W., Buckley F. O. jun., Green R. M. et al. (1978) Prevention of platelet aggregation and adherence to prosthetic vascular grafts by aspirin and dipyridamole. *Surgery* **84**, 37.
7. Wellington J. L. (1978) Expanded polytetrafluoroethylene prosthetic grafts for blood access in patients on dialysis. *Can. J. Surg.* **21**, 420.
8. Jenkins A. (1976) Gore-tex: a new prosthesis for vascular access. *Br. Med. J.* **3**, 280.
9. Loeprecht H., Franz H. E. and Vollmar J. (1978) Experiences with a new alloplastic graft (PTFE) as an arteriovenous shunt for haemodialysis. In: Frost T. H. (ed.) *Technical Aspects of Renal Dialysis*. Tunbridge Wells, Pitman Medical.
10. Collins H. A., Burrus G. and DeBakey M. E. (1960) Experimental evaluation of grafts in the canine inferior vena cava. *Am. J. Surg.* **99**, 40.
11. Wilson S. E., Jabour A., Stone R. T. et al. (1978) Patency of biologic and prosthetic inferior vena cava grafts with distal limb fistula. *Arch. Surg.* **113**, 1174.
12. Fujiwara Y., Cohn L. H., Adams D. et al. (1974) Use of Gore-tex grafts for replacement of the superior and inferior venae cavae. *J. Thorac. Cardiovasc. Surg.* **67**, 774.

13. Clowes A. W. (1980) Extra-anatomical bypass of iliac vein obstruction. *Arch. Surg.* **115**, 767.
14. Rosenthal D., Deterling R. A. jun., O'Donnell T. F. et al. (1979) Interposition grafting with expanded polytetrafluoroethylene for portal hypertension. *Surg. Gynecol. Obstet.* **148**, 387.
15. Donohoo J. S., Gardner T. J., Zahka K. et al. (1980) Systemic-pulmonary shunts in neonates and infants using microporous expanded polytetrafluoroethylene: immediate and late results. *Ann. Thorac. Surg.* **301**, 146.
16. McKay R., de Leval M. R. et al. (1980) Postoperative angiographic assessment of modified Blalock–Taussig shunts using expanded polytetrafluoroethylene (Gore-Tex). *Ann. Thorac. Surg.* **30**, 137.
17. Molina J. E., Carr M. and Yarnoz M. D. (1978) Coronary bypass with Gore-Tex graft. *J. Thorac. Cardiovasc. Surg.* **75**, 769.
18. Yokoyama T., Gharavi M. A., Ying-Chien L. et al. (1978) Aorta-coronary artery revascularization with an expanded polytetrafluoroethylene vascular graft. *J. Thorac. Cardiovasc. Surg.* **76**, 552.
19. Norton L. and Eiseman B. (1975) Replacement of portal vein during pancreatectomy for carcinoma. *Surgery* **77**, 280.
20. DeBakey M. E., Cooley D. A., Crawford E. S. et al. (1958) The clinical application of a new flexible knitted Dacron arterial substitute. *Arch. Surg.* **77**, 713.
21. Sauvage L. R., Berger K., Beilin L. B. et al. (1975) Presence of endothelium in an axillary femoral graft of knitted dacron with an external velour surface. *Ann. Surg.* **182**, 749.
22. Van Lent D., Kuijpers P. J., Skotnicki S. H. et al. (1974) Aorto-iliac surgery: a comparative study between thromboendarterectomy and bypass. *J. Cardiovasc. Surg.* **15**, 352.
23. Minken S. L., Dewelse J. A., Southgate W. A. et al. (1968) Aorto-iliac reconstruction for atherosclerotic occlusive disease. *Surg. Gynecol. Obstet.* **126**, 1056.
24. Irvine W. T., Booth R. A. D. and Myers K. (1972) Arterial surgery for aorto-iliac occlusive vascular disease. *Lancet* **1**, 738.
25. Galland R. B., Hill D. A., Gustave R. et al. (1980) The functional results of aorto-iliac reconstruction. *Br. J. Surg.* **67**, 344.
26. Gordon-Smith I. C., Taylor E. W., Nicolaides A. N. et al. (1978) Management of abdominal aortic aneurysm. *Br. J. Surg.* **65**, 834.
27. Christenson J. T. and Eklof B. (1979) Sparks Mandril, velour Dacron and autogenous saphenous vein grafts in femoro-popliteal bypass. *Br. J. Surg.* **66**, 514.
28. Watt J. K., Gillespie G., Pollock J. G. et al. (1974) Arterial surgery in intermittent claudication. *Br. Med. J.* **1**, 23.
29. DeBakey M. E. Presentation to the International Cardiovascular Society, 1973.
30. Sauvage L. R., Diaconon J., Cengiz M. et al. (1981) The EXS prosthesis: an innovation in Dacron construction for lower extremity revascularisation. In: Greenhalgh R. M. (ed.) *Femoro-distal Bypass.* Tunbridge Wells, Pitman Medical.
31. Louw J. H. (1963) Splenic to femoral and axillary to femoral bypass grafts in diffuse atherosclerotic occlusive disease. *Lancet* **1**, 1401.
32. DeLaurentis D. A., Sala L. E., Russell E. et al. (1978) A twelve year experience with axillofemoral and femoro-femoral bypass operations. *Surg. Gynecol. Obstet.* **147**, 881.
33. Ray L. I., O'Connor J. B., Davis C. C. et al. (1979) Axillofemoral bypass: a critical reappraisal of its role in the management of aortoiliac occlusive disease. *Am. J. Surg.* **138**, 117.

II. Role of Expanded Polytetrafluoroethylene (PTFE) Grafts

Frank J. Veith and Sushil K. Gupta

INTRODUCTION

Gore-Tex or Impra grafts were made available clinically about 5 years ago after encouraging experimental experience in both the arterial and venous systems [1, 2]. Over the past 4½ years, we have used and studied PTFE arterial grafts in more than 600 patients and this experience forms the basis for this section.

Reported patency rates using PTFE grafts in femoropopliteal and tibial arterial reconstructions have varied widely [3–8]. In 1978 we reported comparable early patency when autologous saphenous veins or PTFE grafts were used as femoropopliteal bypasses for limb salvage in similar groups of high risk patients [5]. These promising initial results with PTFE grafts prompted us to use this material for standard extra-anatomical bypasses as well as for a variety of extended extra-anatomical arterial reconstructions and prosthetic bypasses to arteries in the ankle and foot [9]. Our experience with the use of PTFE arterial grafts in these standard and newer operative procedures is summarized below.

Femoropopliteal Bypass

Our present life table patency rates for 220 PTFE femoropopliteal bypasses are shown in *Fig. 3.1.* Over 95 per cent of these operations were for limb salvage so that it is not surprising that 101 grafts were inserted below the knee and 48 grafts were to a blind or isolated segment of popliteal artery with no direct run-off into patent calf arteries. Despite this, the cumulative life table patency at 4 years was 73 per cent. These results are based on 67 cases followed over 2 years and 25 cases followed over 3 years. There are still no meaningful long term or 5-year results with PTFE arterial grafts, and this is an important remaining gap in our knowledge.

There was no significant difference in patency rates up to 4 years whether or not the graft was inserted into an isolated popliteal segment or one with angiographically better run-off (*Fig. 3.2*). These data, like those reported by us earlier [10], are difficult to explain. Nevertheless, these patency rates are based on accurately and completely followed patients and they suggest that PTFE grafts, if used well, may work better than other prosthetics in low-flow situations. The data also support attempts to revascularize a blind popliteal segment even if autologous saphenous vein is not available.

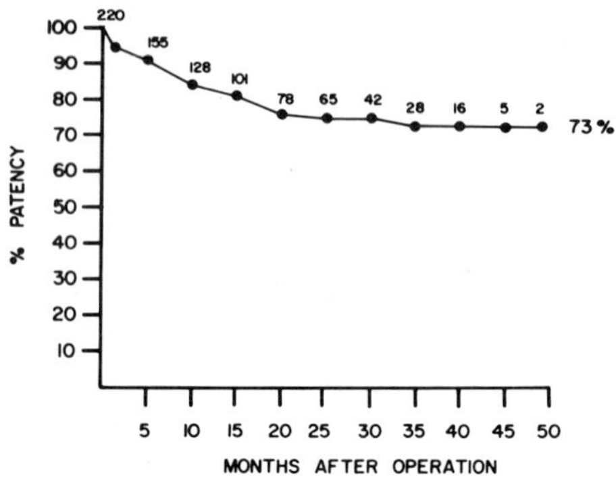

Fig. 3.1. Cumulative life table patency for 220 PTFE femoropopliteal bypasses.

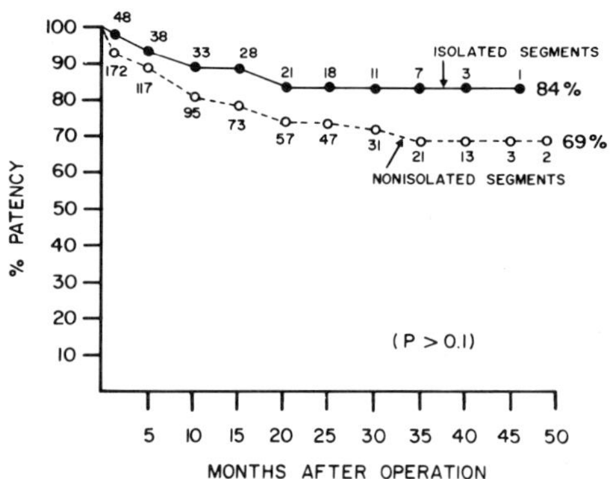

Fig. 3.2. Cumulative life table patency for 48 PTFE femoropopliteal bypasses to isolated segments of popliteal artery and 172 PTFE bypasses to popliteal arteries with better radiographic run-off into calf arteries. The two curves are not significantly different at any point.

Fig. 3.3 shows a breakdown of patency rates for above-knee and below-knee PTFE femoropopliteal bypasses. Patency rates below the knee were not significantly less, a finding also in conflict with commonly held beliefs for prosthetic grafts, but nevertheless one based on hard and accurate data and cases observed over 3 years.

Value of Reoperation

In all the life table data presented in *Figs. 3.1–3.3*, there is one important qualification. As with the upper line in *Fig. 3.4*, the calculations were performed with each patent graft considered patent whether or not a reoperation was required to maintain that patency. If a graft that required a reoperation to restore patency is considered non-patent, the

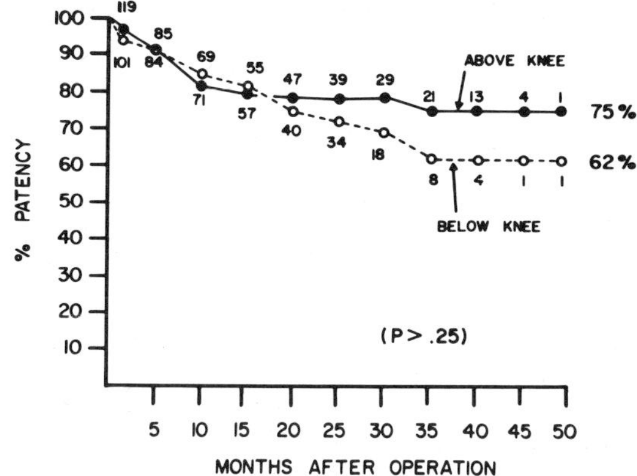

Fig. 3.3. Cumulative life table patency rates for PTFE femoropopliteal bypasses inserted above or below the knee joint. The two curves are not significantly different at any point.

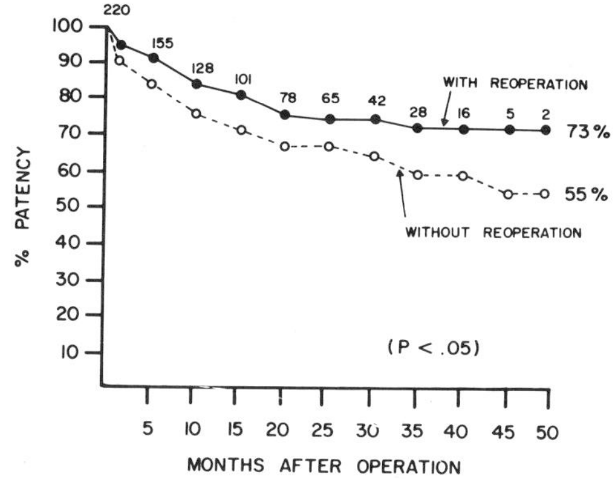

Fig. 3.4. Cumulative life table patency rates for 220 PTFE femoropopliteal bypasses. Calculations upon which the solid line is based are performed with each patent graft considered patent whether or not a reoperation is required to maintain patency. If a graft which closes is considered non-patent whether or not a reoperation restores patency, then results are as indicated by the dashed line.

lower line in *Fig. 3.4* results, with 55 per cent life table patency at 4 years. This brings out two important points. First, appropriate reoperation when PTFE grafts fail in the early or late postoperative period usually restores patency which persists for long periods of time, sometimes for more than 3 years. In fact, PTFE grafts appear to be unique in this regard. The second important point is that this aggressive attitude toward PTFE graft failure with appropriate reoperations produces an important 18 per cent increase in overall late patency rates.

There are many other details about the causes and management of early and late PTFE femoropopliteal graft failures that are important in achieving good results with this graft. These details are fully discussed elsewhere [11] and only a few new or key points need to be emphasized. First, if no anastomotic, inflow or outflow problems are detected by careful intraoperative or preoperative angiography or inspection of the inside of the distal anastomosis, simple thrombectomy may result in over 3 years of patency. Second, we have preliminary data suggesting that aspirin and Persantin may decrease the late failure rate and the incidence of intimal hyperplasia. Third, patch graft angioplasty is still the preferred treatment for intimal hyperplasia. Finally, since publishing our original article [11], additional numbers of cases with longer periods of follow-up confirm the value of appropriate reoperation for early and late PTFE femoropopliteal bypass failure. This is borne out by a 39-month life table patency rate of 61 per cent for all 36 of our patients undergoing early or late reoperation. Operative mortality for these reoperations has been less than 5 per cent.

Axillofemoral and Femorofemoral Bypass

Our life table patency rates for PTFE axillofemoral and femorofemoral bypasses are shown in *Fig. 3.5*. Patency rates of 87 per cent and 81 per

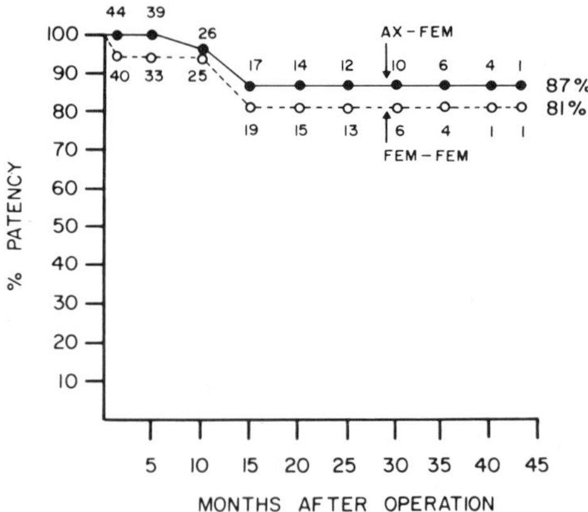

Fig. 3.5. Cumulative life table patency rates for PTFE axillofemoral and femorofemoral grafts.

cent at 43 months are encouraging, but it is not possible to determine whether or not the PTFE graft offers patency advantages over standard Dacron fabric grafts. We continue to use it because it requires no preclotting, is probably easier to reoperate on if it fails, and because it may have less tendency to develop pseudointima and thrombose in low-flow conditions. In this regard, our patency rates with unilateral PTFE axillofemoral grafts are as good as with axillobifemoral procedures. Accordingly, we perform unilateral axillofemoral procedures preferentially unless both limbs are threatened.

Extended Bypasses with PTFE

Significant numbers of patients with axillopopliteal bypasses and small artery bypasses have now been followed for over 2 years and some for over 3, although this group of patients has a high late mortality from associated cardiovascular problems. Of 79 PTFE grafts to vessels below the popliteal artery, there is a 1-year patency rate of 52 per cent and a 2-year patency rate of 40 per cent (*Fig. 3.6*). Results are

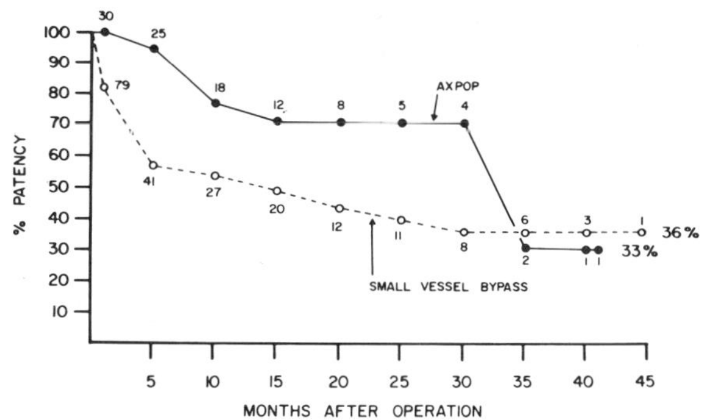

Fig. 3.6. Cumulative life table patency rates for PTFE axillopopliteal bypasses and PTFE bypasses to arteries distal to the popliteal.

somewhat better for grafts inserted in the upper leg but 6 grafts to the ankle or foot have salvaged limbs for over 3 years. Of 24 axillopopliteal or axillo-cross-popliteal grafts there is a 72 per cent 1-year patency rate, a 66 per cent 2-year patency rate and a 33 per cent 3-year patency rate. However, the number of patients followed to 3 years is still so small that the last percentage figure is meaningless.

The operative mortality in more than 100 of these newer operations remains below 5 per cent.

Our present conclusions concerning these newer operations are as follows. They can salvage limbs in significant numbers of patients at 1 and 2 years or more. Morbidity and mortality remain low and we continue to be enthusiastic when other options are not available. Clearly, however, these are not everyday procedures. They require commitment and care in case selection and performance. Their exact role remains to be defined by larger numbers of cases followed for longer periods of time. However, we believe that these operations do have a real place in vascular surgery.

Unanswered Questions

There are several major unanswered questions relating to PTFE grafts in reconstructive arterial surgery. First, what will the long term results be? Four, five and more years of accurate follow-up data from several centres are needed. In addition, bad result reports have to be explained. Certainly some of these may be based on use of PTFE grafts in hopeless circumstances or with poor surgical technique. Second, what is the exact role of antiplatelet drugs in maintaining patency? Third, how do PTFE graft results compare to results with autologous veins and other grafts under varying circumstances. The answers to the last two questions can only be provided by prospective, randomized, controlled studies.

We have been participating in such a cooperative refereed study for over 2 years along with Drs Bergan, Bernhard, Yao, Flinn and Szilagyi. A few remarks about such studies are in order. First, they are difficult to conduct. It is hard to avoid succumbing to prejudices such as the vein's superiority in small vessel bypasses. Also interesting is the large number of patients randomized to the vein group who do not have a usable saphenous vein even after it is dissected out. Despite these problems, more than 300 patients have been entered into the study, and interesting information should result from it. To date all that can be said is that periodic examination of patency data in our own centre has not yet revealed sufficiently clear differences which would justify discontinuation of the randomization procedure.

CONCLUSIONS

Until results from this and similar studies are known, we believe the following philosophy to be reasonable and appropriate for general use of PTFE arterial grafts. Autologous saphenous vein, if available and adequate in the *ipsilateral* leg, should be the graft of choice for arterial reconstructions below the inguinal ligament. PTFE grafts represent an acceptable alternative that can be used when the patient's life expectancy is less than 2–3 years or the vein is unsuitable or unavailable. If a PTFE graft is used, an aggressive attitude with appropriate reoperation for failed grafts will improve overall results.

REFERENCES

1. Matsumoto H., Hasegawa T. and Fuse K. (1973) A new vascular prosthesis for a small caliber artery. *Surgery* **74**, 519.

2. Soyer T., Lempinen M., Cooper P. et al. (1972) A new venous prosthesis. *Surgery* **72**, 864.
3. Burnham S. J., Flanigan P., Goodreau J. J. et al. (1978) Nonvein bypass in below-knee reoperation for lower limb ischemia. *Surgery* **84**, 417.
4. Campbell C. D., Brooks D. H., Webster M. W. et al. (1979) Expanded microporous polytetrafluoroethylene as a vascular substitute: a two year follow-up. *Surgery* **85**, 177.
5. Veith F. J., Moss C. M., Fell S. C. et al. (1978) Comparison of expanded polytetrafluoroethylene and autologous saphenous vein grafts in high risk arterial reconstructions for limb salvage. *Surg. Gynecol. Obstet.* **147**, 749.
6. Haimov H., Giron F. and Jacobson J. H. (1979) The expanded polytetrafluoroethylene graft. *Arch. Surg.* **114**, 673.
7. Hearn A. R. and Charlesworth D. (1978) The early results of reconstruction of the femoral artery with a Gore-Tex prosthesis. *Surgery* **85**, 607.
8. Stansel H. C., Fenn J. E., Tilson M. D. et al. (1979) Surgical principles and polytetrafluoroethylene (PTFE). *Arch. Surg.* **114**, 1291.
9. Veith F. J., Moss C. M., Daly V. et al. (1978) New approaches to limb salvage by extended extra-anatomic bypasses and prosthetic reconstructions to foot arteries. *Surgery* **84**, 764.
10. Veith F. J., Gupta S. and Daly V. (1981) Femoropopliteal bypass to isolated popliteal segments. Is polytetrafluoroethylene (PTFE) graft acceptable? *Surgery* **89**, 296.
11. Veith F. J., Gupta S. K. and Daly V. (1980) Management of early and late thrombosis of expanded polytetrafluoroethylene (PTFE) femoropopliteal bypass grafts: favorable prognosis with appropriate reoperation. *Surgery* **84**, 581.

III. The Glutaraldehyde Stabilized Umbilical Vein Graft: Experience with Lower Extremity Revascularization

Herbert Dardik

INTRODUCTION

After experiencing frustrations with the inability to secure sufficient length and quality of autologous veins, particularly in patients with advanced ischaemia, and then the disappointment in using allogenic vein grafts and modified xenografts, we turned our attention to the umbilical cord vein graft in 1972.

Initial laboratory experimentation demonstrated the predictable rejection that occurred within several weeks of implantation [1]. This was manifest by thrombosis and biodegradation with aneurysm formation. Previous workers [2–4] had also experienced failures using umbilical cord vessels without any type of tanning with aldehydes. Stimulated by the work of Rosenberg et al. [5] and Carpentier [6], we investigated the use of both dialdehyde starch and glutaraldehyde on umbilical cord vessels and then studied the results following animal implantation. In contrast to predictable failure without chemical modification of the graft, we were able to achieve success first in the laboratory and then in a small pilot study reported in 1976 [7–9].

Clinical Series

Our experience with the glutaraldehyde stabilized human umbilical cord vein graft (Biograft, Meadox Medicals, Oakland, New Jersey) now consists of 552 implantations in the lower extremity performed over the 5-year period 1975–80. Our experience with the glutaraldehyde stabilized umbilical vein graft has been categorized according to the site of distal implantation (*Table* 3.1), that is, popliteal ($n = 286$), tibial ($n = 169$) or peroneal ($n = 97$). The best clinical test for any new graft material is in the infrageniculate position, particularly the tibial and peroneal systems. Initially, we limited our use of the umbilical vein prosthesis to the latter, but as we gained experience and confidence, we included all types of lower limb reconstructions. Previous lower extremity vascular reconstructions were performed in 23·8 per cent of the popliteal, 57·4 per cent of the tibial and 33·0 per cent of the peroneal bypass groups. Most of these prior failures were femoral popliteal bypasses employing autologous saphenous veins.

Table 3.1. Clinical data

	No. proc.	*Age (mean)*	*M/F*	*Diabetes*	*Prior vasc. surg.*
Popliteal	286	65	178/108	162 (57%)	68 (23·8%)
Tibial	169	63	114/55	89 (53%)	97 (57·4%)
Peroneal	97	71	69/28	70 (72%)	32 (33·0%)
Total	552				

The indications employed for selecting cases for bypass in this series were based on the following: (*a*) limb salvage, manifest by a pregangrenous state and/or progressive lesions of the foot or leg that would otherwise lead to imminent limb amputation; (*b*) rest pain and/or non-healing lesions, but the limb not imminently at risk; (*c*) disabling claudication; and (*d*) prophylaxis for asymptomatic popliteal aneurysms (*Table* 3.2). Many of these patients presented with combinations of these symptoms and findings. Disabling claudication was an infrequent indication for reconstruction, accounting for only 6 per cent of femoral popliteal bypasses and 5 per cent of the tibial bypasses. Peroneal reconstructions are only employed for advanced ischaemia, including pregangrene, progressive gangrenous lesions that threaten

Table 3.2. Indications

	Gangrene/ pregangrene	*Rest pain Ulcers*	*Claudication*	*Aneurysm (elective)*
Popliteal	188 (66%)	75 (26%)	16 (6%)	7 (2%)
Tibial	132 (78%)	28 (17%)	9 (5%)	0
Peroneal	97 (100%)	0	0	0

the limb and rest pain that is unresponsive to more conservative measures such as lumbar sympathectomy. Additional operations were often required because of the advanced stage of the vascular obliterative process. Although these procedures were usually performed at the time of the primary vascular reconstruction, occasionally staging was felt to be better. Inflow reconstruction, such as iliofemoral bypass and more recently, transluminal angioplasty, were sometimes required as were digital or transmetatarsal amputations, débridement and skin grafting. Lumbar sympathectomy was less often employed, since many of these patients had already undergone sympathectomy or were neuropathic.

Technique

Gentle handling of the graft is critical: this includes both manual and instrumental manipulations. Thickness and thinness of the wall has no relevance to the effectiveness of the material. It has been observed that the thicker grafts will become thinner with manual pressure or with arterial pressure once the proximal anastomosis is completed. External tissue shreds may occasionally be seen. They can either be simply snipped off or ignored. One should not pull on these tissue fragments. Rough handling of the graft can produce discoloration from subadventitial dissection of blood. If this is extensive, then the graft should be discarded. Prior to implantation the graft must be irrigated thoroughly to wash out alcohol and aldehyde residues. Hufnagel [10] has described the use of an undiluted heparin rinse after irrigation and prior to implantation that may, by surface bonding, result in increased thromboresistance at the flow surface. Cranley [11] prefers low molecular weight dextran. We employ the former technique but await further data regarding the need and efficacy of these additional preimplant manoeuvres.

Systemic heparinization is employed using 1·25 mg/kg and is monitored intraoperatively by the activated clotting time test [12]. We usually do the proximal anastomosis first, but the distal anastomosis can be performed initially if the surgeon prefers. It is essential that the tunnelling of the graft be performed through a metallic or plastic tunneller. Damage to the graft can occur if it is simply pulled through the tissue tunnel, due to friction between the outer Dacron mesh and the tissues. An alternative technique is to coat the graft just prior to placement in the tunnel with a sterile water-soluble lubricant. For the distal anastomosis, interrupted suture technique with fine monofilament suture material is employed at the ends of the arteriotomy. A continuous technique is employed along the lateral margins. We endeavour to make this anastomosis approximately 22–25 mm long, which has been shown by intraoperative arteriography to give a smoother and better taper. The interrupted suture method may also preserve the compliance of the graft at the anastomosis. Intraoperative arteriography is routine to identify any technical fault and to demonstrate the run-off, including the pedal arch [13].

The medial approach was employed to gain access to the popliteal and posterior tibial arteries at all levels. The anterior tibial artery was dissected from the intermuscular cleft of the anterior compartment by a long anterolateral incision with complementary fasciotomy beyond the limits of the skin incision. A laterally based incision with partial fibulectomy is preferred to the medial approach for exposure of the peroneal artery throughout its entire course. Close attention to a number of technical details is essential in order to secure success. These include meticulous handling of all tissues and particularly the arteries. If calcification exists, fracturing of these vessels must be avoided. This is particularly liable to occur if excessive traction is employed with Silastic vessel loops or if standard vascular clamps are applied tightly. Intraluminal balloon tamponade may be the safest method to achieve vascular control.

Postoperative graft thrombosis presents the surgeon with several options. He may do a thrombectomy or he may simply ignore the graft thrombosis and permit the situation to continue and observe the clinical course of the patient. Finally, the surgeon may replace the original graft with a new one altogether and in this situation the original graft may or may not be removed. The decision as to which option to select depends on a number of factors. These include the time of thrombosis with regard to how long after implantation of the graft it occurs, the mechanism for thrombosis and finally the extent.

Early thrombectomies (in the immediate or early postoperative period) are usually due to one of two factors: (*a*) technical mishap and (*b*) extremely poor run-off. In the latter instance, intraoperative arteriography is helpful to define this problem and the decision could be made either to ignore the thrombosis and accept the situation as a failure or to consider the possibility of performing an adjunctive arteriovenous fistula [14]. Technical mishaps that might not have been appreciated or recognized on the intraoperative arteriogram might be recognized at re-exploration of the graft. These can be corrected, depending on the exact mechanism, by such techniques as removal of plaque distal to the distal anastomosis with vein patch angioplasty, correction of an unrecognized inflow problem by endarterectomy or proximal bypass. Our management in such circumstances consists of re-exploring the graft distally and securing control of the graft and the distal vessel. After heparinizing the patient, an arteriotomy is established in the distal graft along the axis of the graft overlying the site of the distal anastomosis. If necessary, the opening in the graft is extended across the distal anastomosis at the apex and then distally into the artery itself. Since we ordinarily perform an interrupted suture technique at this level, an unravelled suture line is never a problem. Any firm thrombosis is usually located at this point and can be manually removed. Distal exploration with a balloon catheter is performed and the distal circulation further assessed. At this point the status of the proximal portion of the graft must also be appreciated. Generally there is no pulse, and if none can be restored by simple and gentle manual massage from above, a balloon catheter is introduced from below with great care being taken not to overly inflate the balloon. More often, however, we open up the upper wound and manually compress the thrombus downwards so that the patient's blood pressure will extrude the clot. We will then pass the balloon catheter from below upwards making certain that all thrombus is removed and then proceed with closure of the distal arteriotomy. However, since catheter balloons can be easily compressed by firm thrombus, we do not hesitate to secure control of the upper portion of the graft, doing a small arteriotomy at this point and then proceed with manual extraction of thrombus or irrigation of the entire graft with heparinized solution prior to balloon catheter extraction of any residual thrombus. Once these techniques have been completed the upper arteriotomy can be closed primarily as well as the lower one. If the distal arteriotomy extends across the artery, we will apply a saphenous or umbilical vein patch to prevent stricture. Late graft closures usually present a slightly different problem in that the dissection of the graft may be quite difficult particularly at anastomotic areas. In several instances we have explored the graft remote from the anastomosis and performed very simple balloon catheter extractions. This, of course, is fraught with risk and should be limited only to patients who might otherwise not be candidates for extensive reconstructions. In those patients in whom the dissection can be performed in the anastomotic region, manoeuvres similar to those described for early thrombosis are performed. Many grafts can thereby be salvaged even where the graft has been closed for periods exceeding 4 weeks. In those cases where the dissection of the graft is virtually impossible or if there is concern with regard to the status of the graft, either because of changes following implantation or because of damage following manoeuvres to extract thrombus, we have not hesitated simply to implant a new graft placed at either a similar level or at a more proximal level for the proximal anastomosis and distal to the previously performed distal anastomosis. We usually remove whatever segments of graft are readily seen in the operative field.

The most important feature for Biograft thrombectomy is extreme gentleness in the manipulation of the graft. When using a balloon catheter, overinflation must be avoided. On many occasions it may be preferable, prior to balloon catheter extraction of thrombus, to try to extrude the graft by gentle external massage or by direct irrigation of the graft after performing proximal and distal arteriotomies. Openings in the graft may be made vertically at the proximal and distal anastomotic areas. In the body of the graft a transverse opening is preferable in order to avoid stricture. At the distal anastomosis, if the arteriotomy is carried across the anastomosis into the artery, a vein patch should be applied. If there is concern with the structural integrity of the graft or difficulty with the dissection, one should not hesitate placing a new graft. Finally, it is our routine to perform an intra-operative arteriogram at the time of original surgery. This cannot be overly emphasized. The information obtained will be useful in the event of subsequent thrombosis and is essential to guide the surgeon in making appropriate decisions regarding thrombectomy.

Clinical Results

Operative mortality rates for popliteal, tibial and peroneal reconstructions were 3·5, 3·0 and 4·1 respectively (*Table* 3.3). The cumulative

Table 3.3. Mortality (<30 days)

	No. of cases	*No. dead*	*Mortality (%)*
Popliteal	286	10	3·5
Tibial	169	5	3·0
Peroneal	97	4	4·1

graft patency rates for each of the three types of reconstruction are shown in *Figs. 3.7* and *3.8*. There is no statistical validity for the final 2-year figures since the numbers of cases are small. *Fig 3.9* summarizes the cumulative patency rates for popliteal reconstructions according to location of the distal anastomosis (above or below the knee), the presence or absence of diabetes mellitus and the influence of the run-off. As might be predicted, the presence of diabetes mellitus, poor run-off and reconstructions extending distally initially lead to worse results

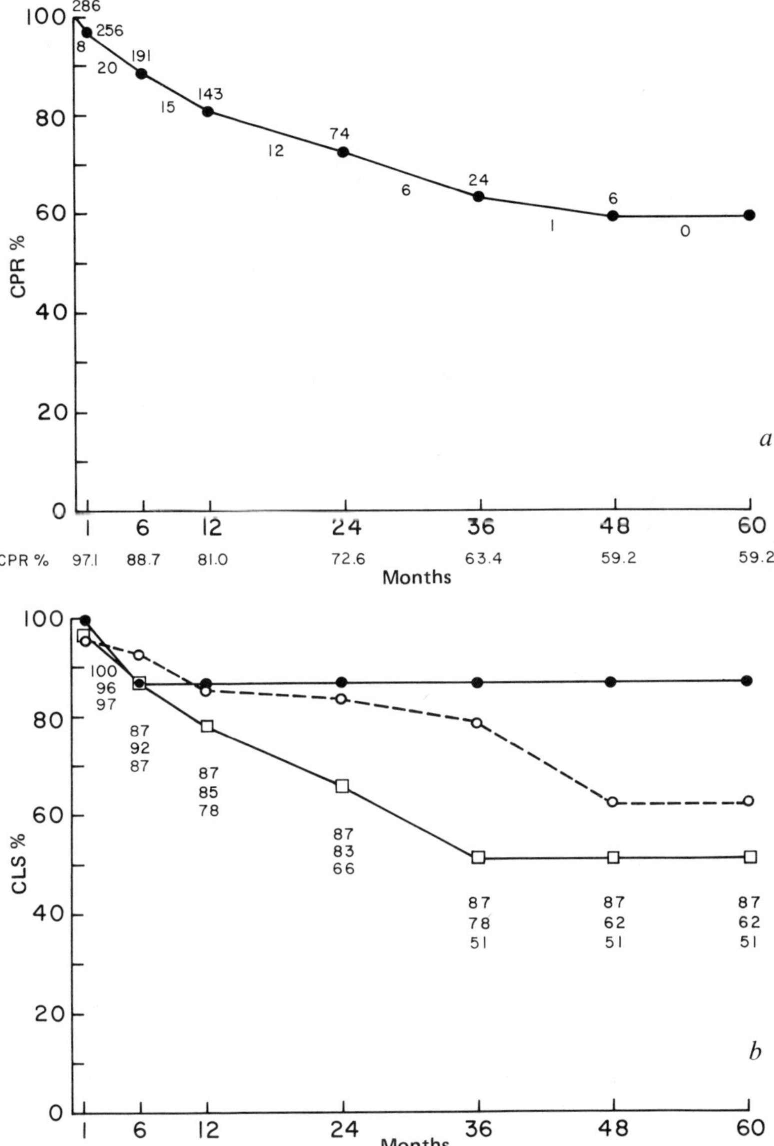

Fig. 3.7.a, Cumulative graft patency rates for all femoral popliteal reconstructions. The number of grafts at risk for a particular time interval is indicated above the curve. The actual number of failures in each time interval is indicated below the curve. *b*, Cumulative limb salvage rates for femoropopliteal reconstructions according to the indication for surgery: ●——● claudication ($n = 16$); ○---○ rest pain ($n = 75$); □——□ gangrene ($n = 188$).

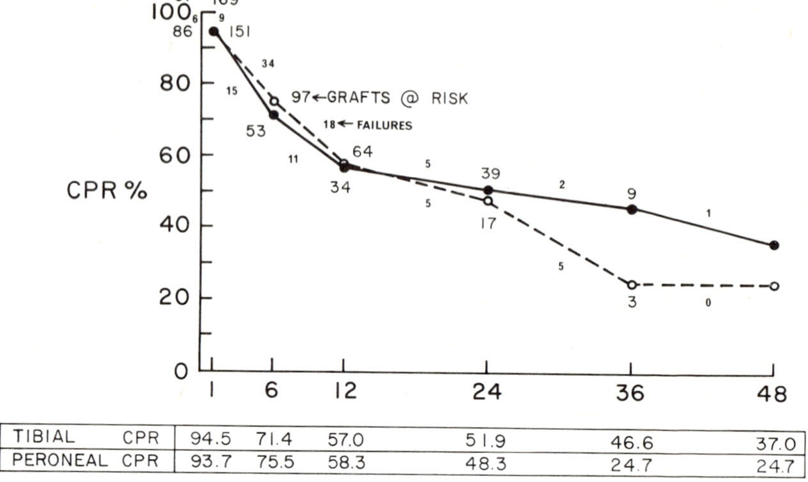

TIBIAL CPR	94.5	71.4	57.0	51.9	46.6	37.0
PERONEAL CPR	93.7	75.5	58.3	48.3	24.7	24.7

Fig. 3.8. Cumulative patency rates for tibial (solid line) and peroneal (dotted line) reconstructions. Grafts at risk for particular time intervals are indicated in the large figures and actual number of failures in smaller figures ●——● tibial; ○——○, peroneal.

than if these factors are not present. However, these differences appear to diminish with time.

Factors that were related to most failures included the quality of the artery into which the distal anastomosis was performed as well as the run-off beyond this vessel. Calcification was associated with a higher incidence of eventual graft closure. The absence of a pedal arch was associated with early graft closure in almost all instances of crural reconstructions. Early failures were usually due to inappropriate case selection with the factors previously identified being present. Late failures were usually due to progressive disease, particularly in the distal circulation. Preliminary investigation employing adjunctive arteriovenous fistulas for remote tibial and peroneal bypasses under circumstances of actual or predictable failure have been encouraging [14]. In some patients an accelerated progression of the atherosclerotic process was also observed in the inflow circulation.

The actual number and percentages of thrombectomies performed for each of the reconstruction groups is depicted in *Fig. 3.10*. Successful thrombectomies were obtained in less than 10 per cent of the popliteal and peroneal reconstructions and 14 per cent of the tibials. Many of the failed thrombectomies would today not have even been attempted.

Fourteen infections (2·5 per cent) occurred in this series of which eleven (2·0 per cent) failed. Ten grafts required removal; in one instance the graft thrombosed and remains *in situ* (*Fig. 3.11*). There were no

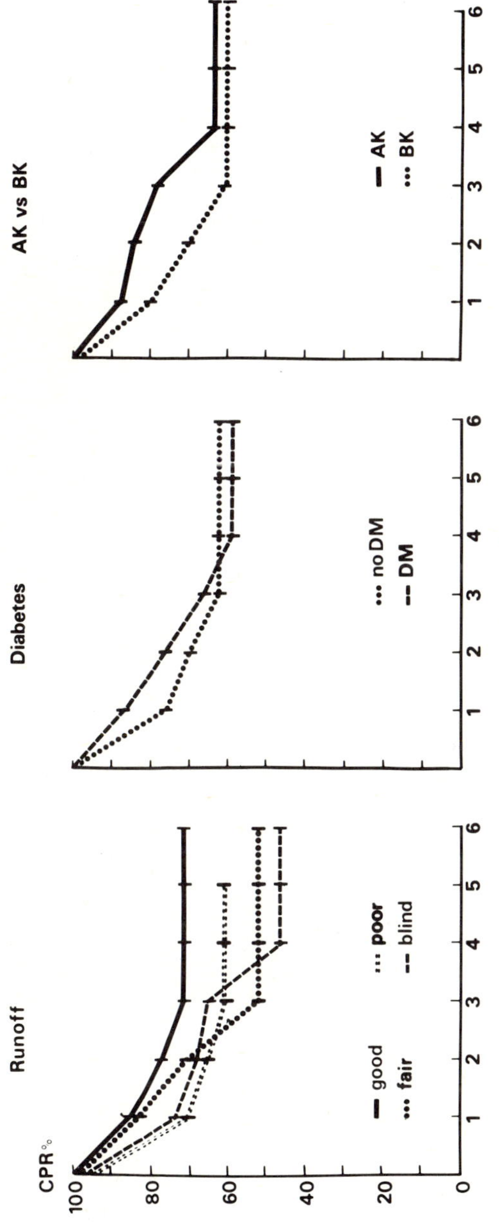

Fig. 3.9. Cumulative patency rates for femoropopliteal reconstructions according to run-off, presence or absence of diabetes mellitus (DM) and location of distal anastomosis (above or below the knee, AK *v.* BK).

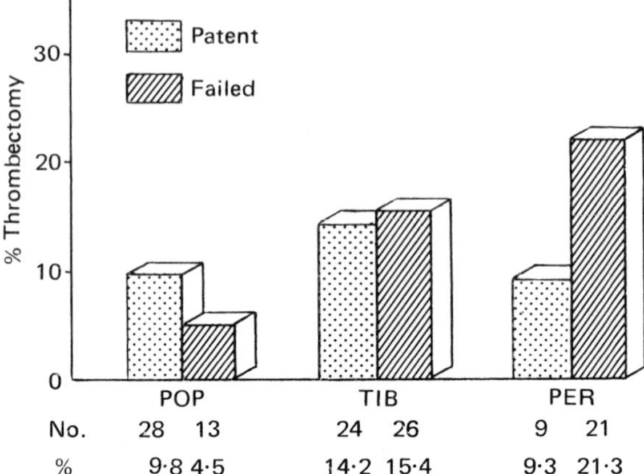

Fig. 3.10. Number and percentage of thrombectomies required for each of the reconstruction groups. Most of the thrombectomies performed that ultimately failed would today not even be attempted based on the results of either preoperative or intraoperative arteriography. POP., Popliteal; TIB., tibial; PER, peroneal.

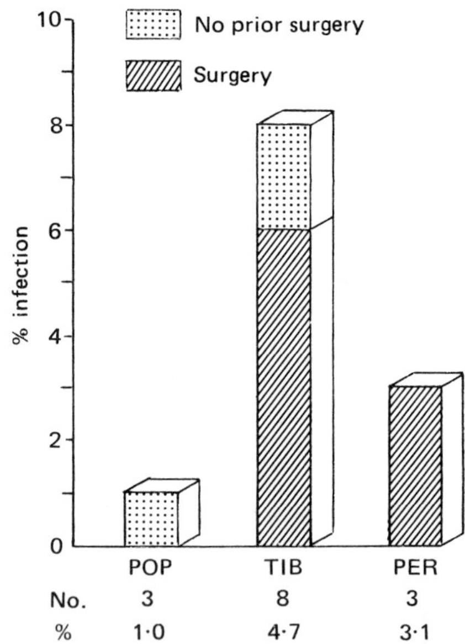

Fig. 3.11. Incidence of infection involving umbilical vein grafts and the results secured following antibiotic therapy and removal of the graft where required. Previous vascular surgery appears to contribute to higher rates of infection in those patients undergoing bypasses to the tibial or peroneal artery. POP, popliteal; TIB, tibial; PER, peroneal. *Incidence* 14 (2·5%): functional, 3; thrombosed (in situ), 1; removed, 10 (drainage 6, sepsis 5, exposed graft 1, bleeding/F.A. 1.) *Failure* 11 (2·0%): AMP, 3; ischaemia, 3; X-ant. bypass, 3; prox-bypass, 1; profundoplasty, 1.

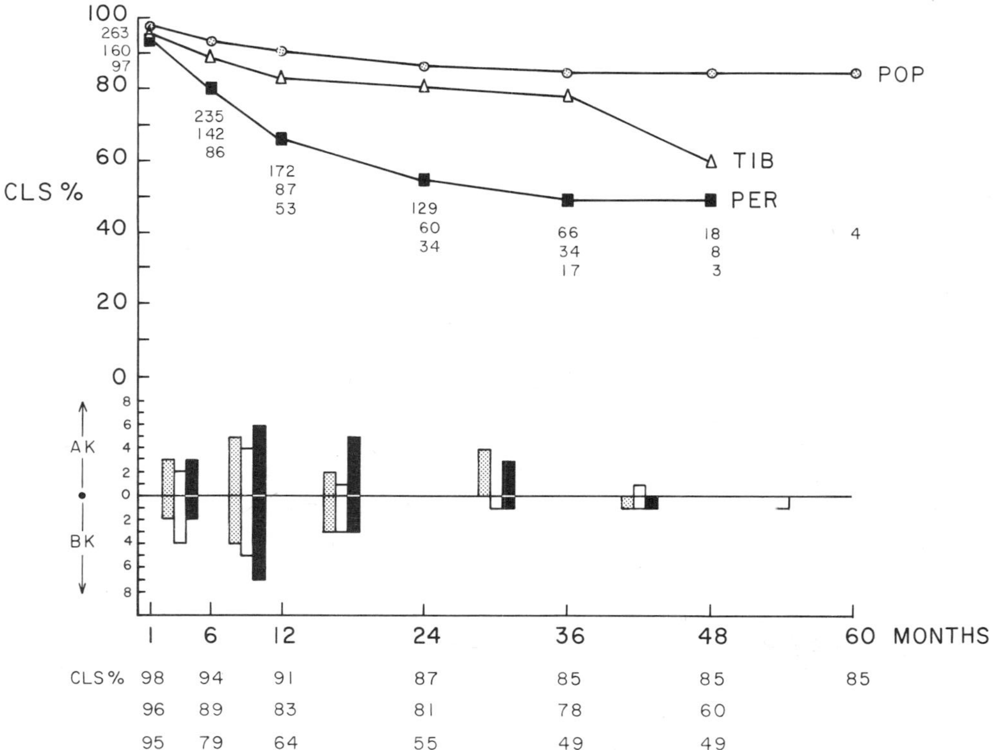

Fig. 3.12. Cumulative limb salvage (CLS) rates following popliteal (POP), tibial (TIB) and peroneal (PER) reconstruction. The actual numbers of amputations are indicated in each time interval in the histogram portion of this figure. Amputations above or below the knee are indicated relative to the horizontal axis.

instances of biodegradation either by aneurysm formation or by myointimal proliferation. Only one graft showed segmental ectasia at 20 months. Three false aneurysms occurred early in the series and were probably due to faulty technique. Cumulative limb salvage is depicted in *Fig. 3.12.* These results confirm the effectiveness even of peroneal reconstruction in securing limb salvage despite later closure of the graft. The actual numbers and types of amputations performed are shown in the histogram in *Fig. 3.12.*

Histopathology

Histological examination of umbilical vein graft specimens showed that they were well accepted by the human hosts and appeared to function with minimal alteration. Extended use of the graft (42-month specimen) did not significantly alter the original preimplant architecture.

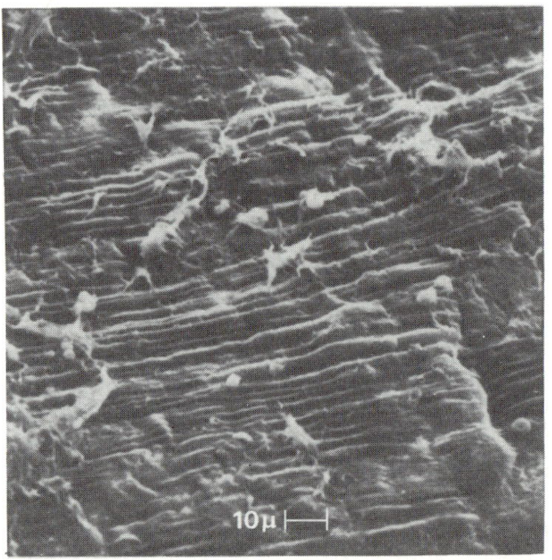

Fig. 3.13. Scanning electron micrograph of a 6-month graft explant showing smooth surface with fibrin and platelets.

There was preservation of the internal elastic membrane confirmed by serial sectioning and use of elastic stains. Electron microscopy demonstrated minimal accumulation of *intracellular* lipid compared to control specimens. Thus, mechanisms which operate for the accumulation of intracellular lipid in living tissue apparently cease to operate in the glutaraldehyde-processed veins. Scanning electron microscopy showed relatively smooth flow surfaces in non-thrombosed graft explants (*Fig. 3.13*).

Critical Surface Tension

Contact angle measurements provide one of the fastest and most sensitive techniques known for identifying changes in surface constitution of any material. Critical surface tension (CST), derived from contact angle data, is a measure of surface-free energy and can be chemically fixed in a biocompatible zone (20–30 dyn/cm) characteristic of endothelized, fully hydrated natural blood vessels. Preimplant CST values of umbilical vein grafts fell into the biocompatible range of 20–30 dyn/cm even after tanning with glutaraldehyde and storage in ethanol. *Fig. 3.14* represents a typical surface tension plot taken from

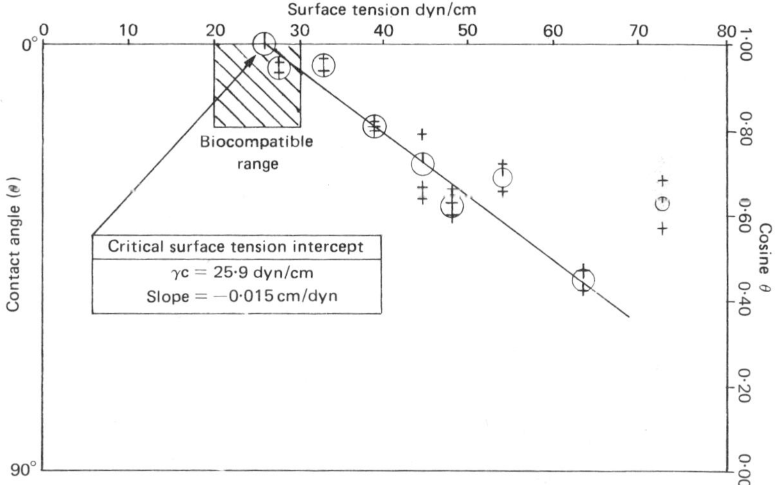

Fig. 3.14. Critical surface tension plot of an 8-month explant specimen. Note that the CST value remains in the biocompatible range of 20–30 dyn/cm even after implantation.

an 8-month explanted specimen. The CST value remains in the biocompatible range. Stability of this parameter has been noted in patent graft samples up to 42 months postoperatively.

Internal Reflection Spectroscopy

Internal reflection spectroscopy (IRS) allows the recording of a diagnostic infrared 'fingerprint' for the interfacial layers of solids and liquids. The technique is sensitive enough to detect and analyse films as thin as 10 Å and to follow changes in the composition, configuration and bonding within such films. Preimplant IRS demonstrates strong protein bands and weak or absent hydrocarbon peaks. Similar patterns were noted in patients with stable atherosclerosis (*Fig. 3.15*). In

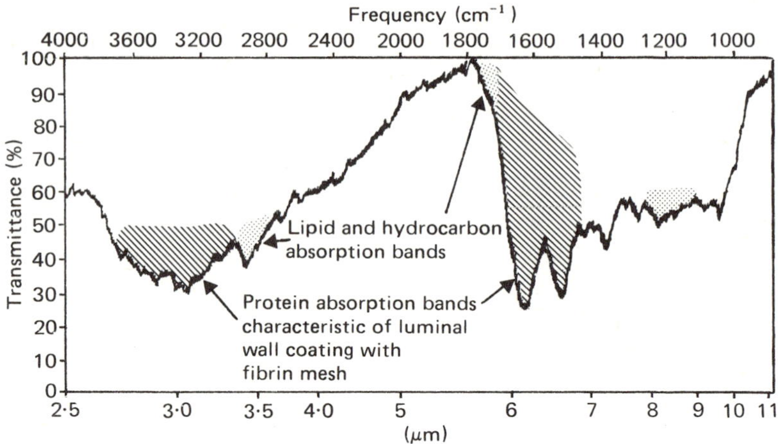

Fig. 3.15. Internal reflection infrared spectrum of the blood flow surface of a patent human arterial graft constructed from a stabilized human umbilical cord vein. This specimen, harvested after 6 months' implantation, was generally overcoated with a thin fibrin deposit in contrast to grafts in other hosts which imbibed lipids into their lumenal walls and remained substantially free of fibrin overlayers.

contrast, some explanted grafts have lipid peaks as demonstrated in the 10-week sample shown in *Fig. 3.16.* This occurred in patients with progressive forms of atherosclerosis. The presence of this lipoidal material does not affect CST. Calcification has to date not been identified in any explanted samples. Lipid levels within grafts appear to be more related to the patient and haemodynamics than to the graft or implant time.

Angiography

Most of the grafts remained identical to their appearance at intra-operative arteriography (*Fig. 3.17*). However, in approximately 20 per cent of the cases, angiographic changes were demonstrable. These changes consisted primarily of a segmented or scalloped appearance (*Fig. 3.18*), but they did not seem to compromise graft function. Several of the patients with these findings have had patent grafts more than 2 years after demonstration of these postoperative angiographic findings. We believe that these changes represent lengthening of the umbilical vein within the outer Dacron collagen tube component of the graft. The degree to which these intraluminal alterations were noted varied from patient to patient.

In only one instance was there evidence of graft ectasia and possibly small aneurysmal formation. The postoperative arteriogram was done

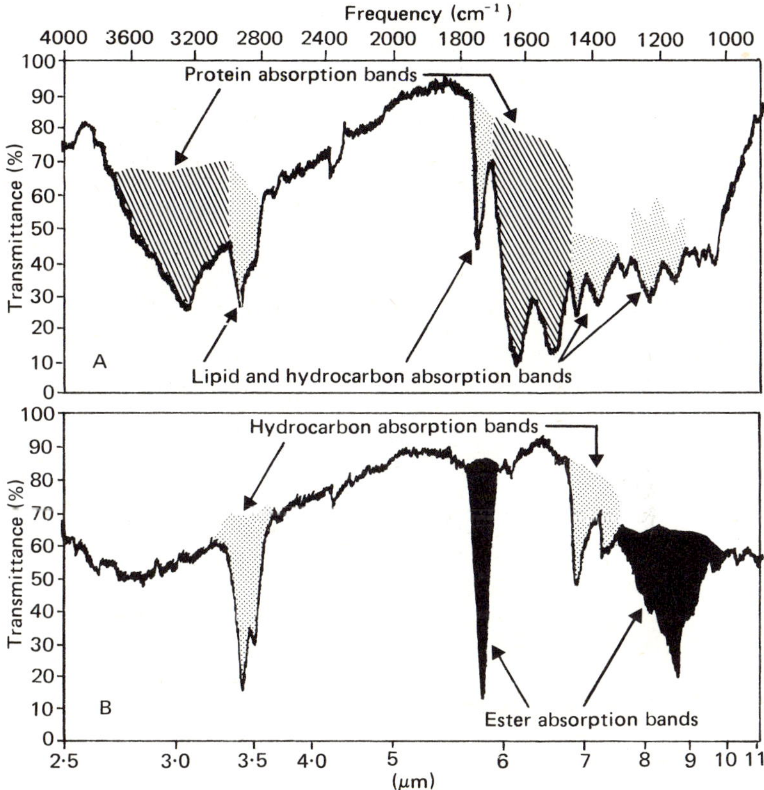

Fig. 3.16. Internal reflection infrared spectra of (*a*) the blood flow surface of a patent stabilized human umbilical cord vein graft harvested after 10 weeks' service in the human arterial system, and (*b*) the oily material that was expressed from this post-implanted vessel by application of pressure. Lipid peaks as demonstrated here occur in those grafts in which there is marked progression of systemic atherosclerosis.

20 months after implantation, and the graft continues to be functional at 28 months. The findings in this particular case may be related to the actual graft preparation technology in that this was one of the first grafts implanted. There has been no other evidence of aneurysmal deterioration. Similarly, we have not seen evidence of intimal hyperplasia within the graft itself, though there have been both angiographic and morphologic findings of intimal hyperplasia at anastomotic areas. These generally occurred at sites of widely disparate diameters between the graft and the host vessel, or in instances where considerable disease was present at the time of implantation, particularly in the femoral artery region.

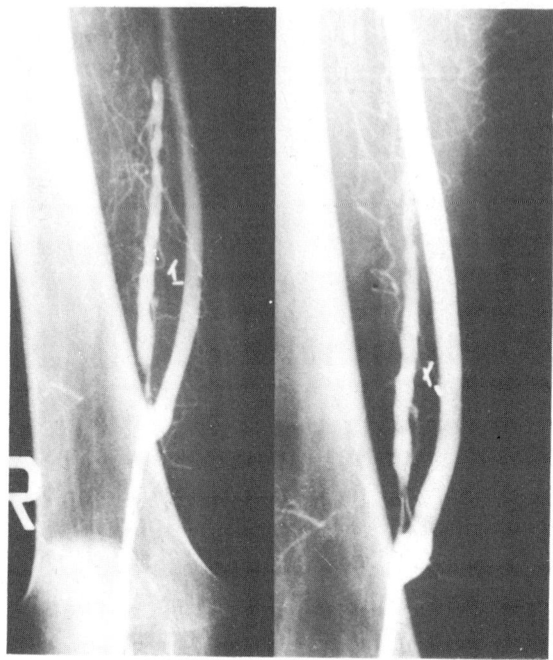

Fig. 3.17. Comparative views of femoropopliteal bypass showing striking similarities between intraoperative arteriogram (*left*) and 32-month postoperative arteriogram (*right*).

DISCUSSION

From its inception and even to the present day, the umbilical cord vein project has been surrounded by scepticism and at times incredulity. Review of our results, however, suggests that in fact the glutaraldehyde stabilized umbilical vein prosthesis can serve as an attractive alternative to the saphenous vein.

The results of the cumulative patency rates obtained in reconstructions of the popliteal, tibial or peroneal arteries were similar to those obtained by us and others using autologous saphenous veins in comparable cases [15–22]. Analysis of the failures in this series indicates that the majority were due to faulty case selection. Using today's criteria, most of these patients would not now be considered suitable for operation—for example, those with absence of the pedal arch and extensive calcification of the run-off vessels. Most graft failures are due to progression of the disease, usually in the distal circulation, but sometimes in the proximal inflow circulation as documented by serial arteriography.

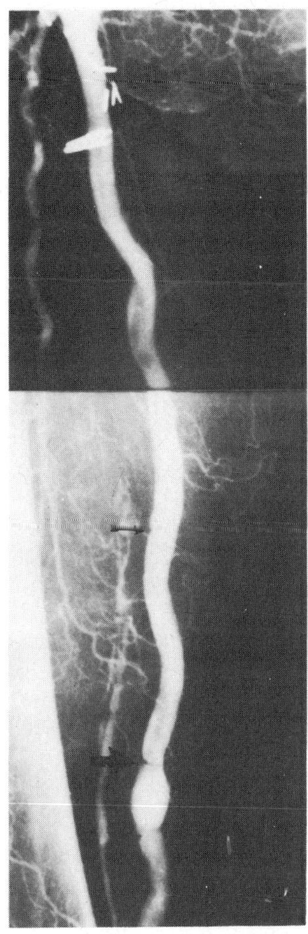

Fig. 3.18. Twelve-month postoperative arteriogram depicting small surface irregularities (small arrow) and focal segmentation (large arrow).

The clinical proving ground for various graft materials employed in the lower extremity has classically been in the femoral popliteal site. We believe that to demonstrate the superiority of one particular graft material over another the most difficult areas of reconstruction should be chosen and for this reason we feel that the peroneal and perhaps in some instances the tibial arteries would be better than the femoropopliteal region. Obviously these patients should only be operated upon to save their threatened limbs, and lacking an adequate autologous saphenous vein, it would certainly be justifiable to use any of the several accepted materials now available. To date, our experience with the glutaraldehyde stabilized umbilical vein continues to be favourable and we believe it provides an excellent alternative to the saphenous vein for reconstruction in the lower extremity.

The postoperative morphological data further confirm the biodurability of this graft material. Evidence of biodegradation has been minimal, without any significant incidence of aneurysmal degeneration, calcification or intimal hyperplasia. Lipid deposition has been noted by light and electron microscopy as well as by infrared spectrographic analysis. This observation, however, is related to the type of lipid metabolism indigenous to the particular patient rather than to the graft itself. High lipid levels in the early postoperative period were manifest in patients with evidence of progressive atherosclerotic involvement in other systems. Many of these patients died early of myocardial infarction or strokes. Late and minimal lipid deposition occurred in patients with stable systemic atherosclerosis. These patients showed no progression.

An interesting phenomenon associated with glutaraldehyde was the increased resistance of this graft material to infection. The low rate of infection in this series is a manifestation of this resistance, as well as the absence of graft dissolution and haemorrhage when graft infection did occur.

Predicting the morphology of these grafts beyond 5 years is, of course, impossible, but based on analogous experience with the glutaraldehyde stabilized porcine heart valves, it is very possible that increasing degrees of fibrosis, calcification and possibly even aneurysmal degeneration may occur. Certainly this represents less of a problem for lower extremity prostheses than cardiac prostheses in that most patients presenting with advanced lower extremity obliterative atherosclerosis requiring reconstructions already have a limited projected life span. We would anticipate that should there be any graft degeneration, replacement is feasible. The more significant problem, however, relates to our inability to prevent disease progression, particularly downstream from the distal anastomosis.

Many graft materials tried in the past have produced less than spectacular success. The next 5 years will be critical in determining the ultimate place of various graft materials in treating patients with vascular occlusive disease. Realistically, it is unlikely that any one of the new materials will accomplish a major breakthrough in securing longer term graft patency and function than that presently achieved. Our hopes and expectations may be unrealistic and outside the bounds of what can possibly be accomplished. The benefits now achieved with the clinical use of various graft materials might therefore be interpreted as having reached a level beyond which even the development of an 'ideal' graft would be unlikely to further improve long term graft patency and durability as determined by standard life table methods. It must be recognized that the exact graft material is less important than surgical expertise, knowledge and judgement. Additionally, one must consider the patient and the biological status of his disease. Although uncontrollable in many aspects, cessation of all smoking and attention to an exercise programme and dietary factors may be among the most critical factors in securing long term success of the operative procedure.

REFERENCES

1. Dardik I. and Dardik H. (1975) The fate of human umbilical cord vessels used as interposition arterial grafts in the baboon. *Surg. Gynecol. Obstet.* **140**, 567–71.
2. Anzola J., Palmer T. H. and Welch C. S. (1951) Long femoral and ileofemoral grafts. *Surg. Forum* **2**, 243–6.
3. Nabseth D. C., Wilson J. T., Tan B. et al. (1960) Fetal arterial heterografts. *Arch. Surg.* **81**, 929–33.
4. Yong N. K. and Eiseman B. (1962) The experimental use of heterologous umbilical vein grafts as aortic substitutes. *Sing. Med. J.* **3**, 52–7.
5. Rosenberg N., Martinez A., Sawyer P. N. et al. (1966) Tanned collagen arterial prosthesis of bovine carotid origin in man. Preliminary studies of enzyme-treated heterografts. *Ann. Surg.* **164**, 247–56.
6. Carpentier A., Blondeau P. and Marcel P. (1968) Remplacement des valves mitrales et tricuspides par des heterogrefes. *Ann. Chir. Thorac. Cardiovasc.* **7**, 33.
7. Dardik H., Ibrahim I. M. and Dardik I. (1975) Modified and unmodified umbilical vein allografts and xenografts employed as arterial substitutes: a morphologic assessment. *Surg. Forum* **26**, 286–7.
8. Dardik H. and Dardik I. (1976) Successful arterial substitution with modified human umbilical vein. *Ann. Surg.* **183**, 252–8.
9. Dardik H., Ibrahim I. M., Sprayregen S. et al. (1976) Clinical experience with modified human umbilical cord vein for arterial bypass. *Surgery* **79**, 618–24.
10. Hufnagel C. A. (1978) Heparin-bonded surfaces in prostheses and biografts. In: Dardik H. (ed.) *Graft Materials in Vascular Surgery*. Chicago, Ill., Symposia Specialists Inc., Year Book Medical Publishers, pp. 191–201.
11. Cranley J. J. and Hafner C. D. (1980) Current status of the umbilical vein graft. In: Bernhard V. (ed.) *Complications in Vascular Surgery*. New York, Grune and Stratton, pp. 597–613.
12. Mabry C. D., Thompson B. W. and Read R. C. (1979) Activated clotting time (ACT) monitoring of intraoperative heparinization in peripheral vascular surgery. *Am. J. Surg.* **138**, 894–900.
13. Dardik H., Ibrahim I. M., Koslow A. et al. (1978) Evaluation of intraoperative arteriography as a routine for vascular reconstructions. *Surg. Gynecol. Obstet.* **147**, 853–8.
14. Ibrahim I. M., Sussman B., Dardik I. et al. (1980) Adjunctive arteriovenous fistula with tibial and peroneal reconstruction for limb salvage. *Am. J. Surg.* **140**, 246–51.
15. Dardik H., Ibrahim I. M. and Dardik I. (1979) The role of the peroneal artery for limb salvage. *Ann. Surg.* **189**, 189–98.
16. Dardik H., Ibrahim I. M., Jarrah M. et al. (1980) Three-year experience with glutaraldehyde-stabilized umbilical vein for limb salvage. *Br. J. Surg.* **67**, 229–32.
17. DeWeese J. A. and Rob C. G. (1977). Autogenous venous grafts ten years later. *Surgery* **82**, 775–84.
18. Ferris E. B. and Cranley J. J. (1979) Use of umbilical vein graft as an arterial substitute. *Arch. Surg.* **114**, 694–7.
19. Cutler B. S., Thompson J. F., Kleinsasser L. J. et al. (1976) Autologous saphenous vein femoropopliteal bypass: analysis of 298 cases. *Surgery* **79**, 325–31.
20. LoGerfo F. W., Corson J. D. and Mannick J. A. (1977) Improved results with femoropopliteal vein grafts for limb salvage. *Arch. Surg.* **112**, 567–70.

21. Naji A., Jennifer C., McCombs P. R. et al. (1978) Results of 100 consecutive femoropopliteal vein grafts for limb salvage. *Ann. Surg.* **188**, 162–5.
22. Walden R., L'Itahen G. J., Megerman J. et al. (1980) Matched elastic properties and successful arterial grafting. *Arch. Surg.* **115**, 1166–9.

IV. The Need for Compliance in Prosthetic Arterial Replacements

D. Annis and R. Clarke

The mechanical properties of arterial prostheses have not been a primary consideration in their design except in as much as they have met the essential requirement of being sufficiently resilient to withstand pressures within them during a lifetime of clinical use. Most emphasis has been placed upon the development of a fabric material with the least thrombogenic surface, and this has led to the production of a variety of woven, knitted and velour grafts of polyethylene terephthalate (PET) or of polytetrafluoroethylene (PTFE). The most recent development in the area of prosthetic artery grafts has been the entry into clinical usage of expanded microfibrous PTFE grafts (Gore-Tex, Impra).

The mechanical properties of all these grafts are wholly different from those of the natural vessels which they are designed to replace. Because PET and PTFE are rigid polymers, grafts made from these materials undergo hardly any deformation in diameter in response to the physiological loading conditions of pulsating intraluminal pressure; the more so when they have been infiltrated with collagenous scar tissue. In contrast, the wall of a natural vessel is elastic and undergoes large deformation for relatively small stresses. When the vessel is subjected to physiological loading *in vivo*, it undergoes a continuous cyclical change in radius, in wall thickness and, to a lesser extent, in length. These changes in dimension fluctuate around average values which represent large extensions of the dimensions of the vessel in its relaxed state (this is clearly illustrated by the considerable shortening and narrowing of the natural vessel together with thickening of the wall which occurs after a length of a vessel is excised). These large strains result in stresses distributed non-uniformly throughout the wall of the living artery [1].

There are therefore fundamental differences between an inelastic prosthesis and the natural artery. Perhaps the only feature which they share is that they are both tubular conduits for blood. Despite these extreme rheological differences, PET and PTFE grafts perform reasonably well when used to replace large and medium-sized arteries.

Unfortunately, the rate of failure increases with a decrease in diameter. Failure of small diameter prostheses may be due to early thrombosis or, later, to the development of an increasingly thickened hyperplastic intima.

It has been suggested by many investigators that the repeated failure of small bore inelastic prostheses is the result in part of the mismatch in mechanical properties between the synthetic and the natural artery leading to disturbances in flow regimens within and distal to the graft. If this is so, then a successful small diameter arterial prosthesis should closely match the mechanical properties of the natural vessel which it replaces. It must be said, however, that the hypothesis of mismatched mechanical properties has yet to be proved. It will require precise knowledge of the rheological properties both of the natural vessels and of the prostheses, a knowledge of the stresses in the system and of the haemodynamic events in the vessel during pulsatile flow. Although there have been a number of very thorough analyses of the rheology of blood vessels [2, 3], as yet there has been no equally thorough analysis of the mechanical properties of different types of arterial prosthesis. It should be possible, however, from the basic principles of fluid mechanics, to predict certain gross effects of such a mismatch upon the haemodynamic parameters.

The anastomosis of a naturally compliant vessel to a rigid synthetic prosthesis must result in a discrepancy between their diameters during much of the cardiac cycle. With each pulse there will be either a sudden narrowing or sudden diversion of the flow boundaries. In conditions of steady flow both these situations are known to produce turbulence, the severity of which depends upon the relative change in diameter and the Reynolds number of the flow across the site of union. When the union is between a natural artery and an inelastic prosthesis the conditions are further complicated by the continuous movement of the arterial wall and by the pulsatile nature of the flow. It seems certain that under these circumstances there will be some disturbances of flow and possibly turbulence at the anastomosis, though the precise nature of that disturbance is still the subject of study.

In the normal arterial circulation a pulse pressure wave travels throughout the length of major vessels in response to each heart beat. The velocity of propagation of the pulse wave is controlled by the elastic properties of the arterial wall. The introduction of a rigid segment of graft in that system increases the velocity of propagation, leading to haemodynamic changes within and distal to the graft. The sudden change in wall stiffness which occurs at the two anastomoses due to the mismatch in mechanical properties of the graft and artery will also lead to reflected waves which will be superimposed upon the normal wave, causing flow disturbances.

Recent investigations [4] into the aetiology of arteriosclerosis have shown a correlation between sites in the artery wall which are exposed to turbulent flow and the incidence of arteriosclerotic lesions. Similar correlations have been observed at sites of high shear stress in the wall of vessels. High shear rates and turbulence are damaging to erythrocytes, platelets and to endothelial cells, and together they are likely to contribute to the formation of thrombus and ultimately to the failure of the graft.

A further cause of failure is frequently observed which may also be related to the mismatch in mechanical properties between the graft and the host vessel. In vessels of small internal diameter late failure is often associated with the development of a slowly increasing hyperplastic intima at or near the anastomosis. A point is reached at which flow is reduced within the vessel and occlusion occurs due to thrombosis. This may be due to the occurrence of high stresses in the wall of the natural artery close to the anastomosis resulting from the restraint on normal pulsatile movement of the artery wall by the inextensible synthetic graft. In particular, these stresses may be concentrated round the stitch holes of the anastomosis.

Evidence to support the mismatch hypothesis is sparse and difficult to demonstrate by rational experiment. Several investigators have attempted to prove the need for elastic walled arterial grafts by comparison of measurements of certain properties of currently available prostheses including tissue grafts as well as the stiff-walled prostheses. They have tried to correlate some index of distensibility with patency rates. Unfortunately such an approach lacks scientific rigour. When comparisons of several different types of graft are made it is difficult to isolate the effects of mechanical properties from those other variables between the grafts, such as their size, their surface structure and their chemical properties. This is especially the case when graft materials may range from rigid PET grafts to autologous vein grafts. A measurement which has often been used to characterize the mechanical properties of arterial grafts is an elastic modulus derived only from the *in vitro* measurement of changes in outer diameter for given increments of pressure. Unfortunately it may be misleading to compare grafts of different types using this empirical modulus since such a comparison does not take into account various differences in fundamental mechanical properties. For instance, if an arterial graft is constructed in such a way that it is anisotropic (that is to say it does not have elastic properties which are identical in all directions), it is likely to lengthen on inflation. However, if only changes in diameter are considered in the elastic modulus, then it will be misleading to use this modulus to make comparisons between an isotropic and an anisotropic prosthesis.

Similarly, if a graft is made from incompressible material (that is one which preserves its volume under loading), inside diameter may be inferred from a measurement of the outer diameter. However, with grafts which are constructed of compressible material (such as one of fibrous knitted or woven construction where a significant part of the wall is open space), then the inner diameter must be either measured directly or calculated from a precise knowledge of the change in volume of the material under loading. It is therefore not valid to compare grafts with different basic mechanical properties using an elastic modulus derived from measurements of pressure and outside diameter, yet this comparison has been made frequently in published work.

The advantage of an elastic-walled arterial prosthesis has therefore not been satisfactorily demonstrated by studies using grafts that are currently available. However, there remains a strong feeling that the performance of small diameter arterial grafts will be enhanced if their mechanical properties are made to closely match those of the natural artery. This has led several investigators [5–7] to produce novel prostheses having elastic walls.

We have developed an elastic-walled artificial artery. This comprises a cylinder with porous walls made up of a matrix of polyurethane fibres, each of which has a diameter of 1–1·5 μm (*Fig. 3.19*). This prosthesis is described elsewhere [7].

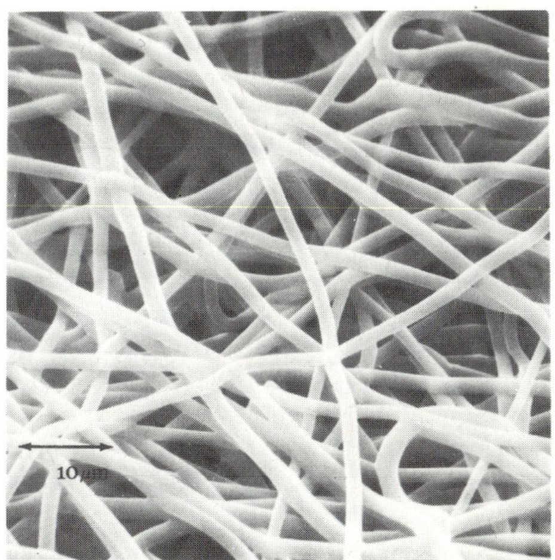

Fig. 3.19. Scanning electron micrograph of the surface of the electrostatically spun graft; fibres approx. 1·5 μm in diameter.

One of the original aims of this development was to investigate the hypothesis that the success of a small diameter arterial replacement depends in part upon a close match of mechanical properties of the graft to host vessel. To this end, we are characterizing the mechanical properties of the graft so that we might compare them with the mechanical properties of natural vessels published in the scientific literature.

To do this we need to obtain a useful relationship between the strains in the graft, that is the changes in diameter, wall thickness and length, and the stresses caused by physiological loading of intraluminal pressure and longitudinal tethering force from surrounding connective tissue. A relationship which relates stresses to strains for a general case is known as a constitutive relation, which comprises a constitutive equation and a number of constitutive constants. The constitutive relation allows the prediction of the changes in graft dimensions for any known state of stress.

The constitutive equation for the Liverpool graft is of the same type as that used by Patel [2] to describe the mechanical properties of the natural vessel. This considers the artery to be an incompressible, anisotropic, homogeneous material which undergoes large deformations for relatively small stresses. The same assumptions have been shown to apply to our graft. The constitutive constants for the graft are obtained from a series of *in vitro* experiments in which values of stress and strain calculated from measurements of forces applied to the graft and the corresponding deformation. The experimental results are used to verify the applicability of the model.

By using results from two models of the same form derived by similar experimental procedures we feel confident that we may draw a valid comparison between the predicted *in vivo* performance of the natural artery and the Liverpool graft. If significant differences exist between the graft and the natural vessel, it will be necessary to modify the properties of the graft until there is a close match between the two.

Whilst this work is still in its early stages, we have achieved some success. In large (>6 mm internal diameter) arterial replacements in animals we have seen a firm but delicate attachment at the anastomoses resulting from the ingrowth of connective tissue into the interstices of the surface of the graft, and, according to the animal species, a variable extent of new intima on the blood surface. Thus, in the dog a completely new intima formed throughout the length of a 120 mm long 6-mm bore graft. More recently we have had fair success with implantation of 4 mm internal diameter grafts as interposition vessels in the common carotid artery of dogs. It is hoped that patency rates of the 4 mm grafts will improve with modifications which lead to a closer match with the natural vessel.

We believe that the development of a successful synthetic graft to replace the smaller arteries of the body will be achieved only when grafts are so designed as to least disturb flow through them. This will only be achieved by a rigorous analysis of the rheological properties of the natural and prosthetic vessels, leading to the development of grafts with mechanical properties which closely match those of the natural artery.

REFERENCES

1. McDonald D. A. (1974) *Blood Flow in Arteries*, 2nd ed. London, Arnold.
2. Patel D. J. (1972) In: Bergel D. H. (ed.) *The Rheology of Large Blood Vessels in Cardiovascular Fluid Dynamics*. London, Academic Press.
3. Doyle J. M. and Dobrin P. B. (1973) Stress gradients in the walls of large arteries. *J. Biomechanics* **16**, 631–9.
4. Fry D. C. (1969) Certain chemorheologic considerations regarding the blood vascular interface with particular reference to coronary artery disease. *Circulation* **39** and **40**, Suppl. IV, pp. IV-38–IV-57.
5. Lyman D. J., Albo D., Jackson R. et al. (1977) Development of small diameter vascular prostheses. *Trans. Am. Soc. Artif. Intern. Organs* **23**, 253–61.
6. Clark R. E., Apostolou S. and Kardos J. L. (1976) Mismatch of mechanical properties as a cause of arterial prosthesis thrombosis. *Surg. Forum* **27**, 208–10.
7. Annis D., Bornat A., Edwards R. et al. (1978) An elastomeric vascular prosthesis. *Trans. Am. Soc. Artif. Intern. Organs* **24**, 209–13.

Edward B. Diethrich

4 Surgery of the Branches of the Aortic Arch

Diminished blood flow through the large vessels arising from the aortic arch, whether due to acquired disease or congenital malformation, has long been recognized as a serious, often fatal condition demanding surgical repair. In the 35 years or so that vascular surgeons have been attempting to ameliorate these deficits, tremendous technical changes have been introduced, simplifying operative approaches, developing improved graft materials, tapping neighbouring vascular systems to re-route blood paths, revascularizing areas heretofore considered taboo and identifying haemodynamic deficits. To keep pace with evolving operative techniques, diagnostics have undergone revolutionary enhancements as well, and the benefits have been a boon to the vascular surgeon.

Regardless of the heights to which our technology has risen to date, lesions of the aortic arch branches, particularly ulcerative atherosclerotic plaques and unrecognized congenital anomalies, still often pose a diagnostic dilemma. The intent of this chapter is to describe the vascular anatomy of the arch vessels and their major divisions, giving particular attention to the availability of collateral pathways. From this foundation, the major pathological disorders afflicting this region, both congenital and acquired, will be discussed with their haemodynamic consequences. Following a brief review of appropriate diagnostic procedures, the chapter will focus on newly developed surgical techniques for the restoration of circulation to the area or the correction of anomalies; however, there will be no discussion of the repair of congenital malformations in paediatric patients since this represents a specialty unto itself.

ANATOMY OF THE AORTIC ARCH BRANCHES

It is important in the study of arch vessel surgery to understand the haemodynamics of the area. For this, a description of the vasculature in the superior mediastinum alone is insufficient. It must be expanded to encompass the major branchings of the arch vessels, particularly into the cervical area, so that collateralization can be appreciated. Moreover, proximal arch vessel occlusive lesions can produce a variety of vascular steals whose symptomatology is as varied as the retrograde flow patterns. To this end, this section is sufficiently detailed to provide an understanding of the haemodynamic consequences of arch vessel lesions.

The aorta ascends from the upper part of the left ventricle into the superior mediastinum for 5 cm, coursing upward, anteriorly and to the left (*Fig. 4.1*). At the level of the second sternocostal articulation, it arches to the left over the trachea and is directed backward and downward on the left side of the trachea becoming continuous with the descending aorta at the level of the fourth thoracic vertebra. At the convexity of the arch, three main branches are given off: innominate (brachiocephalic), left common carotid and left subclavian arteries. Variations at this point are not uncommon, with the innominate artery being absent and the right carotid and subclavian arteries arising independently from the arch. The primary branches may also be reduced in number to two or even one, with the left carotid issuing from the innominate, or more rarely, the carotid and subclavian arteries of the left side arising from the innominate artery. There may also be an increase in primary branches to more than four, with the vertebrals (one or both) arising from the arch or even the internal and external carotids issuing directly from the aorta.

Assuming a usual configuration, the first branch of the aorta is the innominate artery, the largest of the arch vessels. For its 5 cm length, it ascends obliquely upward, posteriorly and to the right to the level of the upper border of the right sternoclavicular articulation, at which point it divides into the right common carotid and right subclavian arteries. The location of this division is of particular importance from a surgical standpoint because it is relatively inaccessible through standard operative incisions.

The left common carotid artery is usually the second branch of the aorta. It arises from the highest point on the arch on a plane posterior to the innominate artery. Its thoracic portion runs through the superior mediastinum to the level of the left sternoclavicular joint where it enters the neck. In the cervical area, the left common carotid and its contralateral vessel follow identical paths obliquely upward behind the sternoclavicular articulation, dividing into the internal and external carotids at the upper border of the thyroid cartilage. The internal carotids supply blood to the anterior portion of the brain and the eyes and send branches to the forehead and nose. The external carotids pass upward and forward, giving off branches to the face as they course backward along the mandible, terminating in the superficial temporal and maxillary arteries. Normally, the external carotids supply no blood to the brain unless there is occlusion of the internal carotid or vertebral arteries. In these cases, the external carotids provide crucial collateral flow. The communication between the external and internal carotid

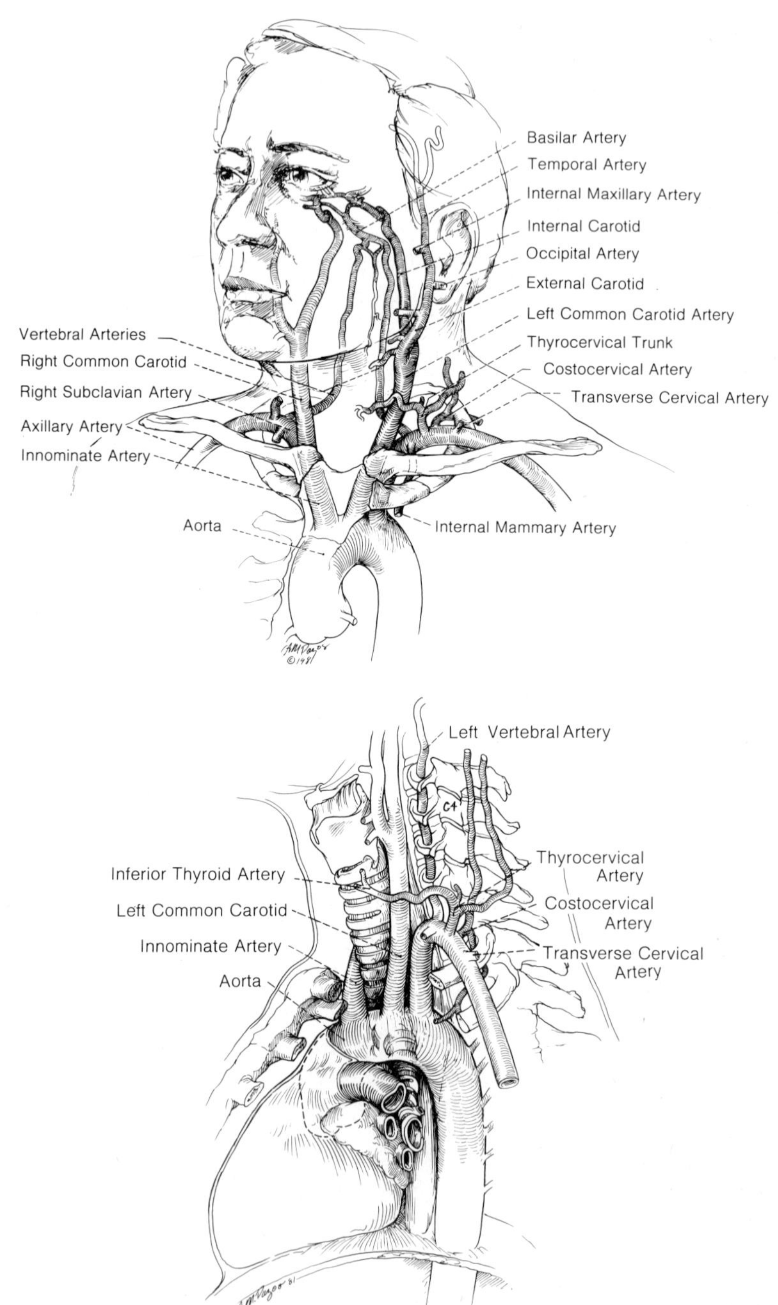
Basilar Artery
Temporal Artery
Internal Maxillary Artery
Internal Carotid
Occipital Artery
External Carotid
Left Common Carotid Artery
Thyrocervical Trunk
Costocervical Artery
Transverse Cervical Artery
Vertebral Arteries
Right Common Carotid
Right Subclavian Artery
Axillary Artery
Innominate Artery
Aorta
Internal Mammary Artery
Left Vertebral Artery
C4
Thyrocervical Artery
Inferior Thyroid Artery
Left Common Carotid
Costocervical Artery
Innominate Artery
Transverse Cervical Artery
Aorta

arteries can be of great importance if the proximal common carotid becomes occluded at its origin on the arch.

The last major arch branch is the left subclavian artery. It arises from the aorta in close proximity to the left common carotid at the level of the fourth thoracic vertebra. It ascends into the superior mediastinum to the root of the neck and arches laterally to the medial border of the scalenus anterior muscle. Here, the first of five branches arises, the vertebral artery, followed closely by the thyrocervical, internal mammary and costocervical arteries. Further on, the transverse cervical, the last branch of the subclavian, arises.

The right subclavian artery, arising from the division of the innominate artery, travels behind the upper part of the right sternoclavicular articulation, passing upward laterally to the medial margin of the scalenus muscle. It then arches slightly as it passes behind the scalenus and courses downward laterally to the outer border of the first rib, where it becomes the axillary artery. The right subclavian has branches similar to those of its left counterpart, although the costocervical trunk arises further along its path than on the left.

Of the subclavian branches, the vertebrals are most significant inasmuch as they are the major conduits for blood to the posterior portion of the brain. They course along either side of the upper cervical vertebrae to join at the lower border of the pons, forming the basilar artery. This vertebrobasilar system then feeds the entire pons and most of the cerebellum.

DISORDERS OF THE AORTIC ARCH VESSELS

Although there are a wide variety of anatomic anomalies of the aortic arch system, only those that interfere with the trachea and/or oesophagus are of practical importance. These conditions, commonly known as vascular rings, are often asymptomatic in infancy but may present problems as the child grows older. Hence, many of the functionally significant vascular rings are identified in childhood or adolescence and repaired electively at that time. For completeness, the more common arch anomalies will be reviewed, inasmuch as some may be encountered in the adult patient, but they comprise a relatively small portion of the surgical procedures undertaken in the arch system.

The common and generally most benign congenital arch malformation, when occurring as an isolated anomaly, is patent ductus arteriosus, an open channel between the left pulmonary artery and the aorta. The symptoms, a thrill palpable over the left sternal border, a

---

Fig. 4.1. (*opposite*) Vascular anatomy of the superior mediastinum and cervical areas.

fistulous-type murmur and bounding peripheral pulses, are classic, and repair by surgical division is simple.

There are a number of arch anomalies which arise from incomplete closure of the embryonic second to sixth arches. Double aortic arch is perhaps the most usual of these, and its obstruction of the trachea and oesophagus becomes manifest in early childhood. A right aortic arch with retro-oesophageal diverticulum or its mirror image produces similar though less severe symptoms. Again, surgery involves simple division of the ductus arteriosus.

Anomalous origins of the pulmonary artery may result from defects in the embryonic sixth arch, causing the artery to originate from a ductus arteriosus or the ascending aorta. The left pulmonary artery may even arise from its right counterpart, producing an anomaly commonly known as vascular sling. Although not a true arch anomaly, this malformation may interfere with tracheobronchial function.

Another abnormal arterial formation occurs when the right subclavian artery originates as the most distal branch of the arch producing a vascular sling which may, on occasion, cause dysphagia because the aberrant artery must course retro-oesophageally to reach its usual right thoracic outlet. Identification of this anomaly, which occurs in about one in 200 people, is usually accidental (*see Case 3*). Surgical division of the anomalous vessel and its reimplantation in the right common carotid artery can be accomplished through a supraclavicular procedure described later in this chapter.

A distinctive acquired pathology is the frequently catastrophic aortic dissection, cleavage of the aortic wall by a medial haemorrhage. This condition and ruptured abdominal aortic aneurysm are the main causes of fatalities from aortic disease. Medial dissection is due almost entirely to sustained systolic hypertension, but intrinsic aortic disease is also contributory. It is uncertain whether intramural haemorrhage resulting from rupture of vasa vasorum or an intimal tear is the initiating mechanism, but in 90 per cent of cases an intimal tear forms a connection between the true and false lumens. The aorta proximal to the arch vessels is involved in approximately 65 per cent of cases, with longitudinal extension possible to the aortic bifurcation and beyond. Another 25 per cent may demonstrate an entrance tear in close proximity to the subclavian artery. A propagating medial dissection may occlude branch vessels by extension, compression or formation of an intimal flap. Owing to the very high risk of mortality from acute dissection, vigorous antihypertensive drug therapy and/or surgical replacement of the damaged aorta constitute current treatment.

Other acquired aortic arch disorders, aside from those traumatically induced, can be categorized as inflammatory or atherosclerotic in origin. The most well-known inflammatory process is Takayasu's arteritis, a non-specific panarteritis involving the thoracic and abdominal aorta with segmental occlusion of the major branches. The disease may progress to coarctation, narrowing, occlusion or aneurysmal dilatation. It has a predilection for women, particularly young Orientals. This type of arteritis is rare in the United States, but is reported world wide. Usually appearing in the second or third decade of life, it runs a protracted course with constitutional symptoms (fever, malaise, night sweats, anaemia, nausea, vomiting, arthralgia) appearing early on. Cerebral symptoms may develop from innominate artery involvement, and upper extremity claudication may evolve from subclavian stenosis. Surgery may be called for to eliminate the systemic symptoms of arterial occlusion, with bypass grafting from an uninvolved segment of the aorta to a distal, non-diseased portion of the occluded artery.

Other types of aortitis, syphilitic, bacterial or non-specific, are usually treated medically unless there is residual damage to the aorta, such as in aneurysmal dilatation necessitating graft replacement.

The preponderance of adult surgical procedures undertaken on the arch branches are for the treatment of what many call the aortic arch syndromes, a collection of conditions which produce segmental occlusion of the arch vessels. Atherosclerosis is responsible for 90 per cent or more of the aortic arch syndromes and is the major cause of acquired vascular disease, culminating in either luminal obstruction or dilatation. The disease has a preference for development in arterial bifurcations, branchings and curves, with the most common sites (in decreasing order) for atheromatous formation in the thoracic and cerebrovascular circulations being the common carotid bifurcation in the neck, the lower basilar and upper vertebral arteries at or near their intracranial junction, several of the major intracranial arterial branchings and the origins of the subclavian, innominate, common carotid and vertebral arteries. Atherosclerotic occlusive involvement of the ascending aorta is uncommon, with the aorta mainly afflicted in its abdominal segment. The arch may be diseased, but dilatation is the usual result in this area, with obstruction, rare in itself, affecting only the abdominal aorta.

Atherosclerotic lesions in the aortic arch vessels are by far the most common causes of aortic arch syndromes. Involvement of the arch vessels is most usual in the left subclavian artery, followed by the innominate and left common carotid arteries. Multiple arch vessel involvement is evidenced in some 40 per cent of patients. In occlusive lesions, symptoms generally appear when the lumen is reduced by 50 per cent or more, in cases of thrombotic occlusion, or if the plaque haemorrhages. Ulcerative lesions may induce embolic symptoms at any time.

Symptoms in the arch syndromes are classically those of cerebrovascular insufficiency of either the vertebrobasilar or the carotid type.

There may also be associated upper extremity ischaemia or microembolic events. Carotid insufficiency produces anterior circulation ischaemia and is evidenced by syncope, dizziness, memory loss, difficulties with thought processes, amaurosis fugax and focal neurological deficits. The posterior circulation is affected by vertebrobasilar insufficiency which is manifested by gait disturbances, ataxia, vertigo, tinnitus, diplopia, visual blurring and paresis. Symptoms vary with the degree and location of obstruction and the potential for collateralization and retrograde flow. Often, proximal lesions can be well tolerated if there is sufficient collateral circulation.

HAEMODYNAMICS OF ARCH VESSEL LESIONS

Collateralization in the mediastinum and cervical areas is a common result of occlusion of a primary arterial channel. Collateral arteries are usually pre-existing pathways in which the direction of blood flow can be altered in response to pressure gradients established by an occlusion. The time for these collaterals to become active following occlusion varies and is dependent on the resistance to flow. The functional integrity of the circulation distal to an occlusion is related to the metabolic activity of the area. Hence, certain segments of the arterial system are better able to compensate for an occlusion.

In the thoracic and cervicocranial areas supplied by the arch vessels, there are numerous collateral pathways available to re-route blood to an area deprived of its primary conduit. Identification and surgical correction of obstructive lesions in these areas are dependent to some extent upon the recognition of these collaterals and the instances in which they are inadequate to supply the tissue in demand.

Proximal innominate artery occlusion can produce collateral flow through any of a number of channels: (i) branches of the left carotid and subclavian arteries; (ii) anastomoses between the costocervical branches of the right subclavian and the first intercostal artery; (iii) communications between the intercostal arteries and branches of the axillary and internal mammary arteries with retrograde flow in the right subclavian artery; (iv) right vertebral artery in a retrograde manner. Left common carotid artery occlusion at its origin can be compensated for from three sources: (i) branches of the external carotid artery; (ii) branches fed by the thyrocervical and costocervical trunks of the subclavian artery; (iii) the ipsilateral vertebral artery via the external carotid arteries. Proximal subclavian occlusions, either right or left, produce collateral flow patterns through: (i) the descending branch of the occipital artery via its communications with the vertebral; (ii) retrograde flow down the ipsilateral vertebral artery; (iii) the ipsilateral external carotid artery via branches of the thyrocervical trunk; (iv) branches of the costocervical trunk; (v) retrograde flow through the ipsilateral internal mammary artery.

Among the major branches of these arch vessels, occlusion of the internal carotid artery near the bifurcation will initiate collateral flow through: (i) circle of Willis via the anterior cerebral and anterior communicating arteries; (ii) basilar artery via the ipsilateral posterior communicating artery; (iii) external carotid artery via the ophthalmic artery and/or the caroticotympanic arteries. Collateral flow to compensate for proximal vertebral artery occlusion comes from: (i) communication of the occipital artery branch of the external carotid with the muscular branches of the vertebral; (ii) the intraspinal vertebral to vertebral anastomoses; (iii) communication of the ascending cervical with the distal vertebral artery.

In times of peak demand or if concomitant atherosclerotic disease is manifest in the normal collateral channels, proximal occlusions of the arch vessels may initiate or enhance retrograde flow, stealing blood from lower resistance vascular beds. Perhaps the most famous of these vascular steals is the subclavian steal syndrome. By definition, this condition of proximal subclavian obstruction (*Fig. 4.2*) causes retrograde vertebral flow which drains the cranial blood volume to the

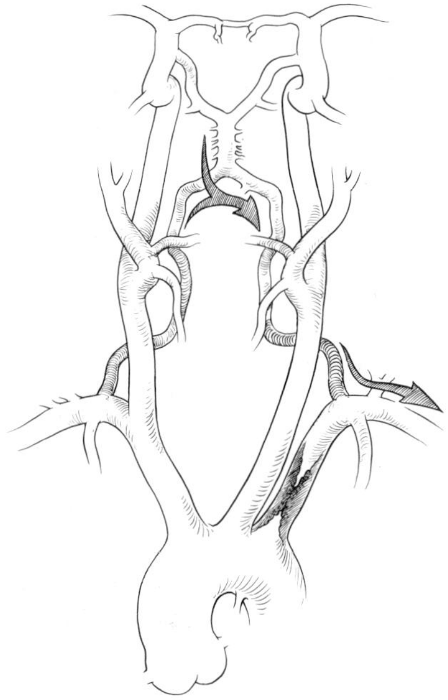

Fig. 4.2. Proximal left subclavian artery occlusion inducing a steal of blood from the cerebral system via retrograde flow in the vertebral artery.

extent that symptoms of vertebrobasilar insufficiency are manifested. Technically, the same symptoms can be produced in any collateral situation in which the vertebral artery is involved should the shunt of blood be significant. Normally, the vertebral system should be able to assist in the collateralization of blood around a proximal subclavian lesion, but in the instance in which atherosclerosis has involved the ipsilateral vertebral or intracranial communicating arteries, there is insufficient blood volume remaining in the cranial system to ward off the effects of ischaemia. Innominate artery occlusion produces a variant of this defect, reversing flow in the vertebral artery and reducing and perhaps reversing flow in the right carotid artery. Vascular steals are potentially as numerous as are the collateral pathways, but few are as haemodynamically significant as the subclavian steal syndrome. Surgical correction of this condition will be discussed later.

DIAGNOSIS OF ARCH VESSEL LESIONS

Any symptoms of cerebrovascular insufficiency or embolic incidents should immediately initiate a search of the thoracocervical vasculature for the causative lesions. While such symptoms may not have a vascular origin, the possibility should be pursued if the symptomatology has been carefully reported and appears to conform to the aortic arch syndrome or the various congenital anomalies.

Preliminary examination should begin with diligent recording of pulses and auscultation for bruits. Not infrequently, subclavian stenoses produce a bruit heard above the clavicle. Carotid stenoses are likewise often audible if they have not proceeded to occlusion. Because proximal arch vessel lesions may often be associated with lesions elsewhere in the cerebrovascular vessels, examination must be over the entire upper portion of the body.

Another physical finding of predictive importance is differential upper extremity blood pressure readings. Proximal arch vessel stenosis with a potential for steal often is attended by a decreased pressure reading on the affected side. This is a distinct diagnostic clue that should not be overlooked.

To further evaluate the haemodynamics of the cervical–cerebral arteries, there is an array of reliable, simple, non-invasive diagnostic procedures available. Oculoplethysmography and carotid phonoangiography are good tests in combination which assess the carotid branches. There is also a new generation of ultrasound equipment which employs spectral analysis of arterial flow, particularly valuable for study of the carotid bifurcation. Forehead thermography, supraorbital Doppler ultrasonography and supraorbital fluoroscein angiography are other tests of use in cranial evaluations.

Despite these valuable screening tools, arteriography remains the only method for accurate definition of suspected arterial lesions. It is often the only means of identifying proximal arch vessel lesions and assessing the availability of collateral flow. It can also guide the decision for staged or simultaneous procedures when multiple lesions are found. However, a relatively new technique, digital subtraction angiography, is showing great promise, and though it does not appear that it will replace angiography, vascular imaging should at least render the use of arteriography even more selective.

ARTERIOGRAPHY

Definitive identification of atherosclerotic lesions or degenerative changes in the aorta and its branches is achieved at present only through radiographic visualization by means of intravascular injection of contrast medium. Indeed, high quality contrast films are mandatory for surgical candidates so that corrective procedures can be planned.

The most commonly used technique for aortography is the percutaneous Seldinger method in which a catheter is introduced through a peripheral artery and threaded into the aorta. Two retrograde approaches may be used, the femoral or brachial. Both have advantages and disadvantages, and the selection of entry is largely the choice of the arteriographer.

Pressure injection of opaque contrast medium into the ascending aorta provides excellent visualization of the thoracic portion of the aorta, the aortic valve (retrograde flow will be seen if it is incompetent) and the arch branches as the medium flows antegrade. The catheter can then be placed at the origin of each arch vessel and films can be made of the innominate, carotid and subclavian circulations in both the mediastinal and cervical areas. A thorough study is a necessity, inasmuch as multiple lesions, collateral flow and vascular irregularities must be identified prior to surgical intervention.

SURGERY

Armed with the results of a carefully performed examination, the surgeon can make a decision for operative intervention based on this clinical picture, the severity of symptoms and the potential for future serious adverse events. Further assessment of the feasibility of repair and then planning for the operative procedures are based on the arteriographic findings.

Mention should be made here of the use of intraoperative pressure gradient determinations in thoracocervical vascular procedures. Arteriograms do not often give a precise definition of the actual decreased blood flow in a compromised segment of the circulation. Hence, in high quality reconstructive surgery, pressure transducers and multiple sampling needles are mandatory. Highly stenotic lesions may induce pressure gradients in surrounding vessels being considered as alternative routes for revascularization, particularly in the presence of extensive involvement or multiple lesions. Measuring pressure gradients also provides information on the extent of collateral circulation already developed, helping the surgeon to judge the extent of revascularization needed and whether or not interposed grafts may be required over simple transpositions. Similarly, once reconstruction has been completed, the pressure determinations should be repeated to be certain that existing gradients have been obliterated and new ones have not been created by the re-routing of blood.

Operative Approaches

Access to lesions of the aortic arch and its branches obviously depends upon the location, nature and extent of disease. Newer techniques avoid extensive thoracotomy and sternotomy whenever possible in favour of supraclavicular incisions and limited thoracic access via the second intercostal space. Re-establishment of circulation in areas affected by proximal atherosclerotic plaques often involves bypass grafting rather than endarterectomy, particularly for extensive or multiple lesions.

To better present the techniques used in aortic arch vessel surgery, two newer, simpler operative approaches will be described, then individual attention will be given to lesions at various sites in the arch vessels and their cervical branches. Illustrative case reports are interspersed where appropriate to demonstrate the indications for and selection of surgical procedures.

Supraclavicular Approach

This approach is employed for exposure of both subclavian arteries and the common carotid arteries (*Fig. 4.3*). The patient is positioned on the operating table with the scapula on the affected side slightly elevated and the head turned away from the surgical site. A supraclavicular incision is made 1 cm above and parallel to the clavicle just lateral to the sternal head of the sternocleidomastoid muscle and extended laterally for approximately 5 cm. The platysma muscle is divided and the scalene fat pad identified. The omohyoid muscle is also frequently divided. The clavicular head of the sternocleidomastoid muscle is

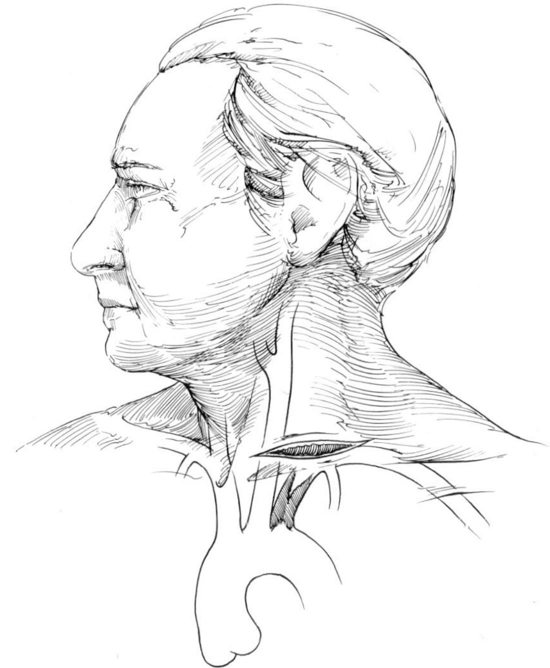

Fig. 4.3. Orientation of the 5 cm lateral supraclavicular incision.

divided. The scalene fat pad is excised and all venous and lymphatic channels ligated. The phrenic nerve is identified in its course over the anterior scalene muscle. The nerve is carefully dissected away from the muscle and slung with heavy silk suture. The anterior scalene muscle is divided near its insertion into the first rib, thereby providing exposure of the subclavian artery.

To disclose the subclavian origin, the thyrocervical trunk is identified and may be ligated at its origin to facilitate mobilization of the subclavian artery. Dissection is carried medially, staying directly on top of the artery. The internal mammary artery is located and divided. Finally, the origin of the vertebral artery is identified. From this point on, the course of the dissection is medial, leading to the origin of the subclavian either on the aorta or at the innominate bifurcation. Now that adequate exposure of the subclavian artery has been obtained, a variety of procedures are possible, and they will be described later.

Limited Right Anterior Thoracotomy

This approach is used for exposure of the ascending aorta. An incision in the right second intercostal space is made 1 cm from the sternum

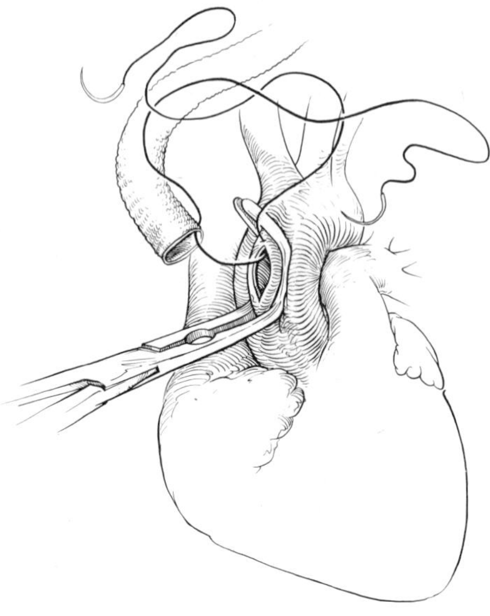

Fig. 4.4 Preparation for anastomosis of a bypass graft to the aorta. An arteriotomy has been opened over a partial occluding clamp on the aorta, and the trimmed graft is being anastomosed end to side to the aorta with 4/0 running monofilament suture.

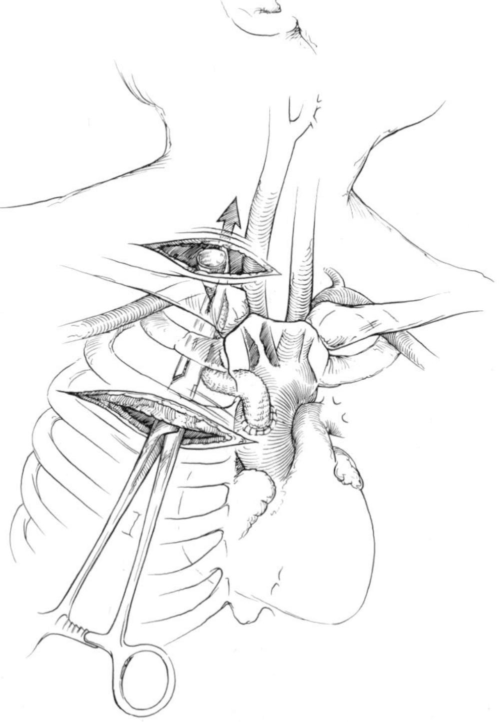

Fig. 4.5. Once the aortic anastomosis has been made, a tunnel is made beneath the clavicle to the supraclavicular incision and the graft is passed superiorly with the aid of a clamp. The diagram shows a right supraclavicular incision, but a similar procedure on the left is possible with the graft tunnelled beneath the sternum and left clavicle to the left incision.

extending laterally for 11 cm. The incision is opened to the pectoralis major muscle, which is spread. Dissection is continued to expose the pleura, which is opened, a self-retaining retractor is placed and the lung is retracted laterally. Fat overlying the aorta is incised and the pericardium is opened to gain access to the ascending aorta.

Once the aorta has been exposed, preparations for placement of a bypass graft are undertaken. The type of graft (single or bifurcated) and its distal anastomosis will be discussed in relation to the lesions being bypassed. To begin proximal graft placement on the aorta, a partial occluding clamp is placed on the ascending aorta's lateral aspect, and a longitudinal arteriotomy is opened over the clamp (*Fig. 4.4*). An 8 mm knitted Dacron graft is selected and trimmed appropriately. Larger diameter grafts may be required if the conduit is to feed multiple vessels. The graft is anastomosed to the arteriotomy site with 4/0 running monofilament suture. At this point the graft is ready to be tunnelled to its distal destination. This approach is then combined with the supraclavicular incision which has been opened primarily, and a tunnel between the two incisions beneath the clavicle is made to accommodate the graft, which is passed superiorly with the assistance of a clamp (*Fig. 4.5*). The graft is now ready for anastomosis to either the subclavian or the common carotid arteries. Bypass to the left side is made in a similar fashion, tunnelling the graft beneath the sternum and left clavicle to emerge at the left supraclavicular incision.

Single Proximal Lesions

The origin of the innominate artery is usually easily accessible through the anterior mediastinum unless the arch rises high into the superior mediastinum. In the past, median sternotomy was used to expose the innominate and endarterectomize any plaque from its origin. Direct endarterectomy of the innominate origin necessitates occlusion of the artery if the obstruction is not total, thereby interrupting cerebral flow. This is tolerable for short periods of time if bilateral disease is not present, but if extensive disease is found, plaque excision could require prolonged occlusion time. If there is arch involvement as well, it is sometimes difficult to obtain a satisfactory end-point distally on the aorta itself, thereby leading to aortic dissection once blood flow is restored.

We have abandoned this approach in favour of simpler grafting alternatives. In most cases of isolated, proximal obstruction of the innominate artery without disease in the carotid–subclavian bifurcation, a single bypass graft can be taken from the ascending aorta via the anterior thoracotomy described to the right common carotid artery exposed through the supraclavicular incision. The graft should be tunnelled along the course of the innominate artery beneath the clavicle and brought up to the lateral aspect of the common carotid for attachment. This will establish an excellent antegrade flow to the cerebral circulation with retrograde flow to the upper right extremity.

However, should the bifurcation at the subclavian origin be involved as well, then the procedure is altered slightly. The right common carotid and subclavian arteries are identified through the supraclavicular approach as described previously. The right anterior thoracotomy is opened to expose the ascending aorta and a bypass graft is taken from the aorta to the right common carotid as detailed above. Following this, a curved occluding clamp is placed just proximal to the subclavian lesion. The vertebral artery and the subclavian distally are clamped. The subclavian is transected and the stump oversewn with 3/0 monofilament suture. The free end of the subclavian is then anastomosed to either the lateral aspect of the bypass graft (*Fig. 4.6*) or to an arteriotomy site opened in the common carotid above the graft insertion.

In the case of ulcerative, proximal innominate artery lesions, direct endarterectomy can be performed if it appears that the lesion can be excised without creating the potential for dissection. Inasmuch as this is often not feasible, it is preferable to perform an aorto–right common carotid bypass with transposition of the subclavian as outlined above. Under these circumstances, the innominate artery must also be ligated above the lesion to prevent further embolization.

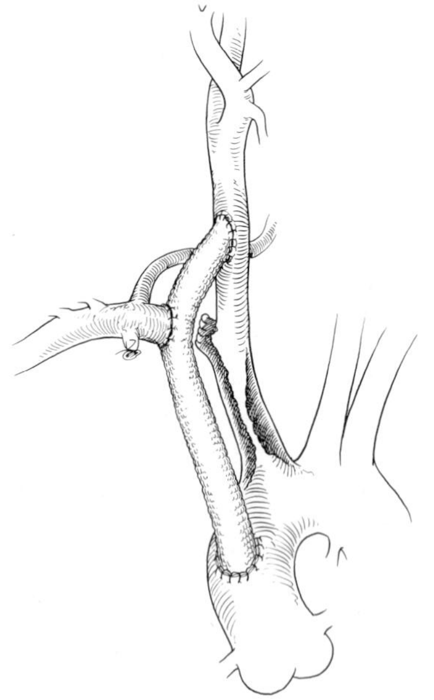

Fig. 4.6 Proximal innominate artery atherosclerosis extending into the subclavian origin is bypassed by a graft from the aorta to the right common carotid with implantation of the divided subclavian artery in the lateral aspect of the graft. Alternatively, the divided subclavian can be anastomosed to an arteriotomy site opened above the graft insertion on the common carotid artery. The proximal subclavian stump is oversewn.

Isolated, proximal lesions of the left common carotid or left subclavian origins can be handled in a similar way through the supraclavicular approach. If no pressure gradient exists in the neighbouring artery, the diseased vessel can be transected, the stump oversewn and the artery anastomosed to its neighbour. Alternatively, a graft can be taken between the two. Should both arteries be involved, a bypass graft can be taken from the ascending aorta through the right anterior thoracotomy, tunnelled beneath the sternum and left clavicle to the left supraclavicular exposure and anastomosed to the left common carotid. The subclavian artery can then be transected, the stump oversewn and the artery anastomosed to the left common carotid artery, if it is free of disease, or to the graft directly, as outlined for lesions on the right side. An alternative approach is to take a separate graft from the left common carotid to the subclavian, but this is not our procedure of choice.

Ulcerative lesions of the left common carotid or subclavian arteries are not uncommonly responsible for transient embolic events in the upper extremity or head. Since access to the origins of these arteries is simpler than with the innominate artery, endarterectomy is feasible, but it carries similar risks of aortic dissection if the lesion extends into the arch. Transposition is the procedure to use if disease is confined to one artery. If both origins are involved, then the graft procedure described above should be used.

Case 1

A 64-year-old Caucasian male had cold-induced blanching of the left third finger for the past 8 years. Over the last 3 years, the frequency and extent of blanching had increased with associated pain. At examination, the entire left hand was involved, with the addition of paraesthesia. Selective subclavian arteriography demonstrated an ulcerative plaque in the proximal left subclavian artery. Transposition of the left subclavian to the left common carotid artery was undertaken via the supraclavicular route. A postoperative thoracic aortogram (*Fig. 4.7*) showed the stump of the ligated subclavian with patency of the carotid-subclavian anastomosis. Symptoms in this patient were completely resolved by the procedure.

It should be noted here that proximal obstructive lesions of either subclavian artery are responsible for one of the more commonly referred to vascular steals, the subclavian steal syndrome. Historically, treatment of this condition involved a complicated sternotomy and endarterectomy of the subclavian at its origin. Later, prosthetic grafts between the common carotid and subclavian gained favour. Our preference for the simpler supraclavicular approach is based on its obvious advantages, and the transposition of the vessel establishes adequate blood flow without the necessity of interposing grafts. Whenever possible, in the subclavian area we elect vessel transposition, provided, of course, that the lesion is an isolated one and no pressure gradient is established by the transposition.

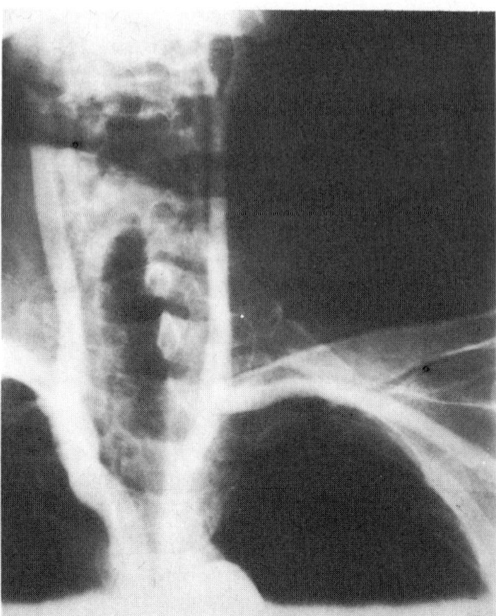

Fig. 4.7. Postoperative aortogram in *Case 1* denoting the patent transposition site with uncompromised flow in both vessels. The stump of the proximal subclavian artery can be seen on the arch (arrow).

Case 2

A 60-year-old male had suffered an injury to his left upper chest and shoulder in a car accident in 1974. In the years following, he developed numbness, tingling and weakness in the left arm. He also demonstrated weakness on the right side when exercising the left arm. Although he was being evaluated for coronary artery disease at the time, a pressure differential was noted between the right and left arms—140/70 right and 90/60 left. At catheterization, selective arch vessel arteriography delineated a high grade, proximal stenosis of the left subclavian artery. There was a left vertebral artery steal with collateral circulation to the distal left subclavian artery, also supplied by the right vertebral artery (*Fig. 4.8*). There was no distribution from either external carotid artery to the vertebrobasilar system. No other lesion was found. At the time of operation, a pressure gradient of 90/60 existed between the subclavian and carotid arteries. Following transposition, the gradient was obliterated. The symptoms were corrected by the carotid–subclavian transposition.

Isolated lesions of the origin of the right subclavian artery in the presence of normal innominate and right common carotid arteries may be encountered. These are treated just as those on the left would be, with transposition or grafting to the right common carotid. Disease in the right common carotid origin without proximal involvement of the innominate can be treated similarly. However, if a pressure gradient exists between the non-diseased artery and the obstructed carotid, then a bypass graft must be taken from the aorta to the right common carotid artery.

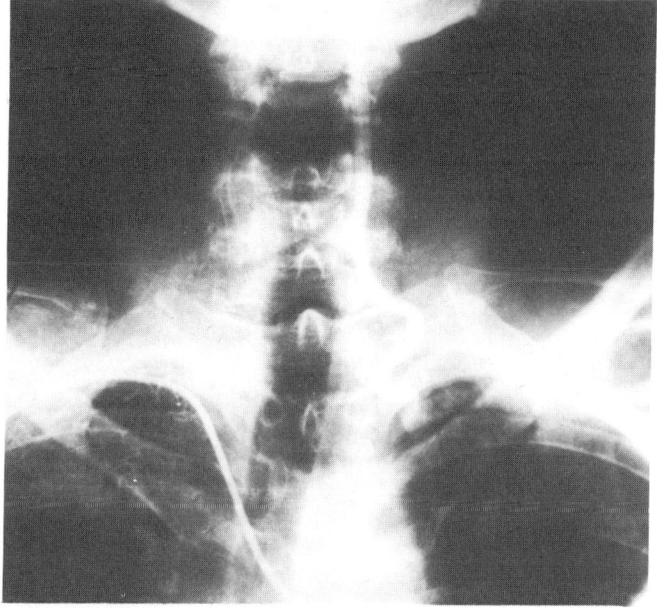

Fig. 4.8. Selective left subclavian artery arteriography shows the enlarged left vertebral artery with subsequent retrograde filling of the distal left subclavian artery.

As was mentioned previously in the discussion of arterial anomalies, an aberrant right subclavian artery sometimes can be found as the cause for subclavian steals even in middle-aged adults. Although symptoms from this aberrancy are more commonly related to the oesophageal constriction by the vascular sling, the complication of vascular insufficiency may be manifested.

Case 3

A 51-year-old female complained of intermittent throbbing in the ears over the previous 7 months. Over the past 2 months, the throbbing had become almost continuous, with the addition of dizziness, headaches and weakness in her right hand grip. The radial pulse was decreased and delayed on the right, and right arm blood pressure was lower—110/90 right, 150/80 left. A grade IV/VI right supraclavicular bruit was also detected. Combined oculoplethysmography/carotid phonoangiography demonstrated a 20 per cent flow reduction in the left internal carotid artery, and an occlusion of the right subclavian artery was suggested by findings of the upper extremity arterial Doppler study. Aortic arch arteriography with selective visualization of the arch vessels denoted an anomalous right retro-oesophageal subclavian artery with proximal atherosclerotic stenosis (*Fig. 4.9*). A delayed film demonstrated a right subclavian steal phenomenon. A left middle cerebral artery aneurysm was also disclosed by cerebral angiography. At operation, the aberrant subclavian was transected through a right supraclavicular approach and reimplanted on the right common carotid artery. Aneurysm repair was then undertaken after having re-established adequate cerebral perfusion via the transposition procedure.

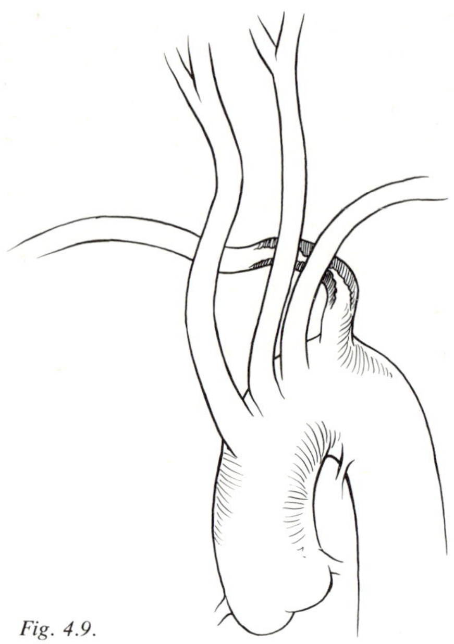

Fig. 4.9.

Multiple Lesions—Proximal and Distal

Multiple proximal occlusions, although uncommon, may be seen. More common are multiple stenoses of varying grades at perhaps two of the arch vessel origins. Whether or not obstruction is total, however, these circumstances make it necessary to take a bypass graft from the ascending aorta out of the superior mediastinum and into the cervical region for revascularization. A single bypass graft may be taken to the right common carotid artery in the supraclavicular area. Alternatively, a bifurcated graft from the ascending aorta to the right and left common carotids may be taken with appropriate transposition or grafting options available to revascularize compromised left and/or right subclavian arteries (*Fig. 4.10*).

For the sake of completeness, another type of bypass procedure for these lesions should be mentioned, and that is the bypass graft between left and right subclavians or left and right common carotids across the anterior neck. Patients do not seem to accept well the pulsating graft across the neck, so this procedure is not our first choice for multiple proximal lesions.

At times, bilateral lesions may be found in the subclavian arteries. The appropriate transposition procedures should be staged unless multiple proximal lesions necessitate bypass grafting from the aorta. In

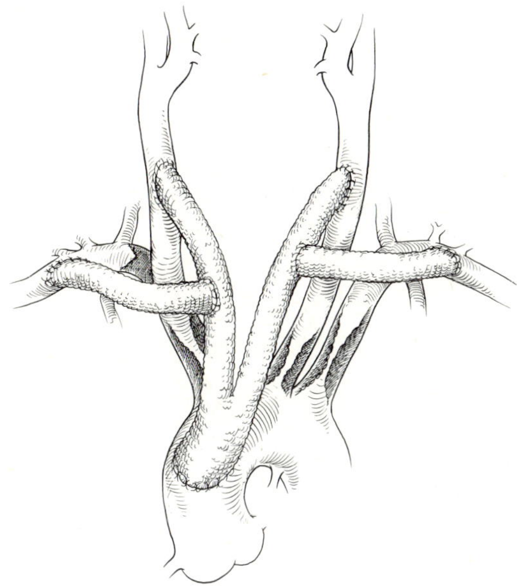

Fig. 4.10. An alternative approach to bypassing multiple proximal lesions in the arch vessels. A bifurcated graft from the aorta to both common carotids has additional grafts taken from it to the subclavians.

the latter instance, right and left subclavian lesions should be done simultaneously.

Case 4

A 73-year-old woman with a history of coronary artery disease, myocardial infarction, arrhythmias and congestive heart failure was seen for evaluation of her cardiac status. In addition to the anginal and cardiac failure symptoms (chest pain, orthopnoea, dyspnoea on exertion, etc.), she had begun to notice intermittent pain and numbness in her upper extremities, worse on the right side than the left. Also, she had begun to experience postural vertigo. Upper extremity pressures were 90/60 right, 80/60 left. A thoracic aortogram revealed 100 per cent occlusion of the right subclavian proximal to the vertebral branch (*Fig. 4.11*). There was also 95 per cent stenosis of the left subclavian proximal to the vertebral artery with steals from the vertebrals on both sides (*Fig. 4.12*). Two procedures to correct the lesions were performed 1 week apart. The bilateral carotid–subclavian transpositions corrected the upper extremity and cerebrovascular symptoms adequately.

In cases of extensive disease, multiple lesions may be found not only proximally but also in the cervical branches of the common carotids. Any of the previously described proximal lesions may be accompanied by lesions at the bifurcation into the internal and external carotid arteries. Proximal revascularization is then only part of the treatment, inasmuch as endarterectomy of the bifurcation must also be undertaken to ensure adequate cerebral flow. Positioning of the distal

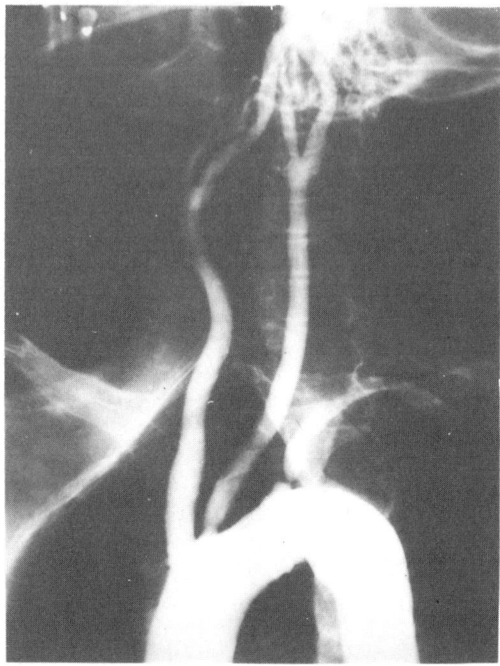

Fig. 4.11. Aortogram in a 73-year-old woman (*Case 4*) with bilateral upper extremity numbness and pain (worse on the right). The right subclavian is completely blocked and the left subclavian is 95 per cent stenotic just above its origin. (Reproduced by kind permission of *American Journal of Surgery.*)

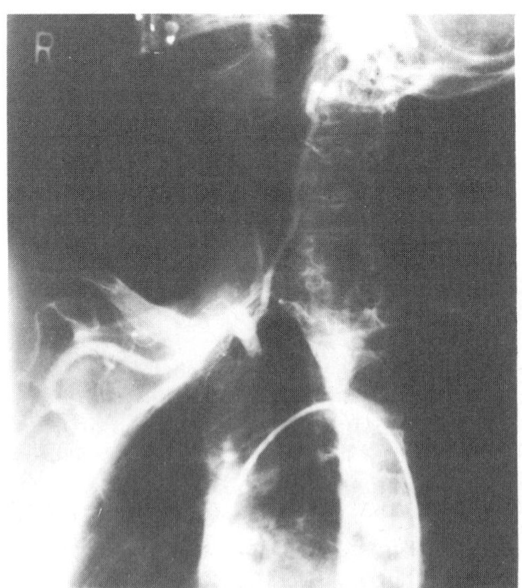

Fig. 4.12. Delayed film in *Case 4* showing the right subclavian filling by way of the vertebral artery. (Reproduced by kind permission of *American Journal of Surgery.*)

anastomosis of the aortocarotid bypass may be taken either at the proximal segment of the common carotid with endarterectomy of the bifurcation or anastomosis of the graft to the endarterectomized portion (*Fig 4.13*). We have utilized both procedures, but preference depends upon the extent of disease at the carotid bifurcation and the favoured method to repair the endarterectomized segment.

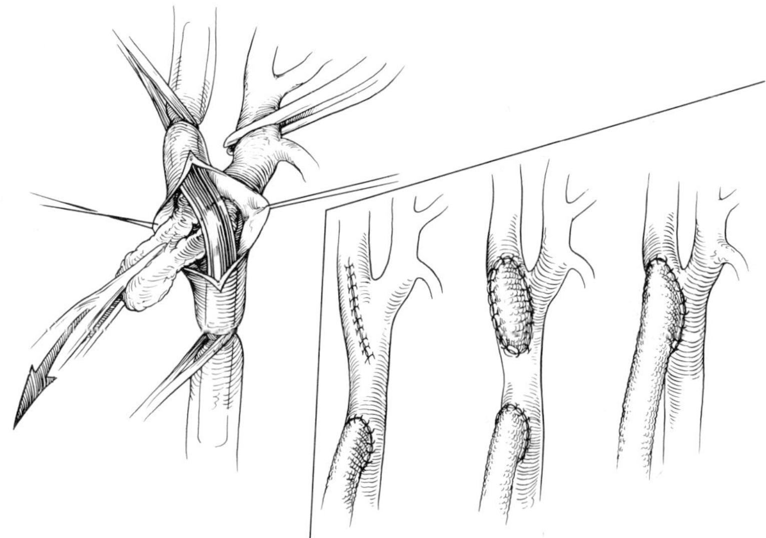

Fig. 4.13. Endarterectomy of the bifurcation in association with bypass grafting for proximal disease should be done. The endarterectomy site may be closed directly, with a patch graft, or it may become the site for insertion of the graft.

Case 5

A 65-year-old hypertensive male with a history of myocardial infarction, stroke and peripheral vascular insufficiency complained of a constant cold sensation in his left hand with numbness. The pain worsened at night. He also noted decreased strength in his left arm as compared to the right. A thoracic aortogram found multiple lesions: the left internal carotid artery was occluded at the bifurcation, as were the origins of the left subclavian and right common carotid arteries. The left common carotid had an anomalous origin off the base of the innominate artery with moderate disease. The right subclavian artery was moderately stenotic.

At operation, three incisions were necessary to accomplish revascularization. Initially, a right oblique incision was made along the anterior border of the sternocleidomastoid muscle to expose the right common carotid. Following endarterectomy of this vessel (the lesion extended to the bifurcation), the ascending aorta was visualized through an anterior thoracotomy incision in the right second intercostal space. A 16 mm bifurcated, knitted Dacron graft was anastomosed to the aorta. The right limb of the graft was tunnelled through the anterior mediastinum to the right common carotid, where an anastomosis was performed along the endarterectomy site. A left supraclavicular incision was then opened, the subclavian isolated and the left limb of the aortic graft tunnelled through the mediastinum to the left subclavian artery for anastomosis (*Fig. 4.14*). The patient's symptoms were completely resolved by the combined procedures.

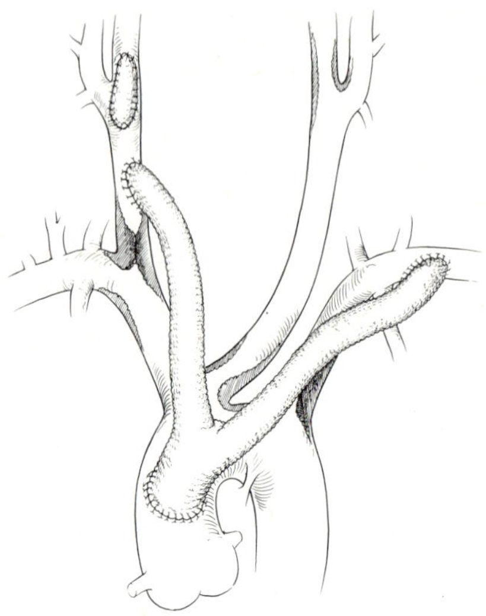

Fig. 4.14. Case 5. A 16 mm bifurcated graft is taken from the aorta to the right common carotid and left subclavian arteries following endarterectomy of the right common carotid artery.

Case 6

A 57-year-old female patient complained of transient loss of vision in the right eye without other associated ischaemic cerebral symptoms. She had a history of recent myocardial infarction. Blood pressure was above normal and differed between the arms—150/100 left and 118/80 right. Carotid pulses were decreased bilaterally. No radial pulse was found on the right; the left radial pulse was diminished. Bruits were heard over both subclavian arteries and bilaterally over the carotid arteries, being greater on the left.

Arteriography revealed occlusion of the origin of the right subclavian artery with complete occlusion of the right common carotid origin as well. Mild disease was found in the left carotid tree. A right supraclavicular incision was made for exposure of the right common carotid and subclavian arteries. The right common carotid was opened and a fresh thrombus was encountered. The clot was removed distally from the internal carotid artery and retrograde flow established. The origin of the innominate artery could be seen, and it was apparent that it was severely compromised by disease. A right anterior thoracotomy was opened in the second intercostal space and the ascending aorta visualized. A 10 mm knitted Dacron graft was anastomosed to the ascending aorta and tunnelled to the supraclavicular incision, where it was anastomosed to the right common carotid just below the bifurcation. The right subclavian artery was divided near its origin, the stump oversewn and the distal portion endarterectomized. The transected subclavian was then joined to the bypass graft with end-to-side anastomosis. The patient made a complete recovery.

The six cases outlined illustrate the wide variety of pathological conditions that can be encountered in aortic arch revascularization. While it is not feasible to describe every potential situation, these general principles of management outlined above apply regardless of the artery involved or the exact site of arterial narrowing. In none of the cases mentioned has the use of a temporary internal shunt been noted. For many years it was routine to use an internal shunt in carotid and subclavian–carotid operations. More recently, we have abandoned the use of shunts except in cases of significant bilateral disease or in instances in which there is insufficient backflow at the time of arteriotomy. The operative techniques currently employed offer the advantage of extremely short occlusion time, thereby assuring that there is no prolonged period of induced cerebral ischaemia during the performance of the endarterectomy or graft anastomosis.

For similar reasons, local or systemic heparinization is not used in the majority of aortic arch revascularization procedures. As shown in *Case 6*, in which an embolectomy of an occluded right common carotid artery was performed, heparin was instilled directly into the common carotid artery following the embolectomy. In the majority of cases, however, heparinization is avoided. With the potential for multiple incisions, particularly in the supraclavicular and cervical areas, we have found that postoperative bleeding can be extremely hazardous, and intraoperative heparinization appears to offer no benefit, except as mentioned above.

POSTOPERATIVE CARE

In all revascularizations in the cervical area, there must be meticulous haemostasis to prevent postoperative swelling. If this is done, there is no need for internal drainage of the supraclavicular or other cervical incisions. In patients with the anterior thoracotomy, one pleural chest tube is usually sufficient.

In the immediate postoperative period, specific attention is paid to the pulses and arterial pressure, particularly in upper extremity revascularizations. Postoperative hypertension is not uncommon in these patients, in whom the baroreceptors have been dissected, particularly in bilateral procedures. This complication can be controlled by either intermittent diazoxide administration or the infusion of nitroprusside. Regardless of the drug used, it is imperative that the pressure is not permitted to drop precipitously or allowed to go below 120 mmHg systolic. Lowering the pressure rapidly in complex revascularization cases can result in occlusion of the grafts and postoperative stroke. It has not been our practice to place revascularization patients on anticoagulant or platelet suppression therapy postoperatively.

Following discharge from the hospital, non-invasive testing is repeated as both a comparison with preoperative data and to provide baseline information for re-evaluation of disease recurrence or progression.

John Lumley

5 Carotid Artery Surgery in Patients with the Stroke Syndrome

The surgical treatment of patients with the stroke syndrome takes its origin from the denervation procedures of the 1930s. Leriche et al. [1] in 1935 performed cervical sympathetic nerve blocks and in 1936 Chao et al. [2] in Peking excised a segment of the internal carotid artery between ligatures in a 47-year-old Russian man and are reported to have reversed the symptoms of the cerebral ischaemia. The purpose of these operations was to overcome spasm of the cerebral vessels, but ligation also prevented embolism from disease of the carotid bifurcation. Cervical ganglionectomy was performed by Barré et al. [3] in 1947 and Johnson and Walker [4] in 1951. An interesting attempt to bypass an occluded internal carotid artery was that of Henschen [5], who transposed a temporalis muscle flap directly on to the cortex. The procedure was reported to have reduced seizures, but there was no angiographic evidence obtained to demonstrate that a new blood supply had been produced. In the early 1950s a number of procedures were introduced to remove or bypass arterial disease in the region of the carotid bifurcation. Carrea et al. [6] in 1951 ligated the external carotid artery and anastomosed its proximal end to the internal carotid artery beyond disease in the proximal part of this vessel. In January 1953, Strully et al. [7] reported an unsuccessful attempt to disobliterate the origin of the internal carotid artery and later in the same year DeBakey carried out the first successful internal carotid artery endarterectomy.

The procedures of Carrea and DeBakey, however, were not reported until later [6, 8], and the paper which provided the greatest impetus to surgery of this region was that of Eastcott et al. [9] in 1954. Their patient, a 66-year-old housewife, had the external carotid artery ligated and the segment of diseased internal carotid origin removed with end-to-end anastomosis of the common carotid and internal carotid arteries. Further cerebral deterioration was prevented in this patient and she has only recently died of non-cerebral causes. The first reported successful carotid endarterectomy was that of Cooley et al. [10] and other procedures undertaken around that time included: resection and homograft replacement of the internal carotid artery [11]; saphenous vein graft replacement of the resected internal carotid artery [12]; and side-to-side anastomosis of the external and internal carotid arteries [13]. The current procedure of choice for disease of the carotid bifurcation is that of carotid endarterectomy. Superior cervical ganglionectomy is still undertaken by some surgeons [14], although there is little physiological evidence that this can influence cerebral blood flow.

More recently developments in the microsurgical field have enabled the introduction of techniques bypassing an established occlusion or severe distal disease of the internal carotid artery. These developments have been pioneered by Yasargil and Donaghy [15] and developed by Chater [16], Reichman [17] and Sundt [18]. Development of this field in the United Kingdom was at first slow, perhaps related to the need for combined training in neurosurgical and microvascular techniques. Such techniques are now, however, becoming standard practice in the neurosurgical field and have been accompanied by a renewed interest in this low morbidity procedure [19].

THE NATURAL HISTORY OF CEREBROVASCULAR DISEASE

During the past 25 years carotid endarterectomy has, as we have seen, become an integral part of the management of patients with the stroke syndrome, this development being based on the prominence of carotid bifurcation atheromatous disease in stroke patients and the premise that transient ischaemic attacks (TIA) are a precursor of the completed stroke. The corroborative evidence for this assumption deserves careful attention. What is not in question is that in the region of 10 per cent of the population of the Western World die of cerebrovascular disease. In the United Kingdom and the United States of America the figure is approximately 11 per cent [20, 21] and in these countries this mortality is only surpassed by cardiovascular disease and malignancy.

It is encouraging that mortality statistics from a number of countries over the past two decades have suggested that the incidence of strokes is declining, but these figures have limitations imposed by change in diagnostic fashion and coding practices in death certification, and the low accuracy of diagnosis. In this respect the figures from the Mayo Clinic [22] are of value, since they utilize the Mayo Clinic medical record linkage indexing system, allowing analysis from 1945. A stroke was considered to include brain infarction due to arterial thrombosis, stenosis or embolism, primary and secondary intracerebral haemorrhage and subarachnoid haemorrhage. The autopsy rate of residents was 58 per cent in 1954, new cases of strokes occurring between 1 January 1945 and 31 December 1974 being based on 1.2 million person-years of observation. These workers noted a reduction in the stroke incidence: for every 100 first episodes occurring per unit of population during the period 1945–49, only 55 occurred in the period 1970–74.

Although the decline was present in both sexes and in all ages, the reduction was more pronounced in the elderly. There was no major change in the age of onset.

It is interesting to note that during the period from 1960 to 1964 the previously declining incidence of intracerebral haemorrhage was reversed. It is possible that this could be related to the long term anticoagulant therapy prescribed for cerebral infarction and TIAs, which was current therapy during this period. Relating the overall decline to the American Heart Association's recommendation in the same year for decreased dietary intake of saturated fat and cholesterol and the introduction of antihypertensive therapy is more difficult. This encouraging decline, from whatever source, does not, however, nullify the persistent problem of this complaint or serve to discourage any effort to prevent or treat the sequelae.

In a large majority of patients the aetiology of the stroke syndrome is atherosclerosis, as demonstrated by an arteriographic series from the Mayo Clinic [23] in which only 28 patients of 5000 studied were suffering from non-atherosclerotic disease and in over half of these patients the disease was sited at the carotid bifurcation. Other lesions occasionally responsible for the neurological symptoms include aneurysms of the brachiocephalic system, these being post-traumatic, micotic, post-radiotherapy and dissecting aneurysms as well as atherosclerotic. Occasionally congenital or acquired arteriovenous fistulas, congenital malformations, kinks, coils and bends occur in the carotid region. These, together with vascular trauma, may give rise to neurological problems. A rare group of arterial conditions that have been sporadically recorded as requiring surgical treatment includes fibromuscular dysplasia, medial wall necrosis and diffuse arteritis, giant cell arteritis, scleroderma, drug-induced stenoses and adjacent inflammatory cervical nodes. Tumours in the region of the carotid bifurcation, e.g. of the carotid body, may also give rise to neurological symptoms.

Cranial and extracranial vessels may be affected by extravascular effects such as hypercoagulability and severe hypertension, conditions giving rise to thrombosis including pregnancy, the pill, idiopathic thrombocytopenia, polycythaemia, sickle cell anaemia, anoxic anaemia and congestive cardiac failure. It is probable that focal neurological sequelae following severe hypertension, or after cardiac arrest, cardiac arrhythmia or extensive trauma, only occur in patients with pre-existing asymptomatic arterial lesions.

Transient Ischaemic Attacks

Despite the established mortality figures and the recognition of the underlying aetiological factors, debate persists as to the relevance and the mechanism of the TIA. The need to perform any prophylactic surgery prior to the onset of irreversible neurological damage is not in question, but the precise relationship of the TIA to the completed stroke is still a matter of controversy. Even its mechanism is uncertain since both a temporary reduction in blood flow and distal obstruction by a microembolus which subsequently disperses may be involved. The earlier theory of arterial spasm [24] has been largely discounted since it was shown by Pickering [25] that retinal arteries, a site of typical TIAs, are among the least responsive in the body.

Denny-Brown [26] explained these attacks by a theory of haemodynamic crisis based on the assumption that, in a patient with an extracranial arterial stenosis, sudden lowering of blood pressure could produce a significant fall of blood pressure in the distal tree. In support of this theory, Denny-Brown and Meyer [27] were able to reproduce TIAs by lowering and subsequently raising the blood pressure in an animal with local cerebral arterial stenosis. Although Kendell and Marshall [28] failed to produce neurological symptoms by lowering blood pressure in patients with a history of TIAs, the reversible nature of strokes after temporary carotid clamping, such as seen in aneurysm surgery or during carotid endarterectomy under local anaesthesia, upholds this theory of a potential mechanism for TIAs.

Recently the microembolic theory, as first suggested by Millikan et al. [29], has gained support, credence being lent to the theory by the report of Fisher [30], who observed retinal emboli in patients with visual TIAs. It seems probable, therefore, that both these factors are involved in the production of TIAs and their existence may be largely dependent on the presence of an adequate collateral circulation. In this context accessory blood flow may occur between the external carotid and ophthalmic artery, the meningeal and cerebral arteries, the occipital and vertebral arteries, the cervical and vertebral arteries and the occasionally encountered rete mirabile of the internal carotid artery. Occasionally, in prolonged occlusive disease of the cerebral vasculature such as Moya Moya disease, anastomoses develop between the middle meningeal and cortical vessels. A persistent trigeminal or hypoglossal artery may occur and, in the case of the latter, cerebral ischaemia secondary to disease of this vessel has been reported by Sutherland and Donaldson [31].

The final pathway of the collateral circulation is the circle of Willis, and anatomical variations of this important anastomotic ring arc not uncommon [32]. When assessing TIAs it is important to be aware that they can be mimicked by a number of other neurological and non-neurological problems. Variable symptoms may result from hypoglycaemia and they may be difficult to distinguish from the symptoms of subdural haematoma, seizures, migraine, Menière's disease and even multiple sclerosis.

Perhaps the greatest controversy about the TIA relates to its natural history. Some of the discrepancy between results may relate to the different populations being analysed. Whereas some may represent a highly selected subgroup of patients from neurological and neurosurgical centres with a specific interest in cerebrovascular disease, others may include patients on anticoagulant therapy and exclude patients who have proved surgically accessible lesions and have subsequently undergone carotid endarterectomy. The definition of the TIA is another possible factor of variance.

Many of these aspects were carefully analysed by Brust [33] in a study of 27 articles on the natural history of TIAs. Although 8 of these reports were based on more than 100 patients, 3 were on less than 20. It was in 2 of these papers that a zero stroke incidence was reported. Follow-up varied from 3 months to over 10 years; some studies began with the first attack, whilst others required all patients to have had at least one attack within 1 or 2 months for inclusion into the group. Brust also found considerable variation in the definition of hypertension in his analysis, as well as the various exclusion factors involved. He concluded that the difference of definition in these patients in terms of patient selection therapy, duration and follow-up, patient age, social and economic status, associated disease and other factors left considerable uncertainty as to what really was the natural history of the TIA. Not one of these studies emerged with conclusive data, and one is still left with figures indicating stroke risks from less than 1, to more than 60 per cent. Perhaps a realistic figure is that offered by Wisnant [34] of a 7 per cent completed stroke incidence in patients with TIAs per year of follow-up.

The TIA, therefore, remains the prime indication for surgical intervention, provided that the results obtained are accompanied by a superior morbidity and mortality to those of the natural history of the disease. The place of surgery in the acute, the progressive or the completed stroke is very limited and is best left for consideration until the results of this form of surgery have been presented. Considerable interest has recently been directed at patients with asymptomatic yet operable disease of the carotid system, and before proceeding to operative techniques, it is worth pausing to consider the various ways in which such lesions are diagnosed in medical practice.

PATIENT ASSESSMENT

Examination of symptomatic and asymptomatic patients may reveal stigmata of generalized vascular disease with symptoms of cardiac and lower limb ischaemia. Pulse deficits and bruits may be present over the orbit and distal vessels together with associated hypertension and blood pressure variation in the upper or lower limbs.

Specific investigations of the carotid system can be divided into those assessing the carotid bifurcation, those related to assessment of the first branch of the internal carotid artery, namely the ophthalmic artery, and tests that can compare parameters at both these levels to estimate the pulse pressure propagation velocity through the internal carotid artery. Directional Doppler velocity meters are used in all these evaluations, although alternative or supplementary techniques are also available.

The first report of the Doppler examination of carotid arteries came from Miyazaki and Kato [35] in 1965. These workers made haemodynamic comparisons of the right and left carotid arteries in patients with hemiplegia. In 1972 Planiol and colleagues [36] demonstrated that it was possible to differentiate between the velocity profiles of the common, internal and external carotid arteries. The internal vessel was particularly characteristic with its high diastolic velocity. Since that time many studies have been undertaken for evaluating the haemodynamics of the common carotid bifurcation by means of Doppler shifted signals [37–39]. Many factors have been included in the waveform analysis but a commonly used ratio is the peak-to-peak velocity/mean velocity, known as the pulsatility index. Less precise information can be obtained by a skilled observer listening over this region. Ultrasonic scanning systems evaluating the carotid bifurcation directly are improving in quality and a combinaion of real time B scanners with directional Doppler velocity meters may produce the most reliable long term results. Non-ultrasonic means of evaluating the carotid bifurcation include carotid phonoangiography [40].

Indirect assessment of the internal carotid artery by the characteristics of its ophthalmic branch are based on the original work of Brockenbrough and his colleagues [41] in 1969. Flow in the periorbital vessels is normally anteriorly out of the orbit, but in the presence of severe carotid artery disease a pressure gradient develops between the external and internal carotid arteries and retrograde flow may result. This retrograde flow may be reduced or obliterated with compression of the ipsilateral or contralateral facial and superficial temporal arteries. The accuracy of this technique varies widely between centres. Lye and colleagues [42] reported 3 per cent false positive and 22 per cent false negative results. In our own study of patients with retrograde flow in one or more periorbital arteries, only 65 per cent were found to have an internal carotid artery stenosis of more than 50 per cent while 15 per cent of internal carotid artery stenoses of greater than 80 per cent were not associated with an observable retrograde flow. Photoplethysmographic pulse detectors can be used as an alternative to ultrasound in detecting supraorbital vessels, but no increase in accuracy over conventional pulse recording devices has yet been claimed.

The application of suction to the sclera to evaluate the intraocular pressure (ocular pneumoplethysmography) is based on the principles of ophthalmodynamometry and measures pressure reduction in the internal carotid artery distal to a stenosis [43]. Peroperative comparison of ocular pneumoplethysmography with directly measured internal carotid artery systolic blood pressure shows very good correlation, but hypertension, bilateral internal carotid artery stenoses and disease of the ophthalmic artery may invalidate results, and local ocular disease is a contraindication to the use of this technique.

The third group of investigations is based on measurement of the pulse rate propagation velocity between the common carotid and ophthalmic arteries. The pulse pressure wave can be assessed in the orbit by measurement of eye volume changes with an oculoplethysmograph. Pulse arrival times on the ear lobe measured simultaneously, through light opacity plethysmographs, enable comparison of arrival times through the internal and external carotid systems of the two sides.

These many and varied investigations are now widely available in vascular centres but the emphasis laid on them varies greatly between institutions. A remarkable development in some countries has been to rely on the accuracy of non-invasive tests alone as an indication for surgery without undertaking subsequent angiography, one centre operating on 25 per cent of cases without additional radiological information [44]. In our own experience, however, comparison of Doppler studies with angiography in 50 patients showed an incidence of 11 per cent false positive and 9 per cent false negative information.

With the imminent arrival of digital angiography, many of these problems are likely to be reduced as, with a single intravenous bolus of contrast solution, it should be possible to obtain good visualization of stenotic disease in all extracranial vessels.

Preoperative radiological assessment of all patients is routine in most centres and it is essential to obtain biplanar views of the carotid bifurcation and of the intracranial circulation. Whether this is obtained by direct carotid puncture or by selective arteriography depends on local expertise and equipment. Concomitant information of the aortic arch and vertebral vessels is also desirable and essential if the patient's symptoms/signs or non-invasive investigations suggest disease in these areas.

CAROTID ENDARTERECTOMY

When selecting patients for cerebrovascular surgery it is important to remember the generalized nature of their disease. In our own patients there is a 20 per cent incidence of symptomatic cardiac disease, this agreeing with the figures of other workers [45], and cardiac problems are the major cause of death on follow-up of both operative and non-operative patients in this group. Hypertension is also a common finding, being of a similar order of magnitude. The incidence of lower limb disease is high, being 28 per cent in our own patients, over half of these requiring lower limb reconstructive surgery. These figures, however, may highlight the screening for peripheral vascular problems undertaken in a vascular unit. Nevertheless, the incidence of diabetic patients has been relatively low as compared with the 15 per cent quoted by Thompson et al. [46] in 1978. Eighty-five to ninety-five per cent of these patients are smokers and often have associated respiratory disease.

Anaesthesia

General anaesthesia is preferred for carotid endarterectomy as this enables the airway to be controlled continuously and oxygen and carbon dioxide levels to be maintained as required. It has also been shown to reduce the cerebral oxygen requirements [47, 48]. The effect of varying anaesthetics on ischaemia has also been demonstrated; in dogs the infarct size is less with light halothane than with deep levels and barbiturate drugs have a protective effect [49]. Hypothermia has been shown to reduce the extent of infarction in experimental animals, but is generally cumbersome to institute routinely. Etheridge [50], however, stated that he used the technique for management of his more difficult cases.

Early workers in the field undertook this form of surgery under local anaesthetic. The initial mortality was in the region of 10 per cent and the introduction of general anaesthesia, hypercarbia and induced hypertension by Wells et al. [51] showed a marked reduction of operative morbidity. Nevertheless, at the same time a clearer understanding of the indications for surgery and the establishment of precise operative techniques were taking place and improvements may not have been entirely due to changes of anaesthesia. With the advent of neuralept analgesia and a better understanding of regional techniques, some surgeons have reintroduced this concept [52, 53]. Hobson and colleagues set out to perform the procedure under regional anaesthesia and if this proved unsatisfactory, because of patient cooperation difficulties or the onset of ischaemic changes on cross-clamping, they abandoned the operation and performed it the following day under general anaesthesia with shunting.

Adequate oxygenation is mandatory as, although this may constrict the blood vessels in normal brain, it is an essential requirement for metabolism of ischaemic cerebral tissue. Induced hypertension has been favoured by many workers in the field, but while it is certainly essential to maintain a stable circulatory system, as autoregulation of blood flow is lost in systolic blood pressure below 60 mmHg, induced hypertension may increase the instance of myocardial problems and it is probably advisable to maintain the patient's blood pressure near his preoperative norm.

Operative Procedure

The patient is placed supine with a small sandbag between the shoulders, the head inclined slightly upwards to empty the cervical venous plexus and the neck rotated and flexed to the contralateral side. Overextension or excessive lateral flexion must be avoided as this may cause kinking of tortuous vessels or compression of the vertebral artery by cervical osteophytes. A head towel is used but leaving the lower half of the ear exposed, the ear lobe being folded upwards under an adhesive drape.

The incision preferred is along the anterior border of the sternomastoid muscle, the length being partly dependent on the level of the carotid bifurcation, but usually extending from just above the clavicle to the mastoid process. The greater auricular nerve and anterior cervical nerves cross the field and occasionally require division, as may the external jugular vein. Care is taken to keep the upper part of the incision posterior to the vascular parotid gland. In the case of a very high bifurcation an alternative approach is obtained by incision along the posterior border of the sternomastoid muscle [54], although in this position the accessory nerve crosses the field and has to be carefully preserved. The carotid bifurcation is approached by deepening the incision through the platysma, sweeping the submandibular lymph nodes anteriorly.

A more extensive proximal or distal exposure can be obtained by dividing the omohyoid or the posterior belly of the digastric muscle respectively. The common facial vein and a varying number of branches of the pharyngeal venous plexus overlying the bifurcation require careful division and ligation. The hypoglossal nerve must be identified and may require mobilization. The descendens hypoglossae can be followed upwards to identify this nerve and the small sternomastoid muscular branch of the occipital artery may require careful ligation and division to aid mobilization. By gently inserting a self-retaining retractor at successively deeper levels the carotid bifurcation is reached. Dissection should be by knife rather than by blunt dissection because of the danger of dislodging any loosely adherent thrombus within the arteries.

The common carotid artery and its two divisions are mobilized well away from the bifurcation and the plane of dissection obtained close to the vessels, adjacent tissue being retracted away from the artery rather than retracting the vessel itself. The common carotid is firstly mobilized and separated from the adjacent internal jugular vein and vagus nerve and a sling passed around it. The internal carotid artery is next mobilized well clear of any disease at its origin, keeping close to the adventitia and thereby avoiding damage to the adjacent carotid sinus and superior laryngeal nerves. If a high coil or kink is present this is best left for mobilization after clamping all the vessels. If local thrombus has been demonstrated arteriographically the internal carotid artery is best mobilized and clamped before the dissection of its parent trunk.

The external carotid artery is mobilized close to the adventitia and distal to its superior thyroid branch which is controlled separately with a double loop of silk; this can then be pulled taught to prevent back bleeding later in the procedure. Occasionally, if extensive disease of the external carotid artery is present, mobilization includes its facial and lingual branches.

The gentleness required during this dissection cannot be overemphasized and the arteries must never be squeezed or suddenly jerked. The carotid sinus nerve must also be left intact, but if mobilization is producing cardiac anomalies, 1 or 2 ml of 1 per cent lignocaine can be injected carefully into the outer wall of the carotid bifurcation to anaesthetize baroreceptor activity. Heparin (5000–10 000 i.u.) is administered intravenously prior to clamping, it being essential to use low pressure vascular clamps on these vessels. The arteriotomy is placed on the posterolateral aspect of the distal common carotid artery and extended across the bifurcation into the internal carotid artery. The interior of the latter must be carefully examined to ensure that the arteriotomy extends into normal distal vessel, the eventual length being approximately 2 cm into both of these arteries.

The merits of shunting during carotid endarterectomy are discussed below, but if a shunt is used it is inserted at this stage. The Javid shunt is preferred: it is first clamped across its centre and the smaller end gently inserted into the internal carotid artery, being threaded along the artery as the vascular clamp is released. Once the bulb has passed into normal vessel, the small ring clamp is applied to its first ratchet. Any obstruction to shunt passage must be recognized and the cause identified; no force must be used. After back-bleeding through the shunt to expel air bubbles, the proximal end of the shunt is inserted in similar gentle fashion into the common carotid artery. Any factors hindering this gentle insertion must be carefully eradicated. Occasionally proximal dilatation is required. After insertion, the clamp across the centre of the shunt is slowly released and, should any air or debris be seen passing along the shunt, it should be immediately reclamped, the lower end of the shunt withdrawn and the procedure repeated. The technique of shunting requires careful attention to detail and the training of all members of the team.

The endarterectomy should be commenced along one cut edge of the common carotid artery. The outermost plane of cleavage which can be freely obtained is followed circumferentially, trying to maintain a single plane throughout. The proximal end of the endarterectomy is cut obliquely with scissors aiming at a gentle chamfer from the common carotid artery to the endarterectomized segment. Provided that the arteriotomy is beyond severe local disease, there is no advantage in dissecting the plane below the arteriotomy. Every effort should be made to leave adherent intima at this lower end. The dissection in the internal carotid artery is carried distally until the thin feathered end of thickened intima is reached and this may require extension of the arteriotomy. It is essential that the distal intimal limit is adherent. If it is carefully followed in this manner, a tacking stitch is rarely required. Such stitches are difficult to insert without cutting into the protruding intimal edge and act as a focus for subsequent thrombus formation.

The external carotid end point is usually just within the origin and can be reached through the common carotid arteriotomy. The atheroma is mobilized circumferentially and the origin everted by gentle forward pressure on its vascular clamp and backward retraction on the common carotid artery wall. On rare occasions it is necessary to place an additional longitudinal arteriotomy in the external carotid artery to obtain a satisfactory end point. On completion of the endarterectomy, the inner wall is flushed with a stream of heparinized saline to identify any residual strands of atheroma. The arteriotomy is closed with a continuous 6/0 vascular suture.

Careful attention to this fine suture line, possibly with the use of magnification, enables the normal calibre of the internal carotid artery to be maintained. If there is any danger of stenosing the distal end point a venous patch is advised, but this is rarely necessary. When a shunt is being used this should be left until the closure is near completion. A second stitch may be started at the proximal end of the incision. On removal of the shunt and reclamping of the vessels the endarterectomized segment is filled with heparinized saline before completing the closure. The first clamp to be removed is that on the internal carotid artery to allow back flushing of any potential debris into the segment. This vessel is then compressed near its origin while the external and common carotid arteries are opened, any debris being flushed into the external rather than the internal carotid system. Gentle pressure is maintained on the suture line for a number of minutes, since fine needle holes in endarterectomized vessels need some initial support, particularly in a heparinized patient. A fine cannula may be left alongside the carotid sinus nerve to allow subsequent installation of local anaesthetic in the event of postoperative instability of blood pressure. After subcutaneous and skin closure a light dressing is applied.

Shunting

Routine operative shunting of blood from the common to the internal carotid arteries was used in early studies [55] and is still advocated by a number of experienced surgeons [46, 56]. In many centres the initial catheters have been replaced by purpose-designed shunts [57, 58]. Routine shunting, however, has been challenged on grounds of technical difficulty and necessity. The problems associated with such shunt introduction include clotting of the shunt. Spielberger et al. [59] considered that 5 per cent of shunts inserted were non-functioning and Pipegrass and Sundt [58] routinely found clot in postoperatively examined shunts, although this problem was largely overcome by their most recently heparin-impregnated version. Shunt insertion may dislodge local thrombus or atheromatous debris and may initiate dissection proximally or distally; air embolism may also occur. The presence of a shunt may reduce the view to the endarterectomy area and require a more extended arteriotomy. The ring clamps or compression snares applied to the outside of the vessel may also damage intervening intima and act as a focus for subsequent thrombus formation.

The use of a shunt has also been challenged on the lack of conclusive evidence that its insertion can reduce the postoperative morbidity. The 'no shunt' surgeons believe that postoperative strokes are due to embolism occurring during the arterial mobilization and that temporary occlusion of the carotid artery during endarterectomy is relatively unimportant [60, 61]. Accepting the disadvantages of inserting a shunt, other workers have attempted to use a more rational approach to the subject by selectively using a shunt in patients who are at high risk of cerebral damage during cross-clamping. The need to identify such a group, however, raises its own problems. A number of methods of assessment have been introduced. For operations carried out under local anaesthesia the level of consciousness can be used for assessment, but under general anaesthesia a different approach is required. Jugular venous pressure was introduced at an early phase [62] but challenged [63], in that the measurement did not indicate local metabolic needs and was influenced by the geometry of the circulation and additional collateral formation. At best the reading was a measurement of the hemispheric oxygen tension rather than focal needs and probably represented an average figure for the whole brain.

Rob [64] considered that a good estimate of collateral hemisphere circulation could be obtained by observing the back flow of the internal carotid artery. The collateral hemisphere pressure can be measured by a transducer placed on the end of a distally inserted shunt or by the insertion of a needle into the distal segment before and after clamping. There has been no uniform agreement on the critical level of stump pressure by workers advocating its use. Moore and Hall [65] considered that a pressure of less than 25 mmHg put patients at risk of cerebral damage, whereas Hays et al. [64] used a stump pressure of 50 mmHg as their critical level. Hobson et al. [52] emphasized that a high stump pressure did not necessarily protect against all strokes, these being sometimes observed in patients with stump pressures of greater than 70 mmHg. These varying reports, together with the conflicting views on the value of EEG monitoring [66, 67], emphasize the difficulty of assessing cerebral flow through collateral vessels.

The value of any of these measurements for the use of shunting has been challenged by Curi et al. [68], who use the technique of carotid compression to assess the potential safety of carotid endarterectomy. These workers consider that if a patient withstands carotid compression on the proposed operative site of longer than 10 seconds without demonstrating clinical symptoms, it is safe to cross-clamp the vessel for the period of the operation, symptoms occurring under 7 seconds being a contraindication to surgery of any form at this level. This report requires confirmatory evidence, but it is possible that such a high risk group could be managed by initial extra–intracranial surgery with low morbidity.

Operative assessment of the endarterectomized vessel may be made by electromagnetic flow measurement, Doppler periorbital studies or angiographic techniques. The latter provide maximum information on the endarterectomized segment but are only advisable in operating theatres equipped to use angiography as a routine.

EXTRA–INTRACRANIAL ARTERIAL BYPASS

This procedure is undertaken under general anaesthesia using endotracheal intubation and headshaving appropriate to the scalp incision. The proposed site of anastomosis is placed uppermost, the patient's body being turned to maintain this position, with appropriate head fixation and towelling. The scalp vessel used is generally the anterior or posterior branch of the superficial temporal artery, the posterior being preferred if the anterior is seen to be providing good collateral channels through the ophthalmic vessel. This scalp vessel may be mobilized from the under surface of a frontoparietal skin flap or, in preference, through a direct incision over it. The dissection is under loup or microscopic magnification using sharp-pointed scissors and leaving the vessel in continuity after mobilization until it is required for anastomosis.

The recipient vessel in this technique is usually a cortical branch of the middle cerebral artery. If a bony flap is raised, then the most appropriate vessel may be chosen, but a much lesser procedure is preferred where a suitable cortical branch is identified through a single large burr hole. Generally, the vessels in the parietal region are larger [69] and a burr hole placed 5 cm superior and 1 cm posterior to the external auditory meatus is a useful starting point. Occasionally this requires enlargement, but rarely to more than double this size, before an adequate vessel is encountered.

The dura is incised in stellate fashion, this usually being in the region of the posterior branch of the middle meningeal artery which approximates to the line of the lateral sulcus at this point. Once a suitable vessel has been identified, subsequent procedures must be undertaken under the operating microscope, if it is not already in use.

A suitable length of cortical vessel is mobilized, this usually being in the region of 1 cm. The area chosen is one with minimal numbers of additional or fine perforating cortical branches. The arachnoid mater is cleared from the area and small microvascular clamps applied to the segment. Incision in the vessel can be longitudinal with a diamond knife or, by gently raising the anterior wall, an ellipse of the vessel may be excised with microvascular scissors. Whatever the procedure used, great care must be taken with this delicate manoeuvre. When the cortical vessel has been prepared, the scalp vessel may be clamped proximally with a low pressure micro-bulldog and divided distally, the distal end being then re-routed deep to any intervening skin bridge or, in the case of a scalp flap, turned directly on to the cortical vessel through the burr hole. Final dissection of the end of the vessel to be anastomosed is carried out under the dissecting microscope, it being necessary to clear at least 5 mm of surrounding tissues and adherent adventitia. The end of the vessel is then cut obliquely, the length being appropriate to the arteriotomy in the cortical artery, this being two to three times the diameter of the latter vessel.

An end-to-side anastomosis is fashioned using interrupted monofilament nylon sutures. As it is not always possible to turn the scalp vessel over to complete the side away from the surgeon, it is preferred to use the standard microvascular technique of placing the initial suture in the wall away from the surgeon then proceeding with alternate sutures on either side of this first stitch. On reaching the first corner, two stitches are inserted and tied beyond this level to stabilize the corner before proceeding to the other end. In this technique the final sutures will be the most easily accessible on the side of the surgeon and the last two stitches may be placed rather than tied in position to briefly open all limbs of the anastomosis and ensure patency before completion. As the superficial temporal and cortical vessels are usually free of any disease process, heparin is not usually necessary and is often contraindicated in neurosurgery. If fine cortical branches of the clamped segment have been left unclamped, there may be a little bleeding into the segment during anastomosis and in this case it may be necessary to insert the sutures under a stream of heparinized saline.

Additional microvascular techniques such as the use of stents and dams depend on surgical preference. On completion of the anastomosis the flow can be confirmed and measured with a Doppler probe placed on the scalp vessel. Conventional electromagnetic flow probes are too bulky for safe measurement in this vessel. The corners of cut dura may be turned in towards the anastomosis and the bone filings and chips can be replaced within the bony defect. If a bony flap or a disc of bone has been removed an area must be nibbled away to allow free access of the scalp vessel before suturing the bone back in position. Temporalis muscle and fascia are loosely approximated around the bypass vessel and a wound drain inserted if a flap has been raised.

Symptomatic occlusive vertebrobasilar disease is usually associated with disease of the carotid bifurcation and can often be alleviated by surgical correction of the carotid lesion. When these symptoms occur in isolation, the vertebral or basilar artery occlusion may be bypassed by an anastomosis between the occipital artery and the posterior inferior or the superior cerebellar artery. The operation is carried out with the patient in a semiprone position, the occipital vessel being dissected from the deep surface of a parieto-occipital skin flap. The cerebellar artery is approached laterally as it passes over the cerebellar hemisphere through a small occipital craniectomy.

Postoperative management of both carotid endarterectomy and extra–intracranial bypass includes regular neurological observations and blood pressure measurement, the latter preferably by continuous intra-arterial monitoring. A quarter of patients undergoing carotid endarterectomy show postoperative hypotension of more than 30 mmHg systolic fall over preoperative levels, provided that the carotid sinus nerve and baroreceptor region have been left undisturbed during the operative procedure. Seventy-five per cent of these changes can be reversed by the installation of a small dose of 1 per cent lignocaine along the carotid sinus cannula left in situ at operation. Postoperative hypertension may be related to carotid sinus damage or may be more sinister, in representing the onset of a neurological deficit. The importance of maintaining the patient's normotension cannot be overemphasized. Facilities for angiography and CAT scanning are desirable to identify possible local endarterectomy problems in the carotid endarterectomy group or complications such as acute subdural haematoma in the extra-intracranial patients. If re-exploration is being considered for any of these complications associated with neurological deterioration, it should be carried out as soon as possible.

POSTOPERATIVE PROGRESS

Carotid Endarterectomy

The remarkable variation in the published and unpublished data with respect to postoperative neurological deficits remains one of the mysteries of this controversial subject; the more so since arterial surgical techniques are well established and patient selection as assessed by examination of current literature seems to be fairly uniform. Thompson and his group [46], operating on a very large number of patients, consistently report operative mortality in the region of 0·7 per cent. These authors routinely use a peroperative shunt. Javid et al. [70], in a series of patients amounting to 1400 at the time of the quoted reference, admitted to a 2 per cent operative mortality, peroperative shunting also being their routine.

Some of the earlier studies without shunting reported a much higher incidence of operative death. Bloodwell et al. [71] reported a 5·6 mortality in 536 patients, but the series included patients with TIAs and completed strokes, while later workers include very few patients with acute neurological preoperative problems and often a number of patients with asymptomatic disease—both these factors markedly influencing survival figures.

A more recent account of a series of 104 consecutive patients undergoing carotid endarterectomy by Baker et al. [72] reported an operative mortality of 0·6 per cent in non-shunted patients. These workers were unable to relate their stroke problems to occlusion times, stump pressure or additional lesions. A less optimistic report was given by MacGowan [73], who reported 7 per cent hospital mortality in 64 patients undergoing 72 carotid endarterectomies. This figure, however, represents the total experience of this surgeon and includes possible learning phase problems. Also of note was the fact that only two of the five deaths were due to neurological problems and many reports specify that mortality relates to stroke problems and do not state whether any of these patients died of non-stroke problems or whether these were excluded. If the latter has not been the case, the incidence of postoperative myocardial infarction has been very low in a group of patients who would normally have been considered a high risk category.

In our own practice an unexpected impression was that the incidence of neurological problems was increasing in spite of our growing experience. Analysis of the author's first 100 endarterectomies included no operative mortality whereas the most recent 100 cases included 2 deaths. More extensive analysis of the 8 severe problems in these 200 patients, however, revealed that all 8 were in patients with severe bilateral disease (this being taken as a greater than 70 per cent stenosis in both internal carotid arteries). This predominance has also been noted in the remainder of the series and in subsequent patients, although the mechanism has not been elucidated. Shunting does not seem to have influenced the problem; arteriography and CAT scans have not always been available for analysis, but when present they have not supported the concept that either thrombosis or intracerebral haemorrhage were the causative factor. The problem has been renamed the 'reperfusion syndrome'. The theory that this was due to oedema of revascularized ischaemic brain has not, however, been confirmed in an animal model.

Re-stenosis across the endarterectomized area is uncommon, this being perhaps surprising when one considers the operative damage inflicted on the vessel wall where one might expect extensive scar formation. The usual result, however, is the development of a new intimal covering over the denuded surface and a myointimal cell proliferation is part of the reparative process. Late re-stenosis is usually atheromatous in nature and located at the proximal or distal end of the endarterectomy, whereas early re-stenosis may be non-atheromatous in nature. Cossman et al. [74] reported 10 episodes of re-stenosis in 7 patients from a series of 361. They noted an association of keloid formation of the operation scar in 2 patients with this early re-stenotic lesion and generally advised against surgical intervention. Stoney and String [75] were also able to differentiate their 32 recurrent lesions into early and late and noted diffuse intimal fibrosis, difficulty of repeat endarterectomy and a tendency to further recurrence.

The late results of carotid endarterectomy are encouraging in terms of recurrent TIAs and strokes. Over 90 per cent of vessels remain patent [76]. The figure for symptomatic relief from the procedure is lower than that for the patency, but a number of long term follow-up studies are now available to show that in the region of 70 per cent of patients remain symptom-free [76, 77]. Thompson [8] found a 5 per cent late stroke morbidity and mortality rate and considered that carotid endarterectomy reduced the stroke rate in patients at risk by a factor of 7 in relation to the natural history of the non-operated disease.

Extra–intracranial Bypass

The operative morbidity and mortality of extra–intracranial procedures has been encouragingly low when one considers the severity of the lesions being treated. Analysis of the author's first 100 cases showed one operative death, in a patient undergoing simultaneous carotid bifurcation surgery and in whom the anastomosis never functioned, and one severe stroke in a patient who was undergoing simultaneous ligation of the internal carotid artery for severe distal stenotic disease. A more recent patient with a similar lesion treated by bypass alone, however, sustained a severe postoperative stroke due to embolism from the unligated internal carotid artery. The most satisfactory way of treating this form of lesion is still in doubt.

Postoperative recovery is usually rapid and is not associated with the marked blood pressure instability seen in the carotid endarterectomy patients. Long term patency of these vessels is over 90 per cent, which is surprising in view of their size. This is probably related to the low intrahemispheric blood pressure providing a substantial pressure gradient across the anastomosis. An interesting feature has been the enlargement of the superficial temporal artery (which may increase in diameter up to fourfold) in the postoperative phase. Long term follow-up is still less than 10 years for most series, but the late stroke rate seems to be of the same order as that for carotid endarterectomy.

As with the developing phases of carotid endarterectomy, the procedure has also been tried in acute and progressive strokes. The risk of haemorrhage into a recent infarct does not seem as high as after carotid endarterectomy, probably related to the relatively lower blood flow into the damaged area through the bypass. The operative intervention, however, does not seem to have influenced the progress of the underlying cerebral disease in either group. An interesting aspect of the improvement noted in these patients has been that of higher cortical function. Changes have been reported after carotid endarterectomy [78]. The improvement, particularly after bypass of bilateral internal carotid artery obstruction, is encouraging, but requires long term documentation. The possibility that there is a place for the procedure in patients with dementia of cerebrovascular occlusive origin is also under investigation.

COMMENT

The technical aspects of carotid endarterectomy and the microsurgical techniques involved in superficial temporal to middle cerebral artery bypass are now well established. The TIA is the primary indication for surgical intervention and both procedures are effective in abolishing the symptoms in a majority of patients and the long term instance of completed strokes is low. The operative morbidity and mortality of carotid endarterectomy, however, does not leave room for complacency, and meticulous technique must be maintained with adequate perioperative blood pressure control and particular care of patients with severe bilateral stenotic disease of the carotid bifurcation.

These risk factors must be carefully considered, and when contemplating surgical intervention in asymptomatic cerebrovascular disease, remember that symptomatic improvement cannot be obtained in an asymptomatic patient. The value of antiplatelet drugs in these patients is still to be fully evaluated and the results of the combined North

American and European controlled trial on the value of extra–intracranial bypass surgery are eagerly awaited. The value of these procedures in asymptomatic lesions also needs further clarification. It has not been our practice to operate on asymptomatic disease and we were consequently able to follow-up prospectively a group of patients with varying degrees of carotid artery stenosis as assessed non-invasively. These figures did show a much higher risk of stroke in severe stenotic disease but, over 18 months, minimal stroke risk in lesser degrees of stenosis [79]. When contemplating surgery on selected patients in the severe group, however, it must be remembered that surgery on these patients produces the vast majority of the peroperative stroke problems.

Non-atheromatous lesions such as coils, kinks, fibromuscular dysplasia and sacular or dissecting aneurysms form only a small proportion of encountered cases. The management depends on their surgical accessibility and their risk to the patient if left untreated. Symptomatic patients with coils and kinks may be treated by local resection or various forms of implantation [80] and fibromuscular hyperplasia by dilatation [81].

Aneurysms of the internal carotid artery and giant aneurysms of its proximal branches form a very specific problem which, although amenable to internal carotid artery ligation and extra–intracranial arterial bypass, is accompanied by difficult management problems. Flow in the bypass is related to the pressure drop across the external and internal carotid arteries and until ligation of the internal carotid artery has taken place there may be no such gradient in an aneurysmal circulation. Timing of internal carotid artery ligation is therefore critical since it could also precipitate infarction before adequate flow has been established in the bypass. In practical terms, ligation or completion of the ligation is left to the postoperative phase using balloons or a screw clamp.

In this survey, emphasis has been given to specific risk factors of carotid and extra–intracranial bypass procedures. Research on these areas continues but each centre must continually assess its own surgical results to ensure that when surgery is undertaken, it puts the patient at far less risk than the natural history of their underlying disease.

REFERENCES

1. Leriche R., Fontaine R. and Froehlich F. (1935) L'enervation sinu-carotidienne est-elle permise en point de vue physiologique? *Presse Med.* **43**, 1217–20.
2. Chao W. H., Kwan R. S., Lyman R. S. et al. (1918) Thrombosis of the left internal carotid artery. *Arch. Surg.* **37**, 100–11.
3. Barré J. A., Phihlippèdes D. and Isch F. (1947) Thrombose de la carotide interne. Etude clinique, arterio- et encephalographique. *Rev. Neurol.* **79**, 442–4.
4. Johnson H. C. and Walker A. E. (1951) The angiographic diagnosis of spontaneous thrombosis of the internal and common carotid arteries. *J. Neurosurg.* **8**, 631–59.

5. Henschen C. (1950) Operative Revaskularisation des Zirkultotorishy Geschadigten Gehirus durch Aulfuge Gestielten Muskellappe. *Arch. Klin. Chir.* **264**, 392–401.
6. Carrea R., Molins M. and Murphy G. (1955) Surgical treatment of spontaneous thrombosis of the internal carotid artery in the neck. Carotid-carotidcal anastomosis: report of a case. *Acta Neurol. Lat. Am.* **1**, 71–8.
7. Strully K. J., Hurwitt E. S. and Blankenberg H. W. (1953) Thrombo-endarterectomy for thrombosis of the internal carotid artery in the neck. *J. Neurosurg.* **10**, 474–82.
8. Thompson J. E. (1973) The development of carotid artery surgery. *Arch. Surg.* **107**, 643–8.
9 Eastcott H. H. G., Pickering G. W. and Rob C. G. (1954) Reconstruction of internal caroid artery in a patient with intermittent attacks of hemiplegia. *Lancet* **2**, 994–6.
10. Cooley D. A., Al-Naaman Y. D. and Carton C. A. (1956) Surgical treatment of arteriosclerotic occlusion of common carotid artery. *J. Neurosurg.* **13**, 500–6.
11. Denman F. R., Ehni G. and Duty W. S. (1955) Insidious thrombotic occlusion of cervical carotid arteries treated by arterial graft. *Surgery* **38**, 569–77.
12. Lin P. M., Javid H. and Doyle E. J. (1956) Partial internal carotid occlusion treated by primary resection and vein graft. *J. Neurosurg.* **13**, 650–5.
13. Wegner W. (1958) Side to side anastomosis between the external and internal carotid arteries in the treatment of carotid insufficiency. *J. Neurosurg.* **15**, 168–75.
14. Bryant M. F. (1974) Anatomic considerations in carotid endarterectomy. *Surg. Clin. North Am.* **54**, 1291–6.
15. Donaghy R. M. P. and Yasargil M. G. (1968) Extra–intracranial blood flow diversion. In: *Proceedings of the American Association of Neurological Surgery.* Chigago, Ill.
16. Chater N. (1976) Patient selection and results of extra- to intracranial anastomosis in selected cases of cerebrovascular disease. *Clin. Neurosurg.* **23**, 287–309.
17. Reichman O. H. (1975) Extracranial–intracranial arterial anastomosis. In: Whisnant J. P. and Sandok B. A. (ed.) *Cerebral Vascular Disease.* New York, Grune & Stratton, pp. 175–85.
18. Sundt T. M., Siekert R. G., Piepgras D. G. et al. (1971) Bypass surgery for vascular disease of the carotid systems. *Mayo Clin. Proc.* **51**, 677–92.
19. Lumley J. S. P. (1979) Extra–intracranial revascularization. *Br. J. Surg.* **66**, 317–23.
20. Registrar General Reports (1975) HMSO, London
21. National Heart and Lung Institute Task Force of Arteriosclerosis. (1971) Washington, DC, United States Department of Health, Education and Welfare.
22. Garraway W. M., Whisnant J. P., Furlan A. J. et al. (1979) The declining incidence of stroke. *N. Engl. J. Med.* **300**, 449–52.
23. Houser O. W. and Baker H. L. (1968) Fibromuscular dysplasia and other uncommon diseases of the cervical carotid artery: angiographic aspects. *Am. J. Roentgenol.* **104**, 202–12.
24. Moniz E., Lima A. and De Lacerda R. (1937) Hemiplegies par thrombose de la carotide interne. *Presse Med.* **45**, 977–80.
25. Pickering G. W. (1948) Transient cerebral palsy in hypertension and in cerebral embolism. JAMA **137**, 423–30.
26. Denny-Brown D. (1951) Treatment of recurrent cerebrovascular symptoms and the question of ‘vasospasm’. *Med. Clin. North Am.* **35**, 1457–74.
27. Denny-Brown D. and Meyer J. S. (1957) The cerebral collateral circulation. Production of cerebral infarction by ischemic anoxia and its reversibility in early stages. *Neurology* **71**, 567–79.
28. Kendell R. E. and Marshall J. (1963) Role of hypotension in the genesis of transient focal cerebral ischaemic attacks. *Br. Med. J.* **2**, 334–8.
29. Millikan C. H., Siekert R. G. and Shick R. M. (1955) Studies in cerebrovascular disease. V. The use of anticoagulant drugs in the treatment of intermittent insufficiency of the internal carotid arterial system. *Proc. Staff Meet. Mayo Clin.* **30**, 578–86.

30. Fisher C M. (1959) Observations of the fundus oculi in transient monocular blindness. *Neurology* **9**, 333–47.
31. Sutherland G. R. and Donaldson A. A. (1972) Persistent hypoglossal artery complicated by internal carotid artery stenosis. *Clin. Radiol.* **23**, 222–4.
32. Alpers B. J., Berry R. G. and Paddison R. M. (1959) Anatomical studies of the circle of Willis in normal brain. *Arch. Neurol. Psychiatr.* **81**, 409–18.
33. Brust J. C. M. (1977) Transient ischaemic attacks: natural history and anticoagulation. *Neurology* **27**, 701–7.
34. Whisnant J. P. (1977) Indications for medical and surgical therapy in ischaemic stroke. In: Thompson R. A. and Green J. R. (ed.) *Advances in Neurology*. New York, Raven Press.
35. Miyazaki M. and Kato K. (1965) Measurement of cerebral blood flow by ultrasonic Doppler technique; haemodynamic comparison of right and left carotid artery in patients with hemiplegia. *Jap. Circ. J.* **29**, 383–6.
36. Planiol T., Pourcelot L., Pottier J. M. et al. (1972) Etude de la circulation carotidienne par les methodes ultrasoniques et la thermographie. *Rev. Neurol. (Paris)* **126**, 127–41.
37. Rutherford R. B., Hiatt W. R. and Kreutzer E. W. (1977) The use of velocity wave form analysis in the diagnosis of carotid artery occlusive disease. *Surgery* **82**, 695–702.
38. Keller H., Meier W., Yonekawa Y. et al. (1976) Noninvasive angiography for the diagnosis of carotid artery disease using Doppler ultrasound (carotid artery Doppler). *Stroke* **7**, 354–63.
39. Gosling R. G. (1976) Extraction of physiological information from spectrum-analysed Doppler-shifted continuous-wave ultrasound signals obtained non-invasively from the arterial system. In: Hill D. W. and Watson B. W. (ed.) *Medical Electronics Monographs,* Monograph 21. Peregerinus, pp. 73–125.
40. Lees R. S. and Dewey C. F. (1970) Phonoangiography: a new noninvasive diagnostic method for studying arterial disease. *Proc. Natl Acad. Sci. USA* **67**, 935–42.
41. Brockenbrough E. C. (1969) Screening for the prevention of stroke: use of a Doppler flowmeter. Information and Education Resource Support Unit, Washington/Alaska Regional Medical Program.
42. Lye C. R., Sumner D. S. and Strandness D. E. (1976) The accuracy of the supraorbital Doppler examination in the diagnosis of haemodynamically significant carotid occlusive disease. *Surgery* **79**, 42–5.
43. Gee W., Mehigan J. T. and Wylie E. J. (1975) Measurement of collateral cerebral hemispheric blood pressure by ocular pneumoplethysmography. *Am. J. Surg.* **130**, 121–7.
44. Doerrler J. (1981) Carotid Surgery without Angiography. Lipha Symposium, Manchester.
45. Baker R. N., Ramseyer J. C. and Schwartz W. S. (1968) Prognosis in patients with transient cerebral ischaemis attacks. *Neurology (Minneap)* **18**, 1157–65.
46. Thompson J. E., Patman R. D. and Talkington C. M. (1978) Carotid surgery for cerebrovascular insufficiency. *Curr. Probl. Surg.* **15**, No. 12.
47. Lyons C., Clark L. C., McDowell H. et al. (1964) Cerebral venous oxygen content during carotid thrombo-intimectomy. *Am. J. Surg.* **160**, 561–7.
48. Larson C. P. (1970) Anaesthesia and control of the cerebral circulation. In: Wylie E. J. and Ehrenfeld W. K. (ed.) *Extracranial Cerebrovascular Disease: Diagnosis and Management*. Philadelphia, Saunders, pp. 152–83.
49. Smith A. L., Hoff J. T., Nielson S. L. et al. (1974) Barbiturate protection against cerebral infarction. In: Langfitt T. W., McHenry L. C. and Reivitch M. (ed.) *Cerebral Circulation and Metabolism*. New York, Springer-Verlag, p. 347.
50. Chung W. B. (1974) Long-term results of carotid artery surgery for cerebrovascular insufficiency. *Am. J. Surg.* **128**, 262–8.

51. Wells B. A., Keats A. S. and Cooley D. A. (1963) Increased tolerance to cerebral ischaemia produced by general anaesthesia during temporary carotid occlusion. *Surgery* **54**, 216–23.
52. Hobson R. W., Wright C. B., Sublett J. W. et al. (1974) Carotid artery back pressure and endarterectomy under regional anaesthesia. *Arch. Surg.* **109**, 682–7.
53. Connolly J. E., Kwaan J. H. and Stemmer E. A. (1977) Improved results with carotid endarterectomy. *Ann. Surg.* **186**, 334–42.
54. Firt P., Hejhal L. and Weiss K. (1971) Remarks on the reconstruction of obliterating atherosclerosis of the internal carotid artery. *J. Cardiovasc. Surg.* **12**, 447–55.
55. Crawford E. S., DeBakey M. E., Blaisdell F. W. et al. (1960) Haemodynamic alterations in patients with cerebral arterial insufficiency before and after operation. *Surgery* **48**, 76–94.
56. Javid H. and Taylon C. (1978) Neurosurgical experience with carotid endarterectomy at University Hospitals (1954-76). *Wisconsin Med. J.* **77**, 65–8.
57. Julian O. C. and Javid H. (1971) Surgical management of cerebral arterial insufficiency. *Curr. Probl. Surg.* March.
58. Piepgras D. G. and Sundt T. M. (1976) Clinical and laboratory experience of heparin-impregnated silicone shunts for carotid endarterectomy. *Ann. Surg.* **184**, 637–41.
59. Spielberger L., Turndoff H., Culliford A. et al. (1979) Hand-held toy squeaker during carotid endarterectomy in the awake patient. *Arch. Surg.* **114**, 103–4.
60. Moore W. S., Yee J. M. and Hall A. D. (1973) Carotid artery back pressure: a test of cerebral tolerance to temporary carotid occlusion. *Arch. Surg.* **106**, 520–3.
61. Collins G. J., Rich N. M., Andersen C. A. et al. (1978) Stroke associated with carotid endarterectomy. *Am. J. Surg.* **135**, 221–5.
62. Viancos J. G., Sechzer P. H., Keats A. S. et al. (1966) Internal jugular venous oxygen tension as an index of cerebral blood flow during carotid endarterectomy. *Circulation* **34**, 875–82.
63. Larson C. P., Ehrenfeld W. K., Wade J. G. et al. (1967) Jugular venous oxygen saturation as an index of adequacy of cerebral oxygenation. *Surgery* **62**, 31–9.
64. Hays R. J., Levinson S. A. and Wylie E. G. (1972) Intra-operative measurement of carotid back pressure as a guide to operatvie management for carotid endarterectomy. *Surgery* **72**, 953–60.
65. Moore W. S. and Hall A. D. (1981) Carotid artery back pressure: a test of cerebral tolerance to temporary carotid occlusion. *Arch. Surg.* **99**, 702–71.
66. McKay R. D., Sundt T. M., Michenfelder J. D. et al. (1976) Internal carotid artery stump pressure and cerebral blood flow during carotid endarterectomy, modification by halothane, enflurane and innovar. *Anaesthesiology* **45**, 390–9.
67. Beebe H., Pearson J. M. and Coatsworth J. J. (1978) Comparison of carotid artery stump pressure and EEG monitoring in carotid endarterectomy. *Am. Surg.* **44**, 655–60.
68. Curi E., Dash S. K. and Lim D. B. (1981) Carotid compression test (CCT). A preoperative criteria for selective shunting during carotid endarterectomy. International Vascular Symposium, London.
69. Chater N., Spetzler R. and Tonnemacher K. (1976) Anatomical localization of optimal middle cerebral branch for anastomosis. In: Austin G. M. (ed.) *Microsurgical Anastomoses for Cerebral Ischaemia*. Springfield, Ill., Thomas, pp. 39–51.
70. Javid H., Dye W. S., Hunter J. A. et al. (1974) Surgical treatment of cerebral ischaemia. *Surg. Clin. North Am.* **54**, 239–55.
71. Bloodwell R. D., Hallman G. L., Keats A. S. et al. (1968) Carotid endarterectomy without a shunt—results using hypercarbic anaesthesia. *Arch. Surg.* **96**, 644–52.
72. Baker W. H., Dorner D. B. and Barnes R. W. (1977) Carotid endarterectomy: is an indwelling shunt necessary? *Surgery* **82**, 321–6.

73. MacGowan W. A. L. (1978) Carotid endarterectomy. A clinical review of 72 carotid endarterectomies. *Proceedings 27th International Congress of the European Society of Cardiovascular Surgery,* Book 2, pp. 363–8.
74. Cossman D., Callow A. D., Stein A. et al. (1978) Early restenosis after endarterectomy. *Arch Surg.* **113**, 375–8.
75. Stoney R. J. and String S. T. (1976) Recurrent carotid stenosis. *Surgery* **80**, 705–10.
76. Wylie E. J. and Ehrenfeld W. K. (1970) *Extracranial Occlusive Cerebrovascular Disease. Diagnosis and Management.* Philadelphia, Saunders.
77. De Weese J. A., Rob C. G., Satran R. et al. (1973) Results of carotid endarterectomies for transient ischaemic attack—five years later. *Ann. Surg.* **178**, 258–64.
78. Perry P. M., Drinkwater J. E. and Taylor G. W. (1975) Cerebral function before and after carotid endarterectomy. *Br. Med. J.* **4**, 215–16.
79. Dean R. A. and Lumley J. S. P. (1981) Asymptomatic carotid artery stenoses: incidence and prognosis. *Br. J. Surg.* **68**, 350.
80. Lumley J. S. P. (1980) Techniques of improving blood flow to the brain. In: Taylor S. (ed.) *Recent Advances in Surgery.* Edinburgh, Churchill Livingstone, pp. 113–33.
81. Morris G. C., Lechter A. and DeBakey M. E. (1968) Surgical treatment of fibromuscular disease of the carotid arteries. *Arch. Surg.* **96**, 636–43.

J. G. Pollock and A. J. McKay

6 Abdominal Aortic Aneurysm

INTRODUCTION

Aneurysmal dilatation of the abdominal aorta was first noted by Antullis 1800 years ago, but only within the past 30 years has effective treatment become a practical reality. Following the first report of successful homograft replacement of the abdominal aorta in 1952 [1], the rapid development and improvement of anaesthetic and surgical techniques has meant that elective surgery for abdominal aortic aneurysms can now be performed with a mortality of 5 per cent or less [2–5].

Many factors have contributed to this success story. Anaesthetic techniques have greatly improved over these three decades. Intensive intraoperative and postoperative monitoring can now provide such detailed information that the major causes of mortality such as renal failure or potentially lethal arrhythmias can be detected and treated effectively. The importance of preventing graft infection has been recognized and appropriate antibiotics are available for use as prophylactic agents.

As the demand for such surgery has increased, suitable arterial substitutes have become available following the earliest report that a woven fabric thread of Vinyon could be used to replace the abdominal aorta [6]. Keeping pace with these developments new suture materials and instruments have been designed and critical analysis of several modes of treatment has led to almost world wide acceptance of the best operative procedure for the various presentations of this condition.

Unhappily, while enormous advances have been made in this comparatively short period, problems remain. Surgeons from all over the world continue to report ever-decreasing mortality figures in surgery for elective aneurysm replacement but no such reduction has been found in patients presenting with a leaking or ruptured aneurysm. Around half of these patients still die despite the aggressive application of the most modern anaesthetic, surgical and intensive care techniques. Furthermore, one recognized authority has recently suggested that this figure may represent an irreducible plateau with subsequent reduction in mortality being outwith the scope of our present armamentarium [7].

The technical challenge of providing a suitable arterial prosthesis and developing surgical techniques to allow its safe placement has been met. In this chapter we will describe our own practice of vascular surgery as it relates to abdominal aneurysms. We will attempt to take stock of the cumulative experience gained during the rapid expansion of vascular surgery. Emphasis will be placed on the importance of case selection since it cannot be considered good medicine to replace successfully a leaking aortic aneurysm only to have the patient die some weeks later with a patent arterial graft but multi-organ failure. The significance of co-existent coronary artery disease will be highlighted. So different is the outcome in the treatment of an intact as opposed to a ruptured aneurysm that we will discuss these two major presentations separately.

INTACT ABDOMINAL AORTIC ANEURYSM

Presentation and Diagnosis

So much has been written on the many ways in which an abdominal aneurysm may present that it might be supposed that very few patients with a large pulsatile swelling in their abdomen would escape detection. Sadly this is not the case. As recently as 1976 a review of 9894 autopsies performed in a Glasgow teaching hospital revealed that almost half the ruptured aortic aneurysms were undetected prior to post-mortem [8]. There is clearly considerable scope for improvement in diagnosis.

The patient with an abdominal aortic aneurysm will most commonly complain of an abdominal swelling—noted by the patient himself or by the family doctor—or of abdominal pain or backache. Indeed the presence of backache due to erosion of the vertebral bodies by an expanding aneurysm may mean that the first referral is to an orthopaedic clinic. More unusually, an aneurysm may present primarily as duodenal hold-up due to stretching of the duodenum over the front of the aneurysmal sac. Rarely an aneurysm may be the underlying cause of hydronephrosis (*Fig. 6.1*).

Given such a presentation, how can the presence and nature of the suspected aneurysm be confirmed? Standard texts emphasize the importance of abdominal examination and various methods have been described to distinguish between the truly expansile pulsation of an aneurysm and the transmitted pulsation of the aorta felt through other abdominal viscera or masses. There is little doubt that an experienced clinician will almost always correctly diagnose an aneurysm when the aortic diameter has reached at least twice normal size. However, despite individual conviction of our ability as clinicians it has been suggested that clinical examination alone may be wrong in up to 15 per cent of cases [9].

A thorough clinical examination remains of critical importance but we need not entirely rely on it to confirm the diagnosis. Typical

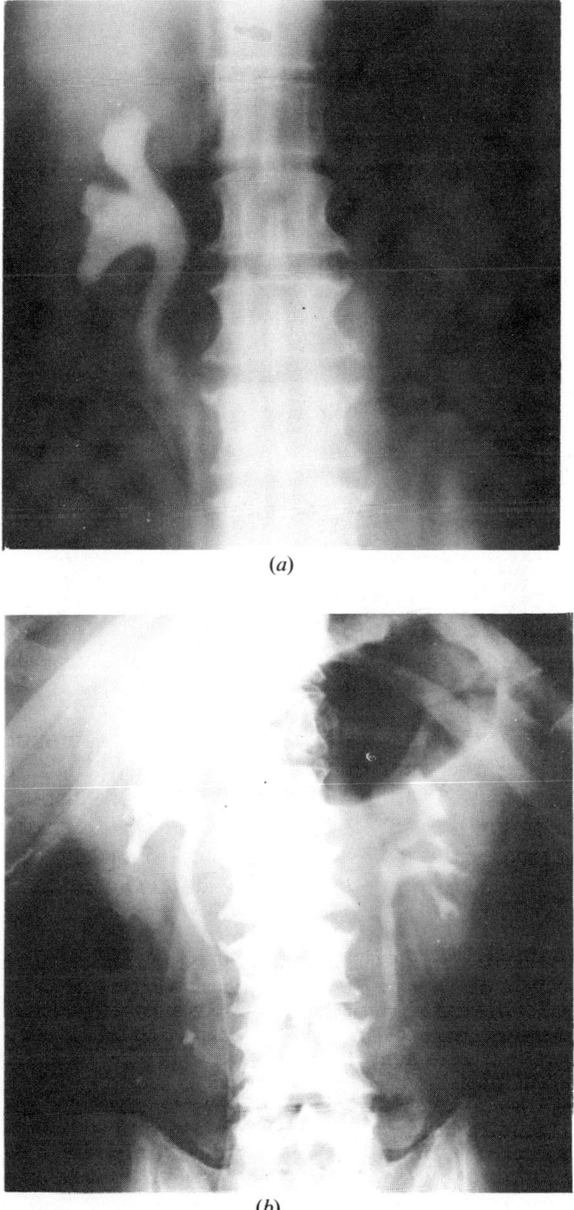

(*a*)

(*b*)

Fig. 6.1. a, Tomogram showing right-sided hydronephrosis in 54-year-old man with abdominal aortic aneurysm. *b*, Postoperative IVP in the same patient showing marked improvement in renal function following excision of aneurysm.

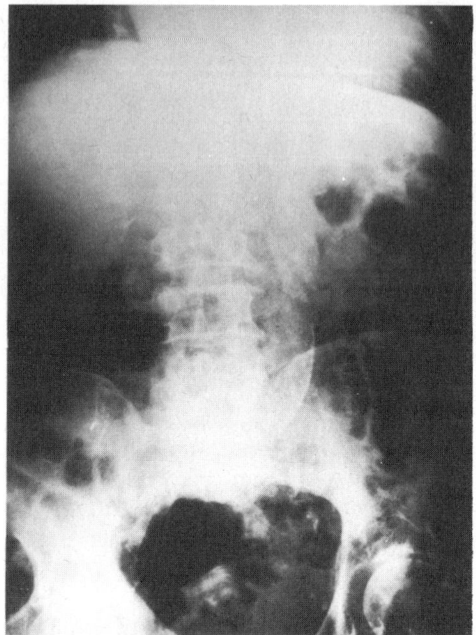

Fig. 6.2.

calcification of the aneurysmal wall will be seen on a straight or lateral X-ray of the abdomen in most cases (*Fig. 6.2*). However, even if calcification is present, this finding alone is not conclusive since calcification may be seen in an aorta that is tortuous but not aneurysmal.

Two modern non-invasive imaging techniques have thus made an important contribution to the accuracy of diagnosis in abdominal aneurysms. We have previously reported on the value of ultrasonography [10] (*Fig. 6.3*) and more recently numerous reports have shown that computerized tomography can give even more detailed information, particularly if an intravenous contrast medium is used concurrently [11, 12] (*Fig. 6.4*) Being non-invasive, these methods have the further advantage that documentation of aneurysmal size can be made regularly so that the rate of expansion of an aneurysm can be recorded if early surgery is not thought to be indicated.

There remains the more controversial issue of the use of aortography in the management of a patient with an intact aneurysm. Although it is invasive and therefore associated with an inevitable morbidity, there is no doubt that aortography can now be performed with relative safety even in the presence of aneurysmal dilatation. Uniquely, it can provide

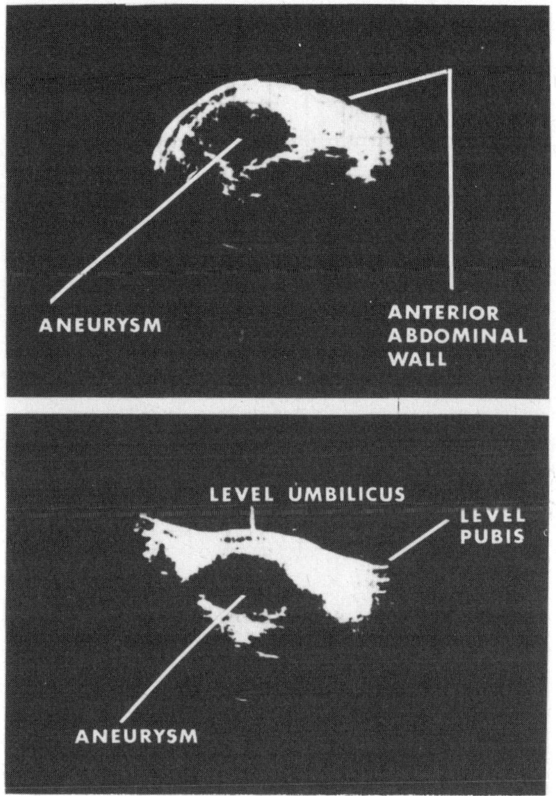

Fig. 6.3

detailed information on both the proximal extent of the lesion and the nature of the peripheral arterial run-off, information which may be invaluable. Perhaps the strongest argument in favour of a routine angiogram in cases of unruptured aneurysm is that the occasional patient with an anomaly of the visceral arteries will be detected preoperatively. In particular renovascular abnormalities important collateral spinal vessels and absence or occlusion of the superior mesenteric artery can be demonstrated. The finding of this last lesion is of particular significance since so often the origin of the inferior mesenteric artery is occluded by the aneurysm and sacrificed at the time of surgery.

Our practice after a thorough clinical examination is to send all patients with a suspected aortic aneurysm for a straight and lateral plain X-ray of the abdomen together with a chest X-ray to ensure that the thoracic aorta is not also aneurysmal. All patients then have an

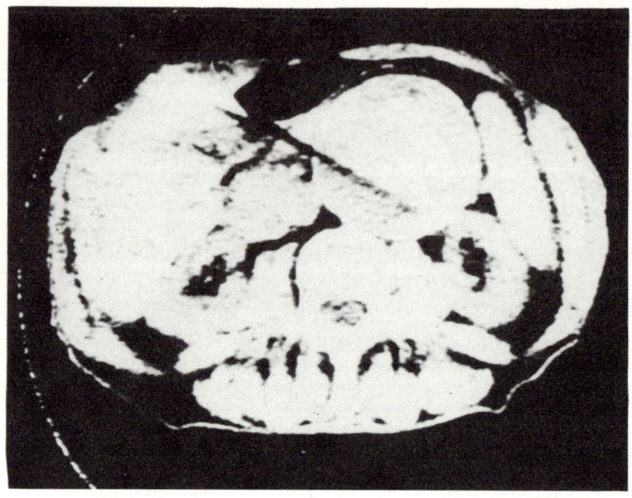

Fig. 6.4

ultrasound assessment of aneurysmal size. Since we consider that the additional cost and relative invasiveness of CAT scanning is not justified in most patients we do not use it routinely. We reserve angiography for those patients in whom the presence of an aneurysm has not been established beyond doubt by non-invasive means. In high risk patients translumbar or retrograde aortography using a Seldinger catheter can be performed under local anaesthesia using iso-osmotic contrast medium.

Preoperative Assessment

When an aneurysm has been diagnosed, a thorough preoperative assessment must be undertaken as for any major surgical procedure. A full cardiovascular examination is made with particular reference to associated cerebral or coronary artery disease (*see below*). Peripheral pulse pattern must be documented by clinical examination aided by using a Doppler ultrasound probe for pulses which are clinically impalpable.

When symptoms are present there is a clear indication for surgery, but the best treatment of an asymptomatic small aneurysm is more difficult. It has become accepted that the risk of rupture increases dramatically when the aneurysm size exceeds 6 cm in diameter [7], but even using monitoring techniques such as ultrasound the rate of growth of aneurysms is somewhat unpredictable and the factors that influence growth are not fully known. However, it has been stated that up to 80 per cent of patients with an abdominal aneurysm will die within a year of diagnosis and 50 per cent of these deaths will be due to rupture [13, 14].

Given this risk of rupture, surgery thus offers the best chance of long term survival for the great majority of patients once aneurysmal disease of the abdominal aorta has been reliably diagnosed. It is therefore our practice to recommend surgery for all aneurysms since we have known rupture occur in aneurysms of 3·5 cm diameter. Similarly, aneurysms of the common iliac artery have a high incidence of rupture. In the elderly frail patient with a small asymptomatic aneurysm or in the patient who is a major surgical risk due to associated coronary artery disease or poor pulmonary function, conservative management will occasionally be the sensible choice.

There are now many publications stating that age is no barrier to elective aneurysmectomy [15] and in essence we agree with this opinion, having successfully operated on several patients in their 90s with gratifying results. In assessing age, however, the physiological age of the patient is far more important than chronological age. Each patient must be assessed individually and the risks of surgery balanced with the possible benefits in the knowledge that application of aggressive surgical treatment has led to a continuing decline in mortality figures for elective surgery despite an increasing proportion of elderly patients. In our own centre the mortality for the last 100 elective abdominal aortic aneurysm replacements was 4·0 per cent. It may be thought that such a figure can scarcely be reduced, but we believe that this is not the case. The aim in vascular surgery should be to continue to reduce mortality figures until they approach the irreducible minimum.

Much work has been done on detailed analysis of the causes of death in elective patients [4, 5, 16, 17]. Several important factors have emerged and it is in these areas that improvements can still be made.

Myocardial Infarction

Postoperative myocardial infarction is the single commonest cause of both early and late mortality following elective aneurysm surgery, accounting for up to 40 per cent of all deaths [17]. Aorto-coronary bypass surgery is now an established and relatively safe surgical procedure [18] and should be considered for selected patients. Indeed in some centres the frequency of fatal postoperative myocardial infarction after aneurysm resection has led to a policy that all elective cases have coronary angiography performed preoperatively [19]. Although long term follow-up results are at present not available, the early signs indicate that this policy has been associated with a lowering of elective mortality [20].

With finite resources there is a limit to the number of coronary arteriograms that can be performed. In the United Kingdom the number of patients undergoing aorto-coronary bypass grafting is increasing annually and to add to that workload would stretch the system perhaps beyond capacity. We therefore cannot perform coronary angiography in all elective cases but strongly support its use for selected patients. Certainly in the young patient with a history of myocardial ischaemia or previous infarction coronary angiography should be performed as part of the preoperative assessment. In the absence of a definite history of angina pectoris or previous myocardial infarction coronary arteriography is not undertaken but an exercise ECG can easily be performed and useful information obtained.

The timing of aorto-coronary surgery remains to be established. In most centres—including our own—the cardiac surgery takes precedence and the abdominal aneurysm is then dealt with around 6 months later. However, concurrent aorto-coronary, and abdominal surgery has now been performed in several places and clearly we await the results of these comparative studies with some interest.

Renal Function and Fluid Balance

As part of the careful preoperative assessment renal function must be specifically examined. There is evidence that even mild degrees of chronic renal failure may significantly increase the risk of elective surgery despite careful monitoring of fluid balance [16]. As well as routine urea and electrolyte estimation, all patients should therefore have a 24-hour urine collection for creatinine clearance measurement. If this is less than 50 ml per minute very serious thought should be given to the advisability of surgery. In many centres routine intravenous pyelography is advocated to provide preoperative evidence of normal bilateral renal function without mechanical obstruction. This investigation will also identify the rare occurrence of a horseshoe kidney.

Pulmonary Function

Inevitably, in an elderly operative population the incidence of chronic obstructive airways disease will be high. This is particulary true in the West of Scotland, with an alarmingly high level of chronic bronchitis and emphysema. It is worth while assessing respiratory function preoperatively, and if this can be improved then the time spent so doing is time well spent. Very occasionally respiratory function will be so poor that elective surgery may not be advisable. We feel sure that although prophylactic antibiotics are essentially used to prevent graft infection, they have also made a contribution to the reduction of postoperative chest complications.

Prevention of Infection

Graft infection should be a rare occurrence but when it occurs it has disastrous consequences. The theoretical danger of resistant organism growth led many vascular surgeons to abandon the use of prophylactic antibiotics when sterile prostheses became available. However, analysis of the results of surgery has shown that in the absence of antibiotic cover infection makes a major contribution to morbidity [5]. In keeping with modern practice we begin antibiotic cover at the time of induction of anaesthesia and continue with it for 24–48 hours. For many years we used a synthetic penicillin specifically aimed at *Staphylococcus aureus* infection; however, recent analysis of infected grafts has shown that many other organisms can be implicated in more than half the cases. Accordingly we now use a third generation cephalosporin given intravenously. In addition, we actively look for any source of infection and nasal, throat and perineal swabs are taken from all patients. A skin infection at any site precludes surgery. Specimens of sputum and urine are routinely sent for culture before and after surgery. Very thorough skin preparation with an iodine based antiseptic is used and adhesive skin drapes are used principally to isolate the perineum from groin incisions.

All central venous and arterial lines are removed as soon as is reasonably possible since they may provide entry sites for organisms. Similarly the urinary catheter is removed on the immediate post-operative day.

Intraoperative Considerations

Monitoring

Major advances have been made in the development and application of monitoring techniques which have made an important contribution to the safety of this major surgery. Most of the responsibility for intraoperative monitoring rests with the anaesthetic team and close cooperation between anaesthetist and surgeon is essential at all times. The following monitoring techniques are employed in every patient.

Electrocardiogram

Continuous ECG visual monitoring allows the earliest possible detection and treatment of any arrhythmia. For example, these patients are particularly susceptible to the development of a low junctional rhythm and characteristic Canon V waves assist in establishing this diagnosis. In addition to standard limb leads, a V5 chest lead is used routinely to assist in detection of subendocardial ischaemia as revealed by ST segment depression on this lead.

Central Venous Pressure (CVP)

The CVP is usually measured via a catheter introduced into the right atrium through an internal jugular vein although the choice of site for placement of the central line is often dependent on the personal preference of the anaesthetist. Measurement of CVP affords a means of assessing fluid balance and, in particular, allows assessment of the patient's tolerance of a deliberate fluid load.

Arterial Pressure

The radial artery can be cannulated with very little risk to the patient. Continuous arterial waveform oscilloscopic visualization allows beat-to-beat monitoring of stroke volume as well as continuous monitoring or arterial pressures. Furthermore, arterial blood gas analysis is thus made readily available at any time during the procedure.

Urinary Output

All patients have a urinary catheter *in situ*. The urinary output is controlled by maintenance of a satisfactory CVP and diuretics are not generally required. When it is necessary to cross-clamp the aorta above the renal arteries, then mannitol 20 g is given prior to cross-clamping. It is rare for such suprarenal clamping to last longer than 10 minutes and renal ischaemia is not often a problem. If there is any question of prolonged renal ischaemia then the kidneys can be protected not only by using mannitol but also by the use of regional anticoagulants and cooling.

Other Monitoring Methods

Pulmonary artery wedge pressures can be measured by using the Swan Ganz balloon-tipped pulmonary catheter [21]. We do not routinely use this catheter but recognize that it provides a more sensitive indicator of left ventricular dysfunction, particularly in patients with arterial hypertension and coronary artery disease. We believe that the central venous pressure measurement of right heart function is adequate for most cases but the Swan Ganz catheter is of particular value in, for example, a patient who has suffered previous left ventricular failure who then requires urgent surgery for an abdominal aortic aneurysm.

Operative Methods

Aortic surgery should not be tackled without adequate assistance and, if at all possible, two assistants should be present at least until the initial dissection is completed. The incision should be large enough to allow full access to the entire abdominal aorta. Our preference is for a vertical midline incision skirting the umbilicus, but many surgeons favour a transverse abdominal incision, claiming that these heal particularly well with a low incidence of wound dehiscence or late herniation. The surgeon's aim should be to perform the minimum dissection necessary and thereafter to insert the simplest prosthesis possible. When clinical examination together with Doppler ultrasound or arteriography have shown an acceptable distal arterial tree then it is often possible to insert an aortic tube graft (*Fig. 6.5*), and we strive to perform this procedure if at all possible.

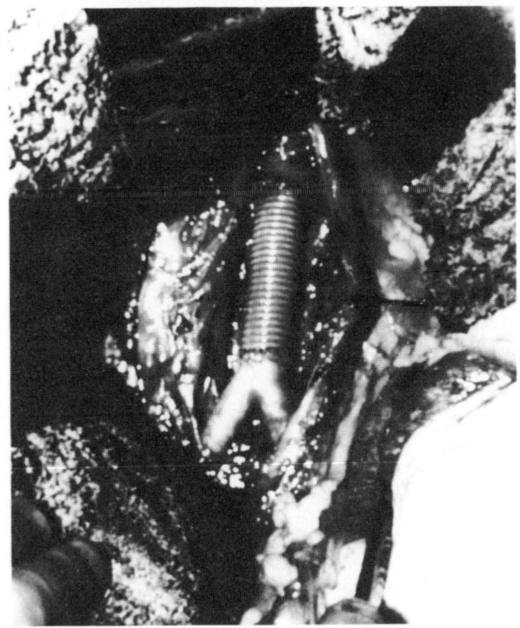

Fig. 6.5 Aortic tube graft in position after resection of aneurysm.

If access to the upper limit of the aneurysm is inadequate, the surgeon should not hesitate to divide the left renal vein since this does not seriously prejudice postoperative renal function. Such division and ligation should be made as far to the right as possible, thus leaving adequate collateral venous return from the left kidney. Very occasionally there is a post-aortic renal vein or the left iliac vein may ascend on the left side of the aorta and cross over at a higher level. The venous pattern is more complex when horseshoe kidney is present [23] and the surgeon should be aware of such venous anomalies.

Having gained proximal control of the aneurysm the lower extent of the sac should be identified and the iliac vessels inspected. Although it is obviously attractive to perform the complete operation in the abdominal cavity, the iliac vessels may be difficult to mobilize adequately and if they are also aneurysmal or diseased, then it is safer to take the lower limbs of the graft to the femoral arteries. On many occasions the pelvic veins will be found to be closely adherent to the iliac arteries, and with the aneurysm sac still *in situ,* a tear in one of these veins can be extremely difficult to control even with adequate assistance. This area of dissection is among the most critical in the entire operative procedure. It is often unnecessary and indeed it may be foolhardy to attempt to mobilize the iliac arteries fully and control of the vessels can be achieved by a limited dissection at a suitable point on each vessel well away from the confluence of the common iliac veins, where they are particularly vulnerable. The vessels can then be controlled by double ligation in continuity.

Although in theory ligation of the iliac arteries might be thought to jeopardize pelvic blood flow, in practice we have not found this to be a problem. In order to preserve pelvic blood flow we would only ligate both iliac vessels below the iliac bifurcation if forced to do so by aneurysmal disease. If only one vessel is ligated pelvic flow is maintained retrogradely from the perfused femoral vessels. If distal iliac ligation is necessary, every attempt is made to re-anastomose the inferior mesenteric artery.

Having completed the initial dissection if the patient is stable, and the blood loss has been minimal, our preference is to use a knitted Dacron graft which is, of course, pre-clotted. Although much has been written on fairly lengthy and complicated techniques for pre-clotting the Dacron material, we have had no cause for concern with the method outlined below.

Approximately 40 ml of blood is taken either from the inferior vena cava by direct venepuncture or from the aneurysm itself, the graft is filled and then completely immersed in this non-heparinized blood, until clot forms. Any further dissection required can be undertaken at this juncture, for example the subinguinal tunnels can be prepared.

The patient is heparinized (5000 i.u. intravenously) and the aorta and distal vessels cross-clamped. In a typical infrarenal aneurysm no attempt should be made to dissect and excise the aneurysmal sac but rather the sac is opened longitudinally, cleared of thrombotic and arteriosclerotic material and lumbar vessel bleeding controlled by direct suture. Care must be taken to clear the proximal aorta of all thrombotic and arteriosclerotic debris since when flow is re-established this material is a ready source of emboli.

If a bifurcation graft is being inserted the body of the graft must be cut to the correct length so that the bifurcation is not compromised as the graft crosses the sacral promontory. Suction is used to clear the graft of blood clot and a strong needle is used for the proximal anastomosis, our preference being Ti-cron 2/0 or 3/0 inserted as a continuous suture. Silk should not be used.

Various modifications of the simple end-to-end anastomosis have been reported, including the use of a protective sleeve of Dacron, and others emphasize the merit of invaginating the prosthesis into the proximal aorta so that the anastomosis lies approximately 1 cm proximal to the cut end of the aorta [17]. We do not routinely use either of these manoeuvers but do modify the preparation of the aorta so that the anastomosis can be performed as easily as possible. The level of cross-clamping is critical in this regard and every effort should be made to leave an adequate cuff of aorta to allow a swift and safe anastomosis to be completed.

The proximal anastomosis is tested prior to starting the first of the distal anastomoses. Particular diligence is required at this stage to ensure that the posterior half of the proximal anastomosis is entirely leakproof since adequate inspection of this area becomes especially difficult when the lower anastomoses are completed. After completion of the first lower anastomosis the open limb of the graft can be used to flush the proximal aorta and body of the graft of any thrombus or debris. Thereafter the aortic cross-clamp is left in place but the completed limb opened and backbleeding is allowed to occur until blood flows down the open limb. When all air and clot has thus been safely removed the open limb is clamped at the bifurcation and the cross-clamp is slowly released from the aorta to allow single limb perfusion. The second limb of the graft is then sutured in the same way, taking care to expel all air and any blood clot prior to final opening of the residual clamp. These manoeuvres are simple but important and must be performed faithfully. The surgeon must be quite certain that air and blood clot have been removed completely before the circulation is finally opened.

When the graft is *in situ* and if the lower limbs have been taken to the femoral vessels, oversewn iliac arteries must be inspected. Despite ligation back-pressure can cause significant bleeding from this site and having seen this occur we now doubly ligate or transfix these vessels. If the inferior mesenteric artery is patent at the time of dissection then every effort should be made to preserve this vessel with a cuff of aortic wall and this is then re-implanted into the prosthesis.

Although close cooperation between the surgeon and anaesthetist is required at all times, there are two periods during the procedure which require particular mention. First, the initial cross-clamping of the aorta may be associated with subendocardial ischaemia and at this point the patient is particularly prone to develop left ventricular failure. Secondly, on completion of the first of the lower anastomoses the aortic clamp is released and hypotension inevitably occurs, as the circulation to one limb is reopened. It is essential that the patient be in positive fluid balance prior to this stage, perhaps by as much as 500 ml. It may be necessary to open the aortic clamp only partially or to re-apply it for a variable length of time until an adequate blood pressure can be maintained. The use of an aortic clamp with a long ratchet has proved to be of considerable benefit in allowing progressive de-clamping (Pollock-Stille).

Opening the limb leads to an inevitable acidosis and while the degree of acidosis is variable, bicarbonate is given routinely at this time. Similarly, on opening the second limb of the graft a more minor episode of hypotension should be anticipated. The level of this hypotension is particularly critical in the patient with an aortic aneurysm since no collateral distal circulation will have developed in the majority of cases, unlike the situation which exists in the patient with distal occlusive disease where an extensive collateral circulation exists.

With the graft in position, the adequacy of distal flow should be assessed and no patient allowed to leave theatre if the patency of the graft is in doubt. Clinical observation of limb colour, venous filling, temperature and the presence of peripheral pulses is inadequate in this context. Several ancillary aids are now available and their use will undoubtedly become more widespread and reduce the need for subsequent surgery owing to graft occlusion.

Electromagnetic Flow Meters

It is known that feeling the pulsation in an artery is not an accurate means of assessing the adequacy of flow through that vessel. However, the electromotive force (EMF) produced by the passage of blood through a magnetic field can be readily measured peroperatively and this EMF bears a linear relationship to the velocity of blood flow. Flow abnormalities can be readily detected by this means and a dampened waveform will be obtained if flow is inadequate (*Fig. 6.6*). Observation of such an abnormality may well induce the surgeon to re-explore an anastomosis and search for a possible technical error. Until recently the EMF probes that have been available have been rather cumbersome to use and have often required the presence of a flow technician in theatre. Improved flow probes are now available and the results are easily interpreted without expert technical knowledge [23] so that their use may well become more widespread.

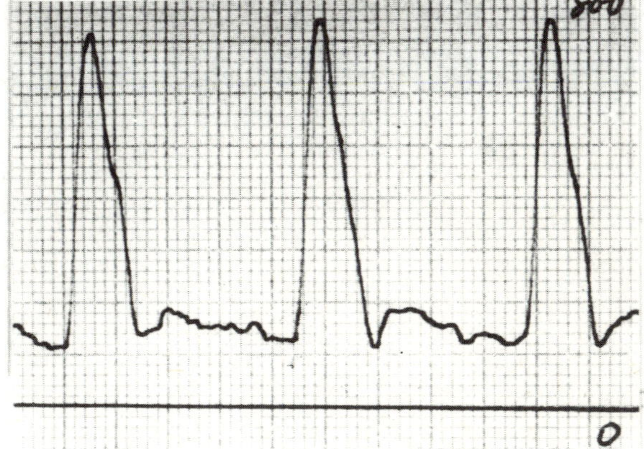

Fig. 6.6. (a)

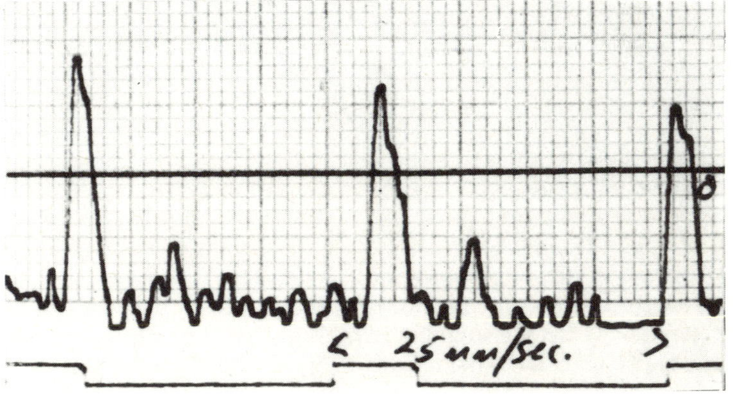

Fig. 6.6. (b)

Fig. 6.6. a, Almost normal arterial waveform. *b*, Waveform obtained following aorto-femoral reconstruction. Clinically the vessel felt normally pulsatile, but EMF probe revealed no flow. *c*, Right hand waveform shows distal obstruction, left hand waveform shows mild proximal stenosis.

On-table Arteriography

It is rarely necessary to use arteriography following excision of an abdominal aortic aneurysm, but where doubt exists as to the adequacy of limb perfusion and no correctable error can be found, we would not hesitate to obtain an angiogram. Although there is evidence that arteriography used routinely leads to detection of the more common causes of technical failure and their subsequent elimination [24], its use is perhaps more appropriate in non-aneurysmal aorto-iliac or femoro-popliteal reconstruction.

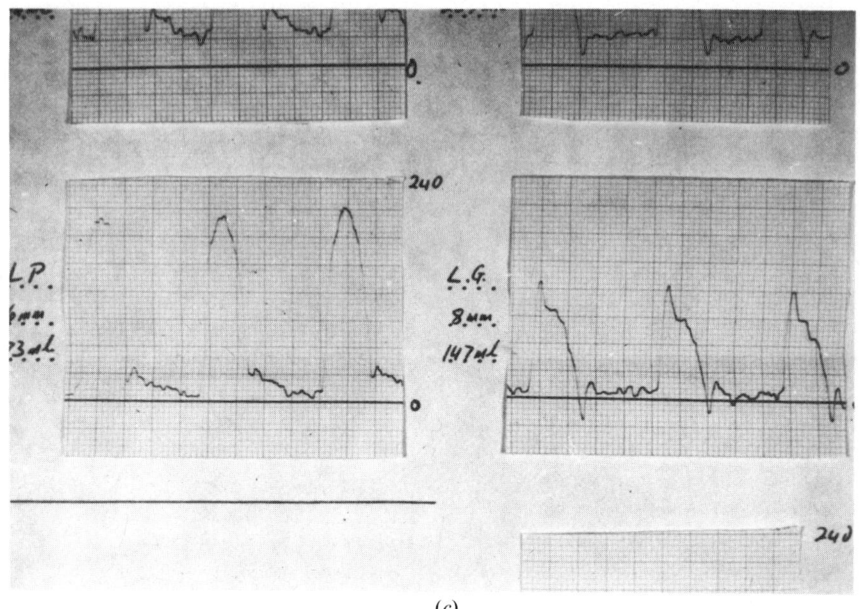

(*c*)

(*cont.*) *Fig. 6.6. c,* Right hand waveform shows distal obstruction, left hand waveform shows mild proximal stenosis.

Pulse Volume Recorder

This segmental air plethysmograph is perhaps the most significant recent development in the field of per- and postoperative assessment of graft patency. It has the singular advantage that the print-out obtained can be easily read by nursing and medical staff both in theatre and when the patient returns to the ward. If the PVR is available peroperatively then the adequacy of distal perfusion can be readily detected. As yet the PVR has been assessed as a research tool but has not become widely available for clinical use.

Doppler Ultrasound

The use of a simple ultrasound pencil probe allows detection of impalpable distal pulses, and in the more recent machines a sonogram can be produced. The probe can be used both in theatre and also for postoperative peripheral pulse assessment.

Our experience is limited to the use of EMF meters and Doppler ultrasound and we rely on these together with a careful choice of procedure, a meticulous surgical technique and clinical assessment of graft patency. The old cliché that the time to do an operation properly is the first time, bears repeating in this context. No matter the sophistication of monitoring methods, the major contribution to patient management is made by the appropriate application of precise surgical skill. Despite a recent suggestion that the time for peak calf blood flow may be delayed for some hours following aorto-iliac reconstruction [25], there is no place for the surgeon who allows the patient with a clearly ischaemic limb to return to the ward on the ill-founded hope that the circulation will somehow improve. Finally, it is good clinical practice to document the peripheral pulse pattern clearly in the case sheet before the patient leaves theatre.

Postoperative Care

The time when the patient is being transferred from the operating theatre back to the recovery area or ward is a potentially dangerous period. The adequacy of post-extubation ventilation must be established and the anaesthetist or respiratory technician should be on hand during this period of transfer. At this time the monitoring of the patient is often inadequate and even an ECG tracing may not be available. The transfer should therefore be effected as quickly as possible. In many centres the initial 24–48 hours postoperative period is spent in an intensive care unit where the detailed intraoperative monitoring can continue. We do not routinely use the intensive care unit in our own hospital for this purpose but the patients are intensively cared for by our own specially trained nursing and medical staff. Naturally, if there is a specific problem with ventilation or in particulary high risk patients we occasionally do make use of the respiratory intensive care facilities.

Postoperative care is intensive for the first 24 hours. Body temperature must be maintained. After a lengthy operation, and particularly with unidirectional flow theatres, hypothermia is almost inevitable. The value of several on-table heating devices in preventing the occurrence of hypothermia is being assessed and at the present time we use a thermostatically controlled water underblanket. Postoperatively conventional bedding is supplemented by the use of the so-called space blanket to restore body temperature to normal as quickly as possible. Hypothermia must be corrected to prevent acidosis, peripheral vasoconstriction and possible cardiac arrhythmia. Occasionally, in addition to the simple measures outlined above, use can be made of the alpha-blocking agent droperidol and also chlorpromazine, both for their vasodilatory properties and also to prevent shivering.

Blood pressure and CVP are monitored and measurements recorded every 15 minutes. Blood gas analysis is performed regularly and oxygen therapy adjusted accordingly. It is particularly important that serum potassium is maintained in the normal range to prevent arrhythmia in this critical phase.

Following recent work on the best means of providing analgesia [26], we have begun to use a continuous morphine infusion to achieve pain relief. Experience has shown that by administering morphine in this way a lower total dose can be given over the initial 24-hour postoperative period, thus minimizing the risk of respiratory depression while maximizing analgesia. Pain relief must be adequate and rigid regimens that provide sporadic pain relief should be abandoned. Excessive pain causes sympathetic stimulation with inevitable hypertension and tachycardia together with peripheral vasoconstriction.

Particular attention is paid to fluid balance. Although operative blood loss will normally be replaced before the patient leaves theatre, an early postoperative haemoglobin value should be obtained and intravenous fluid requirements adjusted according to the CVP and urinary output, which is monitored hourly. Urinary output must be not less than 30 ml per hour, and if this level is not maintained additional intravenous fluids are initially administered, using the CVP as a guide to the level of hydration. In general we deprecate the use of diuretics in the early postoperative phase and would only use them in the face of a rising CVP and continuing lack of adequate diuresis. Additional fluid is usually given in the form of whole blood, reconstituted dried plasma or dextrose/saline solutions. Excessive amounts of albumin should not be administered at this stage.

The peripheral pulse pattern is documented and thereafter the lower limbs inspected regularly. As mentioned previously, a Doppler ultrasound or PVR, if available, provides an objective means of assessment.

On the immediate postoperative day, if all parameters are stable, the urinary catheter, arterial and central venous lines are removed, and the ECG monitoring discontinued. Although there is a theoretical fear of gastric dilatation following aortic surgery, some recent work suggests that the use of a nasogastric tube could be safely discontinued in the elective situation [27], and this has been our practice.

Continuing postoperative care then revolves around early mobilization, regular examination and prevention of complications. Cognizant of the high risk to our patients of thromboembolic disease, like many other surgeons we began to use prophylactic subcutaneous heparin some years ago. However, in a trial situation we encountered an unacceptable level of bleeding and have therefore abandoned its use routinely and reserve it for particularly high risk patients.

Intestinal ileus is still an occasional problem but modification of surgical technique has led to a substantial reduction in the number of cases where ileus is prolonged. We no longer use a plastic intestinal bag for the small intestine during aortic dissection but merely wrap the bowel in moist cotton towels. Loops of bowel are meticulously replaced in an orderly fashion after thorough cleansing of the peritoneal cavity and closure of the posterior peritoneum. However, it is vital that postoperative intestinal obstruction when it does occur should not be assumed to be due to ileus. With such extensive dissection, mechanical obstruction can arise and must be diagnosed and treated swiftly or patients become rapidly catabolic. If this situation does develop, nitrogen balance should be restored by making early use of parenteral nutrition.

As mentioned above, renal failure is now recognized as a major cause of morbidity and mortality and fluid balance is scrutinized in detail to prevent its occurrence. Where acute tubular necrosis does develop, we do not hesitate to make use of renal dialysis where necessary since elective surgery would presumably not have been undertaken in a patient with a poor long term prognosis.

Despite having to sacrifice the inferior mesenteric artery on many occasions, we have rarely found intestinal ischaemia to be a major problem. It should be suspected when bloodstained diarrhoea develops together with pyrexia and leucocytosis, often in the absence of marked abdominal signs apart from some left-sided tenderness. Conservative management with the restriction of oral fluids and antibiotic therapy is usually adequate and a mucosal cast may be passed around the tenth postoperative day. Only in the severely ill patient who fails to respond to a conservative regimen should laparotomy and possible colectomy be considered. Selective mesenteric arteriography may be valuable in establishing this diagnosis and excluding other causes of colonic bleeding.

Other aspects of postoperative care, including the specific management of diabetes mellitus and prevention of infection, are adequately covered in standard texts. Careful nursing has an important role to play in preventing postoperative complications and nursing staff must be supported in the enforcement of a rigid ward discipline both to allow early detection of any potential source of infection and to prevent the occurrence of cross-infection.

Lastly, it is vital that the medical, nursing and paramedical staff all encourage the patients in the early postoperative period. After major surgery all patients are under considerable strain, to which is added the seeming hostility of an intensive care environment. The importance of simple considerate human communication must not be underestimated in the management of the apprehensive postoperative patient.

RUPTURED (EMERGENCY) AORTIC ANEURYSM

The first question to be answered in relation to the treatment of a patient with a ruptured aneurysm is, who should perform surgery? In theory, since this presentation is associated with the worst mortality, the surgery should be performed by the most experienced vascular surgeon in the area. In practice, however, transfer to such a person may either be impossible or not in the patient's best interest. Emergency surgery is therefore performed by the local general surgeon with 'an interest' in vascular surgery. It is worthwhile to note that published data reveal the figure for the operative mortality following surgery for a ruptured aneurysm to be around 50 per cent. Inevitably these reports emanate from hospitals and clinics where vascular surgery is either performed exclusively or as a major interest. It seems likely that the surgeon who is faced with 'the occasional aneurysm' will achieve rather poorer results than the published figures, which are scarcely encouraging in themselves.

If the mortality figures are to be improved (and there has been no substantial change detectable over the past 10 years), more surgeons must be adequately trained to cope with the emergency situation, transfer of the patient must be effected more safely, or—above all—the diagnosis made before rupture occurs.

Much work has been done on the merit of a mobile medical team who are available at short notice to arrange for the transfer of severely ill patients—often with septic shock—to a central intensive care unit [28]. It may be that such a mobile 'shock team' could be employed in the treatment of patients with a leaking abdominal aneurysm. The patient would then arrive for theatre in the best possible condition with accurate base line monitoring data. Others have recommended that the patients should be transferred in a pressurized suit [12].

Whether these methods of transfer are available or not, it is important that the receiving team of surgeons initiates resuscitation prior to transfer. There is seldom need for the hurried despatch of a patient without the establishment of base line monitoring measures. For the team of surgeons that finally has to manage the patient there are two critical questions. First, is the diagnosis of a leaking abdominal aneurysm correct, and secondly, is surgery indicated?

Presentation and Diagnosis

Abdominal aortic aneurysms present as an emergency either when sudden expansion of the aneurysm causes severe abdominal pain or backache or—more dramatically—when the aneurysm actually ruptures.

In a typical presentation the, usually elderly, patient complains of sudden, severe abdominal pain and rapidly develops all the features of shock. A number of such patients die before they ever reach hospital but in many cases the leaking aneurysm seals for some time and there follows a period of relative cardiovascular stability. It is at this stage that most patients reach hospital. Occasionally blood loss is clearly continuing and the level of shock deepening. In such cases immediate surgery is obviously indicated. Fortunately this is relatively unusual and there is more commonly time for a fairly rapid but thorough examination followed by an ordered assessment of the best treatment. The diagnosis is confirmed by the history and clinical examination together with plain abdominal radiography. An expansile swelling is usually palpable, but if the degree of hypotension is marked a pulsatile mass may not be readily felt. A chest X-ray must not be omitted lest thoracic extension of the aneurysmal sac is missed. When blood is drawn for urea and electrolyte measurement blood sugar analysis and serum amylase level should also be ascertained. A full cardiovascular examination must be made and in particular any history of claudication sought. Although aneurysmal disease is commonly localized to the infra-renal abdominal aorta, the finding of associated occlusive distal disease is important with regard to the surgical approach. If the patient is stable and theatre is immediately available, then any patient in whom the diagnosis is in real doubt should have an abdominal ultrasound scan

Somewhat surprisingly the diagnosis continues to be missed all too frequently and it is therefore important that clinicians who see relatively few vascular emergencies remember aortic aneurysm as one cause of an acute abdomen. Furthermore, an abdominal aneurysm may present in several other ways.

In a recent report on the presentation and treatment of 254 aneurysms, 12 were found to have presented in a rather atypical fashion [30]. Of these unusual presentations, most common perhaps is the peripheral arterial embolus. While the great majority of peripheral arterial emboli are due to recent myocardial infarction, valvular heart disease or arrhythmia, a significant number—some suggest up to 10 per cent of all emboli—originate in an aneurysmal sac. The embolic material may be aggregated platelet thrombus or dislodged atheromatous plaque. Whatever the nature of the embolus the lesson for clinicians is clear—beware the embolus with no obvious source. Any examination of the peripheral vascular system must start with a thorough abdominal examination, not with feeling for the femoral pulses.

There are less than 100 documented cases in the literature of an aneurysm presenting as an aorto-caval fistula. Classically, such a patient presents with severe abdominal pain and congestive cardiac failure with progressive renal failure and lower limb ischaemia.

Not surprisingly, the build up of thrombus within an abdominal aneurysm will occasionally cause complete occlusion of the aorta and the patient will present with typical features of aortic obstruction.

We have seen many patients in whom an abdominal aneurysm presented as a pulsatile swelling in the groin with pain along the femoral nerve distribution. This happens when the aneurysm ruptures into the psoas muscle and the haematoma then tracks to the groin.

Lastly, an abdominal aneurysm may rupture into the third part of the duodenum and the patient presents with projectile haematemesis. The bleeding in such patients is so severe that fresh blood may be passed per rectum, and unless one is aware of the presence of the aneurysm, a lower colonic source of bleeding may be wrongly sought.

Preoperative Assessment

A proportion of patients may arrive in hospital profoundly shocked, the diagnosis will be certain and immediate surgery clearly indicated. In such cases no time should be wasted in effecting transfer to theatre and time should not be spent inserting central venous or arterial monitoring lines. The sooner the source of bleeding is controlled the better, even if the surgeon's fist is the only means of doing so. Fortunately, that sort of surgical emergency is the exception.

When the diagnosis has been established, the indications for surgery should be considered. Lest the time spent below discussing the contraindications to surgery become misleading, it should be stated clearly at the outset that almost all patients with a leaking abdominal aneurysm require surgery. Although almost half will not survive, the quality of life in those who do more than justifies the attempt at aortic replacement. Despite an abundance of statistics showing the risk factors associated with this surgery, it is extremely difficult not to operate on all but the most profoundly ill patients.

None the less, emergency aortic surgery is arduous and time-consuming and extremely expensive both in human and financial terms. It is now rare for an infra-renal aneurysm to be technically inoperable and with such major improvements in postoperative life support systems it is tragically possible for a patient to live for many days or even weeks before finally dying with a still patent arterial graft. It is therefore worth while to look objectively at the identifiable risk factors that constitute relative contraindications to surgical intervention:

Age

In itself age is not a contraindication to surgery, but if a patient is over 80 years all other factors must be favourable before surgery is advisable. Some workers have reported a 100 per cent mortality in patients over 80 [16] and in our own centre no patient over 80 years has survived emergency aneurysm surgery in the past 3 years. In that same period there have been no deaths in those under 60, half of those aged 60–70 have died and 66 per cent of the over 70s died following surgery.

Time from Rupture

If the patient has been transferred from another hospital then the preoperative assessment must include obtaining information on the time of rupture, the level of hypotension and the volume of urinary output since the time of rupture. Sustained hypotension has been reported to be associated with a mortality of 75 per cent [16].

Coronary Artery Disease

Many patients will have had a previous myocardial infarction or suffer from angina pectoris. Clearly such patients are at greater risk from major surgery and could have a poorer long term prognosis. They are therefore automatically in the high risk category.

It is technically possible for almost all patients with a ruptured abdominal aneurysm to have the source of bleeding controlled and aortic replacement performed. However, the astute clinician will take all the above risk factors into consideration and it is then a matter of fine surgical judgement to know when surgery is not indicated. It is truly the experienced surgeon who can make the most difficult decision of all—when not to operate.

When the decision to operate is made, basic investigations as for any major surgical procedure should be carried out and the patient transferred with all speed to theatre. Prophylactic antibiotics must not be forgotten. If at all possible the senior surgeon should interview the immediate family and explain the gravity of the situation and the nature of the surgery to be performed.

Intraoperative Considerations

Ideally monitoring should be as for an elective case. In practice, when blood loss is continuing the only measure required is to open the peritoneal cavity and establish control of the source of bleeding as quickly as possible. In this extreme emergency time spent in the insertion of CVP and arterial monitoring lines is time wasted. These things can all be done when control has been achieved. Muscle relaxants should be withheld by the anaesthetist until the surgeon is entirely ready to make the skin incision, for the sudden loss of muscle tone may be sufficient to produce fresh bleeding. If control of haemorrhage is otherwise impossible, a large Foley catheter can be inflated and the balloon impacted proximal to the neck of the aneurysm, thus providing time for a more ordered dissection. It is occasionally necessary to gain haemostasis by approaching the aorta across the lesser sac or by a transdiaphragmatic route [31]. Control is then obtained by clamping the descending aorta.

In the majority of cases bleeding will have stopped prior to surgery and the neck of the aneurysm can be dissected sufficiently to allow proximal control. Dissection must be kept to an absolute minimum. Haematoma is left undisturbed and the initial plane of aortic dissection should be as far away from the apparent source of haemorrhage as possible. In the so-called inflammatory aneurysm the duodenum must not be separated from the aneurysmal wall as any attempt to do so will often lead to opening the small bowel [32].

All the principles of surgery outlined for the elective case apply even more forcefully in the emergency situation and, in particular, the shorter the operation can be made with safety, the better for the patient.

A woven Dacron graft is usually employed to minimize the blood loss by dispensing with the need for pre-clotting and minimizing the ooze through the prosthetic material. Systemic heparinization is impractical but regional heparinization of the distal arterial tree is often possible. The posterior wall of the aneurysm sac is left *in situ*. If the rupture has been posterior, the anterior spinal ligament may constitute the posterior wall of the sac. If there is doubt about the distal run-off or any suggestion of embolization, then balloon catheter thrombectomy [33] should be performed to clear the distal circulation. It is good practice to punch the groins when the iliac clamps have been removed to allow expression of loose fresh clot and restoration of back-bleeding prior to completion of the lower anastomoses. The residual aneurysm sac is used to cover the graft when it is in position, thus preventing direct contact between Dacron and loops of small bowel. If such adherence between small bowel and the prosthesis does occur, then fistula formation is possible [34] with an almost uniformly fatal outcome.

It is clear that if detailed monitoring is necessary for the patient undergoing elective surgery it is all the more critical in the emergency situation. It is especially important that fluid balance is maintained and blood loss adequately replaced. Massive replacement transfusion may be required and if a clotting defect is suspected a full coagulation screen should be undertaken and fresh frozen plasma used to replace depleted coagulation factors as required. Unlike the elective case, we normally send our emergency patients to the intensive care unit to allow a period of assisted ventilation together with continuing intensive monitoring. When respiratory function is adequate without ventilation and the patient is cardiovascularly stable, the patient returns to our own wards where postoperative care does not differ materially from the elective situation, except that the complications discussed earlier are of course more frequent after emergency surgery.

As mentioned earlier, one of the most frustrating aspects of vascular surgery is successfully to replace a leaking abdominal aneurysm after considerable expenditure of effort and time only to be faced with a well-perfused patient who cannot be weaned from the ventilator. There is no easy solution to this problem nor to the question of when assisted ventilation should be withdrawn. Each case must be treated individually, but, having undertaken surgery, every possible effort—including renal dialysis if necessary—must be made to provide the prospect of a full recovery.

REFERENCES

1. Dubost C., Allary M. and Olconomos N. (1952) Resection of an aneurysm of the abdominal aorta. Re-establishment of continuity by preserved human arterial graft with result after five months. *Arch. Surg.* **64**, 405.
2. Volpetti G., Barker C. F., Berkowitz H. et al. (1976) A twenty-two year review of elective resection of abdominal aortic aneurysms. *Surg. Gynecol. Obstet.* **142**, 321.
3. Hicks G. L., Eastland M. W., Deweese J. A. et al. (1975) Survival improvement following aortic aneurysm resection. *Ann. Surg.* **181**, 863.
4. Young A. E., Sandberg G. W. and Couch N. P. (1977) The reduction of mortality of abdominal aortic aneurysm resection. *Am. J. Surg.* **134**, 585.
5. Gordon-Smith I. C., Taylor E. W., Nicolaides A. N. et al. (1978) Management of abdominal aortic aneurysm. *Br. J. Surg.* **651**, 834.
6. Voorhees A. B. jun., Jaretzki A. and Blakemore A. H. (1952) The use of tubes constructed from Vinyon 'N' cloth in bridging arterial defects. A preliminary report. *Ann. Surg.* **351**, 332.
7. Thompson J. E. and Garrett W. V. (1980) Peripheral arterial surgery. *New Engl. J. Med.* **302**, 491.
8. McGregor J. C. (1976) Unoperated ruptured abdominal aortic aneurysms: a retrospective clinicopathological study over a 10-year period. *Br. J. Surg.* **63**, 113.
9. Robisek F. (1981) The diagnosis of abdominal aneurysms. *Surgery* **89**, 275.
10. McGregor J. C., Pollock J. G. and Anton H. C. (1976) The diagnosis and assessment of abdominal aortic aneurysms by ultrasonography. *Ann. Coll. Surg. Engl.* **58**, 388.
11. Pond G. D. and Hillman B. (1981) Evaluation of aneurysms by computed tomography. *Surgery* **89**, 216.
12. Young A. E., Lea Thomas M. and Wright C. H. (1980) Assessment of abdominal aortic aneurysms by computed tomography. *Br. Med. J.* **1**, 765.
13. Gliedman M. L., Ayers W. B. and Vestal B. L. (1957) Aneurysms of the abdominal aorta and its branches: a study of untreated patients. *Ann. Surg.* **146**, 207.
14. Szilagyi D. E., Smith R. F., DeRusso F. J. et al. (1966) Contribution of abdominal aortic aneurysmectomy to prolongation of life. *Ann. Surg.* **164**, 678.
15. O'Donnell T. F. jun., Darling R. C. and Linton R. R. (1976) Is eighty years too old for aneurysmectomy? *Arch. Surg.* **111**, 1250.
16. Gardner R. J., Gardner N. L., Tarnay T. J. et al. (1978) The surgical experience and a one to sixteen-year follow-up of 277 abdominal aortic aneurysms. *Am. J. Surg.* **135**, 226.
17. Thompson J. E., Hollier L. H., Patman R. D. et al. (1975) Surgical management of abdominal aortic aneurysms: factors influencing mortality and morbidity—a 20-year experience. *Ann. Surg.* **181**, 654.
18. McIntosh H. T. and Garcia J. A. (1978) The first decade of aorto-coronary bypass grafting 1967-77: a review. *Circulation* **57**, 405.
19. Hertzer N. R. (1980) Fatal myocardial infarction following abdominal aortic aneurysm resection. Three hundred and forty-three patients followed 6-11 years postoperatively. *Ann. Surg.* **192**, 667.

20. Hertzer N. R., Young J. R., Kramer J. R. et al. (1979) Routine coronary angiography prior to elective aortic reconstruction. Results of selective myocardial revascularisation in patients with peripheral vascular disease. *Arch. Surg.* **141**, 1336.
21. Swan H. J. C., Ganz W., Forrestor J. et al. (1970) Catheterisation of the heart in man with use of a flow directed balloon tipped catheter. *N. Engl. J. Med.* **283**, 447.
22. Barrie W. W., Pollock J. G. and Reid W. (1975) Abdominal aortic surgery and horseshoe kidney. *J. R. Coll. Surg. Edinb.* **20**, 127.
23. Cronestrand R. (1977) Blood flow studies in vascular surgery. In: Hwang N. H. C. and Normann N. A. (ed.) *Cardiovascular Flow Dynamics and Measurements.* Baltimore, University Park Press.
24. Dardik H., Ibrahim I. M., Koslow A. et al. (1978) Evaluation of intraoperative arteriography as a routine for vascular reconstructions. *Surg. Gynecol. Obstet.* **147**, 853.
25. Eklof B., Neglen P. and Thomson D. (1981) Temporary incomplete ischaemia of the legs induced by aortic clamping in man. *Ann. Surg.* **193**, 89.
26. Rutter P. C., Murphy F. and Dudley H. A. F. (1980) Morphine: controlled trial of different methods of administration for postoperative pain relief. *Br. Med. J.* **280**, 12.
27. Gilmour D. G. and Pollock J. G. (1982) Prospective studies on the value of nasogastric aspiration in elective aortic surgery. (in prep.)
28. Ledingham I. (1977) In: *Recent Advances in Intensive Therapy.* Edinburgh, Churchill Livingstone.
29. Lewis D. G., MacKenzie A. and McNeill I. F. (1973) The use of the G suit in the control of bleeding arising from hypocoagulation. *Ann. R. Coll. Surg. Engl.* **52**, 53.
30. Olcott C., Holcroft J. W., Stoney R. J. et al. (1978) Unusual problems of abdominal aortic aneurysms. *Am. J. Surg.* **135**, 426.
31. Buxton B., Reul G. jun. and Cooley D. A. (1978) Transdiaphragmatic approach to the descending thoracic aorta for proximal control during surgery on the abdominal aorta. *Am. J. Surg.* **135**, 726.
32. Bloor K. and Humphreys W. V. (1979) Aneurysms of the abdominal aorta. *Br. J. Hosp. Med.* June, p.568.
33. Fogarty T. J., Cranley J. J., Kranse R. J. et al. (1963) A method for extraction of arterial emboli and thrombi. *Surg. Gynecol. Obstet.* **116**, 241.
34. Cranston D. and Vowles K. D. J. (1980) Aorto-duodenal and subsequent aorto-colonic fistula following operation for ruptured aortic aneurysm. *Br. J. Surg.* **67**, 649.

G. P. Noon and D. Short

7 Reoperation for Recurrent Arterial Occlusive Disease of the Lower Extremity

INTRODUCTION

The direct surgical attack on arterial occlusive disease has become a common reality within the past three decades. Experience has shown that arteriosclerosis, the major cause of arterial obstruction, is frequently segmental in nature and predictable in location. As surgical techniques for dealing with arterial occlusive disease have become standardized, many patients have safely undergone successful arterial reconstructions. However, long term follow-up has revealed a group of patients who require further surgical intervention to relieve persistent or recurrent symptoms of peripheral vascular insufficiency. Reoperation is often technically more difficult than the initial surgery. Furthermore, it may be difficult to discern whether recurrence of symptoms is due to failure of the previous reconstruction to correct the haemodynamic abnormality or progression of the underlying arteriosclerotic process. Lastly, a whole new group of complications peculiar to vascular surgery has arisen, many of which are technically difficult to correct.

This chapter will review the patterns of disease in aorto-iliac and femoropopliteal occlusive disease. Initial evaluation of the patient, leading to the first operation, will be discussed, focusing on factors that may obviate the need for future surgery. Although the arteriosclerotic process is unpredictable in any given patient, candidates must be selected for surgery on the basis of what is known about the natural history of the disease. The specific operation chosen should correct the significant symptom-producing lesions, keeping in mind co-existing arterial disease elsewhere and possible future progression. Finally, candidates for reoperation will be discussed with specific regard both to preoperative evaluation and options for procedures and techniques required for 're-do' surgery.

HISTORY AND PHYSICAL EXAMINATION

Aorto-iliac

Rene Leriche, in 1923 and again in 1940 [1, 2], described a syndrome of upper thigh weariness, impotence, pale lower extremities, atrophy of the leg muscles and absence of trophic changes associated with obstruction of the lower abdominal aorta and iliac arteries. The obstruction may extend from below the renal arteries to the common femoral arteries but usually is localized around the aortic bifurcation. In later stages, this condition may also produce calf claudication, rest pain and gangrenous changes in the distal extremity.

Physical examination will reveal weak or absent femoral pulses, muscle atrophy with poor capillary filling and frequently an abdominal bruit. Later on, loss of hair, trophic nail changes and skin changes of impending or frank gangrene may appear.

Femoropopliteal

Isolated segmental obstruction of the superficial femoral artery almost always occurs at the adductor canal. Since there are few branches of the superficial artery, this thrombosis usually propagates back to the orifice of the profunda femoris artery. Occasionally, sufficient collaterals exist to keep all but a narrow segment of the superficial femoral artery patent. Clinically this situation presents as intermittent calf claudication.

Physical examination with isolated superficial femoral artery obstruction reveals strong femoral pulses with absent, or sometimes weak, popliteal and pedal pulses.

As will be stressed later, the profunda femoris artery is a very important source of collateral circulation when superficial femoral artery obstruction occurs. [3]. Also, the distal popliteal artery and its branches are often spared by the arteriosclerotic process [4].

The occurrence of trophic and gangrenous changes late in the course of aorto-iliac or femoropopliteal disease is the result of progressive arteriosclerosis in important collaterals or in proximal or distal circulation. These changes should always alert the examiner to a multilevel, obstructive process [5].

Peripheral Vascular Laboratory

The peripheral vascular laboratory has been helpful in the evaluation of patients with suspected peripheral arterial disease. It allows one to make objective measurements to confirm clinical findings. These measurements are reproducible and serial studies can document subtle deterioration of arterial flow. In cases with multilevel disease, it is now possible to demonstrate which is haemodynamically the most significant obstruction. This problem may be poorly resolved by physical examination or arteriography.

Both pulse volume recordings [6, 7] (plethysmography) and Doppler perfusion indices [8, 9] may be used to quantitate segmental perfusion. The use of the Doppler probe has become more popular, however, becuase of the convenience of this small instrument, and because ischaemic symptoms induced by exercise correlate better with ankle pressure than with plethysmographic measurements of flow [10].

In normal individuals, the blood pressure is higher in the ankle than in the arm. Because of the variation in the blood pressure between individuals, or different measurements in the same individual, the ratio of ankle pressure to arm pressure (ankle pressure index) is more useful than the absolute pressure in the ankle. This index is greater than 1·0 in normal individuals and values less than 1·0 indicate obstruction to flow. Values in the 0·8–1·0 range indicate obstruction while those of 0·5–0·8 indicate complete occlusion. Claudication usually occurs in the 0·5–0·6 range while rest pain occurs below 0·3, implying severe multilevel occlusion [9, 10]. Particularly in patients with sclerotic vessels that cannot readily be compressed, the figures above may not be accurate. None the less, for most patients they do represent a useful guide to the severity of ischaemia.

Evidence of diminished thigh pressures implies obstruction in the aorto-iliac segments. Normal thigh pressures with diminished calf pressures is evidence of obstruction in the femoropopliteal segments. Decreased thigh pressures with further disease in the calf is evidence of multilevel obstruction and is frequently associated with very low ankle pressures indices.

Arteriography

Since its introduction by dos Santos [11] in 1929, abdominal aortography has become a relatively safe, standard technique which is used routinely in the evaluation of patients with peripheral vascular occlusive disease. Although a vast experience was accumulated in our institution using translumbar aortography, with a low incidence of complication [12, 13], most arteriography is now accomplished using the Seldinger technique [14].

Specific attention should be directed to several anatomical areas of interest. The aorta just below the renal arteries as well as the renal arteries themselves should be clearly delineated. This is important not only in planning the proximal extent of reconstruction but also to identify any renal artery obstruction that might require simultaneous correction for renal salvage or control of hypertension.

Many reports stress the difficulty of assessing aorto-iliac disease by single plane aortography. Oblique films may be used to demonstrate obstructing posterior plaques in aorto-iliac segments which appear relatively normal on anteroposterior films [15, 16]. Arteriographic findings, physical examination, non-invasive laboratory studies and operative examination are all used to determine the extent of involvement.

The orifice of the profunda femoris artery should be clearly seen on arteriography. The incidence of failure to appreciate significant stenosis of the profunda femoris artery on anteroposterior films has been reported to be as high as 50 per cent [15]. This has led some investigators to recommend routine biplane views of the common femoral bifurcation. If the take-off of the profunda femoris cannot be seen clearly, oblique views should always be taken to display the anatomy of this important collateral vessel, especially if it is felt to play a significant role in the patient's problem.

Finally, satisfactory views of the superficial femoral, popliteal artery and distal branches should be available. These are helpful not only in planning distal bypasses but will show the presence of severe, non-bypassable distal disease which may only be helped by lumbar sympathectomy.

Combined Non-invasive Studies with Arteriography

Clearly the results of non-invasive studies can be used to complement arteriography in determining the significance of visible stenoses at different levels. Studies of haemodynamics show that if several levels of obstruction exist, little improvement in the flow will result from correcting the least significant obstruction [17]. Furthermore, in some cases, non-invasive evidence of severe obstruction in areas that look relatively normal on arteriography may alert the surgeon to lesions which may jeopardize the results of surgery, either by failure to relieve symptoms initially or by early graft occlusion.

INDICATIONS FOR SURGERY

The natural history of arteriosclerosis in the lower extremities has been documented in numerous studies [18–21]. Claudication alone in the majority of cases is compatible with prolonged survival, free from fear of limb loss. Factors that increase the risk of amputation include severe claudication (more than one block), smoking, distal arterial involvement and diabetes mellitus (perhaps because of increased distal disease). By contrast, patients with rest pain and impending or actual tissue loss have a high amputation rate. Because arteriosclerosis is a generalized process, these patients may have severe disease in other arteries. When followed long term, they most commonly die of stroke or myocardial infarction and inevitably carry an increased surgical risk [19, 21].

Patients who cannot work or whose lifestyles are unacceptably altered by progressive or disabling claudication are potential candidates for arterial reconstruction. Patients with mild, stable claudication who are minimally inconvenienced are instructed to exercise regularly to improve collateral circulation and are not operated upon. Most patients in this group will remain stable, although in some the symptoms may actually improve [21]. It is unjustifiable to risk loss of limb or life in such patients whose disease process is so relatively benign.

Patients with ischaemic pain, ischaemic skin changes or gangrene are all considered candidates for surgery if their general condition permits. Although some may seem poor operative risks, many will otherwise come to amputation, an operation with as high a mortality rate as definitive arterial reconstruction.

PREOPERATIVE PREPARATION

Efforts to prevent graft infection must begin in the preoperative period. The greatest threat of graft contamination comes from the patient's own skin flora, especially the staphylococcus. Showers with povidone-iodine soap are given the night before and the morning of surgery, concentrating on cleansing the areas in the operative field. We prefer to use a depilatory preparation to remove hair, but if shaving is employed, it should be done as close to the time of surgery as possible.

Finally, antibiotics with anti-staphylococcal activity should be given prophylactically. Presently we prefer a cephalosporin because of cidal activity, relative safety and low incidence of allergy. It is given before the start of surgery to establish an adequate blood and tissue level at the time of surgery. If the procedure is prolonged, doses should be administered intraoperatively to maintain a bactericidal blood level during the procedure. Patients are kept on antibotics for 48–72 hours postoperatively.

SURGERY

Aorto-iliac Disease

Although the occasional patient with very localized disease might be a candidate for endarterectomy, our procedure of choice for aorto-iliac occlusive disease is bypass surgery. This operation generally has the highest reported patency rates, is the easiest for most surgeons to perform and is more versatile than endarterectomy [22–26]. It is particularly relevant to note that, should late graft failure occur, the graft may often be cleared by operating on the groin whereas failure following endarterectomy will require abdominal exploration.

Several important technical factors should be stressed if the need for future reoperation is to be avoided. The proximal anastomosis should be near the renal arteries. This area of the aorta is relatively spared from the arteriosclerotic process, making the anastomosis easier. Even when the lower abdominal aorta is relatively uninvolved, one should avoid the temptation to do a low aortic anastomosis. Progression of arteriosclerosis in the aorta can encroach upon the proximal anastomosis, resulting in total graft occlusion. Our preference is for an end-to-side anastomosis except under certain circumstances. Aneurysmal disease of the aorta is an absolute indication for end-to-end anastomosis. Also, with total occlusion of the aorta up to the renal arteries it is easier to endarterectomize this segment and anastomose it to a graft if the aorta is first transected. Although some groups claim higher patency rates with end-to-end anastomosis, we feel that construction of the anastomosis high into an unobstructed segment of aorta is more important in determining patency than whether it is constructed end to side or end to end. Furthermore, as a general concept, it is better to employ a reconstruction which does not disrupt the native circulation. Should graft occlusion occur or graft sepsis necessitate graft removal, the native circulation may still maintain viability of the distal extremities.

The level of the distal anastomosis is dictated by the pattern of disease. Obstruction restricted to the aorta and common iliac arteries may be bypassed at the external iliac arteries. Critics of aorto-iliac bypass point to possible progression of disease in the external iliac and common femoral arteries causing graft failure. However, as proponents of endarterectomy point out, disease restricted to the aorta and common iliac arteries generally occurs in a younger group of patients who may live 10–15 years without distal progression of disease [27]. Long term follow-up studies from our institution show equal patency rates of aorto-iliac and aortofemoral grafts at 15 years in properly selected patients [26]. Bypass to the iliac arteries avoids incisions in the groin, with the attendant risks of seroma, lymphocoele, false aneurysm and infection. A comparison of reported patency rates following aorto-iliac and aortofemoral bypass and endarterectomy is listed in *Table* 7.1.

In the presence of demonstrable arteriosclerosis of the external iliac or common femoral arteries, either on arteriogram or by palpation at laparotomy, the limbs of the graft are anastomosed in the groins. The distal arteriotomy is begun on the common femoral artery and in all circumstances should afford a view of the profunda femoris orifice. If the superficial femoral artery is patent, the anastomosis extends down on to the proximal superficial femoral artery. If the profunda orifice is stenotic, consideration should be given to endarterectomy or profundaplasty because this will be the only outflow vessel, should superficial femoral artery occlusion occur in the future.

Table 7.1. A comparison of reported percentage patency rates of aorto-iliac bypass, aortofemoral bypass and endarterectomy

Author	*Procedure*	*1 yr*	*5 yr*	*10 yr*
	Endarterectomy [28]	93	74	
Barker	Endarterectomy (limbs) [29]		89	69
	Endarterectomy [30]	71	55	
	BPG	85	71	
Linton/Darling	AI endarterectomy (limbs) [31]	99	95	
	AF endarterectomy	98	88	
	AI BPG	97	96	
	AF BPG	88	74	
	Endarterectomy (limbs) [32]	95	74	
	BPG	91	68	
Szilagyi	Endarterectomy [33]	91	92	
	BPG	100	82	
Butcher	Endarterectomy [34]	89	72	
	Endarterectomy [33]		82	60
	AF BPG		91	71
Kouchoukos/Butcher	AI endarterectomy [35]	96	68	
	AI BPG	70	70	
	AF endarterectomy	72	50	
	AF BPG [36*]	58	52	
	AI endarterectomy			91
	AF endarterectomy			71
	Endarterectomy [37]	98	90	67
	BPG	92	77	41
	Endarterectomy [38]	88	63	
	BPG	65		
	Endarterectomy [39]	100	96	
	AI BPG [40]		90	83
	AF BPG		83	71
	AF BPG [41]	95	79	65
	AF BPG [42]		80	
	AF BPG [43]		82	66
Darling	AF BPG [24]		88	75

AI, Aorto-iliac; AF, aortofemoral; BPG, bypass graft.
* *See* discussion section of this paper.

If the superficial femoral artery is occluded, the anastomosis is carried down the proximal profunda femoris artery, acting as a patch graft angioplasty. Endarterectomy or extended profundaplasty may be required in the presence of severe disease. Even if no significant occlusion exists, extension of the anastomosis on to the profunda might prevent future graft occlusion should progressive arteriosclerosis occur at the orifice. Careful attention should be given to the length of the graft limbs. If cut too short, the tension on the distal sutures may tear the native vessel, contributing to false aneurysm formation. Failure to appreciate how crimped grafts lengthen when distended by blood may lead to cutting the limb too long. This may result in kinking and ultimate occlusion of the limb.

Although one-third of patients with aorto-iliac occlusive disease have distal disease, the proximal disease is corrected first. Most patients will have some relief of symptoms by proximal reconstruction even in the presence of superficial femoral occlusion. Long term patency rates for aortic grafts are higher than those for femoropopliteal bypass, especially with diminished femoral inflow. We rarely combine aorto-iliac reconstruction with femoropopliteal bypass except in situations where the threat of gangrene is so grave that we feel it unwise to await the improvement of aorto-iliac reconstruction alone. We recognize that other workers would proceed to distal bypass more frequently.

For arteriosclerotic occlusive disease of the aorto-iliac segments the use of unilateral grafts is rare. Experience has shown that even if only one side appears significantly obstructed, symmetrical, contralateral obstruction almost invariably develops.

Femoropopliteal Disease

Occlusion of the superficial femoral artery is the most common manifestation of peripheral vascular disease. With isolated occlusion of the vessel, patients may be minimally symptomatic. When combined with proximal or distal disease, however, this condition may produce severe symptoms or cause loss of the limb. Surgery is recommended for claudication only when it is severely debilitating and the anatomical situation promises a high probability of success. Patients threatened with limb loss are approached much more aggressively.

It should be stressed that patients being considered for bypass to the popliteal artery or its distal branches must all be evaluated for aorto-iliac disease. If evidence exists on physical examination, arteriography or non-invasive studies of inadequate femoral inflow, aortofemoral reconstruction is performed first. This may require local or extended profundaplasty to ensure adequate flow to the profunda femoris artery. This procedure alone may relieve all of the symptoms of ischaemic pain or claudication in the lower extremity.

Bypass surgery is almost universally employed for femoropopliteal occlusive disease. Proximally, the bypass is constructed from the common femoral artery. It may also be anastomosed to a limb of a previous aortofemoral graft or to a short endarterectomized proximal segment of superficial femoral artery. Sometimes, if the available vein graft is short, it might be necessary to anastomose proximally to the superficial femoral artery further down. This is not ideal because subsequent occlusion of the superficial femoral artery from progression of disease will cause graft occlusion. This risk must be balanced against the desire to use available autogenous vein, generally accepted to be the best graft.

The site for the distal anastomosis is dictated by the anatomical abnormality as demonstrated by arteriography. Patency rates for grafts anastomosed above the knee joint are generally reported to be higher than for those anastomosed below the knee, regardless of the type of graft used. However, this segment of the popliteal artery is often more involved by the arteriosclerotic process. The distal anastomosis is generally placed above the knee if the distal popliteal artery and its branches are satisfactory.

Intraoperative arteriography should be employed routinely to identify technical mishaps which may lead to early graft occlusion [28]. Kinking or twisting of the graft, stenosis of the anastomosis, dissection or embolization of clot or debris into the distal circulation may all produce graft failure and are best corrected at the time of original procedure.

Although there is general agreement that autogenous saphenous vein of good quality is the optimal graft to the popliteal artery and its branches, there is considerable disagreement as to the best substitute when such a vein is unavailable, as is discussed in detail elsewhere in this book.

For patients requiring bypass to the popliteal artery above the knee, we routinely use a prosthetic graft. In our experience, 10- and 15-year patency of Dacron grafts is equal to vein used above the knee. Presently we are evaluating the use of polytetrafluoroethylene (PTFE) grafts above the knee. Early reports [45, 46] of 1-year patency compare favourably with our 1-year 90 per cent patency using Dacron velour. In addition, this graft requires no pre-clotting and may be used in a heparinized patient.

For bypass below the knee, autogenous vein is preferable to a prosthesis. If saphenous vein is unavailable, arm veins of adequate quality may be used [47, 48]. If these are unavailable, homograft vein, modified umbilical vein [48, 49] or PTFE may be used. There is a considerable discrepancy in the literature regarding long term patency with these materials.

Long bypass to the proximal or distal calf vessels may be required for limb salvage. These procedures are often tedious, with patency rates generally lower than for any other common vascular reconstruction [50, 51]. Limb salvage rates are higher than patency rates because temporary patency might allow some wounds to heal or collaterals to develop by the time of graft occluson, averting progressive rest pain, gangrene and amputation. There appears to be no greater morbidity or mortality associated with this procedure than with primary amputation alone [52–54], although early graft failure may result in a higher level of amputation [55].

Systemic anticoagulation with heparin is employed intraoperatively. This is especially important in patients with poor run-off. If thrombosis occurs in small or segmentally occluded distal vessels while proximal flow is temporarily occluded, it may be impossible to re-establish the distal flow. Obviously, if porous grafts are used, they must be preclotted.

Use of heparin does not obviate the need for flushing of the graft. Small particles of dislodged clot or debris can still be embolized into the distal circulation and flushing should be employed in a thorough and systematic fashion before all suture lines are completed.

Lumbar Sympathectomy

Although some studies show that lumbar sympathectomy increases flow acutely in arterial reconstructions of the lower extremities [56–58], we do not routinely use it as an adjunct to aorto-iliac or femoral popliteal surgery. Studies show that the increased flow is mainly to skin and not muscle [57]. We reserve sympathectomy for cases with skin changes, vasospasm or severe distal disease. When no arterial reconstruction is possible, it may offer the only hope of limb salvage as an isolated procedure in patients with diffuse disease.

Profundaplasty

The significance of the profunda femoris artery in patients with superficial femoral artery occlusion has been stressed by many [3, 59, 60]. Efforts at limb salvage by isolated profunda reconstruction have resulted in reported success rates of from 45 to 95 per cent [60–65]. Several reports stress the importance of good inflow, rich profunda collaterals and an open popliteal artery segment in predicting success for profundaplasty [61, 64, 65]. These same anatomical findings also offer the greatest promise of success for femoropopliteal or femorotibial bypass. Bypass operations generally offer greater initial success rates than profundaplasty with comparable morbidity and mortality rates. Long term, however, profundaplasty may offer an equal or better success rate than bypass operations, especially when these are carried below the knee. It is important to remember that failure of a femoropopliteal graft may leave the patient's limb more ischaemic than before the reconstruction. Failure of profundaplasty seldom worsens the condition and femoropopliteal bypass is still possible, with no alteration in the chance for success. The decision to use femoropopliteal bypass or profundaplasty hinges upon the question of whether it is better to choose initially higher success rates with lower long term potential or to accept lower initial success rates with better long term results. For patients with severe profunda disease we generally recommend attempting profundaplasty first. With localized or minimal profunda disease, femoropopliteal bypass is attempted first.

Extra-anatomical Bypass

Although some authors recommend the use of extra-anatomical bypass, such as axillofemoral and femorofemoral bypass, as an elective procedure for aorto-iliac occlusive disease, long term patency rates [66–68] are generally not as good as those for anatomical reconstruction [69, 70]. The major advantages of extra-anatomical bypass are that it may be performed with local anaesthesia and avoid the operative and postoperative morbidity of an abdominal operation. We reserve the use of extra-anatomical bypass for very ill patients who cannot tolerate a general anaesthetic, or to maintain perfusion of lower extremities after removal of an infected aortic prosthesis.

REOPERATION

The events leading to reoperation after previous vascular surgery of the aorto-iliac or femoropopliteal segments fall into two basic categories: (*a*) progression of arteriosclerosis in native arterial segments, proximal or distal to the reconstruction and (*b*) complications of the previous surgical procedure. Such complications may occur early (within 30 days) or late. Early complications are most commonly haemorrhage (e.g. suture line leak), graft occlusion (usually the result of technical error) or infection. Late complications include graft occlusion, false aneurysm or infection.

The events leading to the need for reoperation are well described in the literature and are to some extent predictable and dependent upon the original procedure and the extent of the disease [71–75]. The preoperative evaluation and surgical treatment for re-do surgery varies somewhat with that described for original procedures.

Signs and Symptoms

The most common symptoms that occur after failure of a previous reconstruction are related to limb ischaemia. If vascular procedures are performed without disruption of the native circulation, failure may not worsen the original situation. However, sudden occlusion of a reconstruction may precipitate symptoms far more severe than those present before the original procedure. This may be because previously developed collaterals have ceased to function or were physically disrupted at the time of surgery. In the former circumstance symptoms may lessen with the passage of time, in the latter, emergency surgery may be necessary to salvage the limb.

Physical examination may give a clue as to the cause of recurrent ischaemic symptoms. Stenosis or occlusion of a previously reconstructed segment will produce diminution or loss of pulses, distal to the reconstruction. Recurrent ischaemia in the presence of full pulses at the site of reconstruction suggests distal disease.

False aneurysms are expanding haematomas which produce symptoms by compression of surrounding structures or by rupture. They are most common in the groin and may be recognized by the patient as a painful, pulsatile mass. When associated with an aortic anastomosis, they may produce symptoms by compression of adjacent viscera or by erosion into the bowel, producing gastrointestinal bleeding. While large false aneurysms in the groin should be easy to diagnose on physical examination, sometimes large graft limbs may be confused for true or false aneurysms. The expanding nature of aneurysms provides the best clue in distinguishing them from normal graft configurations.

Graft infection is the most dreaded of all complications. The symptoms produced are related to sepsis, graft thrombosis with distal ischaemia or rupture with haemorrhage. It may present as a localized suppurative process, or as total graft involvement. Patients may complain either of intermittently draining groin wounds and feel otherwise perfectly well or they may present with low grade, intermittent fevers or high spiking temperatures with septicaemia. Bleeding into the retroperitoneum, into the gastrointestinal tract or externally from a groin wound may occur. Because the clinical manifestations are often subtle, a high index of suspicion for this condition in patients with previous graft implantation should be maintained.

Peripheral Vascular Laboratory

The vascular laboratory perhaps finds its most useful role in evaluating patients with peripheral vascular occlusive disease following reconstructive surgery.

By using non-invasive techniques, patients can be assessed in the early postoperative period and serially thereafter. The results obtained are objective and reproducible, so deterioration of function after vascular reconstruction may be accurately detected both early and late.

Reconstruction of aorto-iliac segmental occlusion should result in normal or near normal segmental thigh pressures and, in the presence of minimal distal disease, normal ankle pressure indices. These correspond clinically to strong femoral and pedal pulses. In the presence of superficial femoral artery occlusion, pedal pulses usually do not return, but ankle pressures should increase in the presence of sufficient collaterals. If persistently low ankle pressure indices occur, then further reconstruction for relief of distal ischaemia may be needed. Followed serially, patients who exhibit good segmental thigh pressure with deteriorating ankle pressures should be suspected of having progression of distal disease. If symptoms of ischaemia return in these patients and objective evidence exists of adequate femoral inflow, attention should be turned to improvement of collateral flow (i.e. sympathectomy or profundaplasty) or consideration given to femoropopliteal or distal bypass. In patients with a previous femoropopliteal bypass, diminishing ankle pressures with normal thigh pressures may warn of impending graft occlusion. Likewise, diminishing thigh pressures in a patient with a previous aorto-iliac reconstruction may be a harbinger of failure of that procedure. Timely intervention in these two circumstances may avoid total graft thrombosis.

Arteriography

As with initial vascular reconstruction, arteriography plays an important role in the preoperative evaluation of patients for re-do surgery. If occlusion is suspected, the infra-renal abdominal aorta, aorto-iliac segments and femoropopliteal segments may all need scrutiny to resolve the cause of failure and to plan the operative approach. False aneurysms and graft deterioration are best demonstrated arteriographically. Unsuspected areas of involvement may be detected which alter the plan of surgical treatment.

Several aspects deserve special mention in 're-do' situations. The arteriograms taken prior to the initial procedure should be studied before repeating them. To search for distal run-off where none existed previously is fruitless. An exception to this would be in circumstances where inflow was so poor that adequate views of distal run-off were never taken. Sometimes, when acute graft occlusion has occurred, it is not possible (because of thrombus and altered collateral flow) to get arteriograms that demonstrate the anatomy well enough to draw conclusions about the cause of graft failure or feasibility of reconstruction. Under these circumstances, it is better to proceed directly to surgery and thrombectomize the occluded segment. Intraoperative arteriography at this time may then demonstrate the cause of graft failure and dictate the proper solution.

EARLY GRAFT OCCLUSION

Aorto-iliac

Early graft occlusion (within 30 days) is usually the result of a technical mishap and should be corrected as soon as possible. The technical difficulties associated with 're-do' vascular surgery are minimal at this early stage. The errors which commonly contribute to graft occlusion are: (*a*) obstruction due to twisting, kinking or stenosis of the graft; (*b*) failure to appreciate the degree of distal run-off obstruction; (*c*) intimal dissection. These problems may be demonstrable on arteriography, but often are not because no contrast material flows through the area of interest. Patients undergoing re-exploration for graft occlusion should have the abdomen, both groins and both legs prepared for surgery, because successful revision may require surgery in any or all of these areas.

Proximal graft obstruction will produce poor inflow and may result in total graft occlusion. This may be due to stenosis of the suture line or kinking of the graft. Abdominal re-exploration is necessary in this circumstance and the graft may be revised or replaced. If adequate thrombectomy of the limbs produces brisk back-bleeding, the new graft may be sutured to the limbs of the old graft.

Occlusion of one graft limb may be due to twisting or kinking. This will also require abdominal exploration to reposition or replace the limb of the graft. The entire graft should be inspected to ensure that kinking does not jeopardize flow in the other limb, leading to later contralateral occlusion.

In the absence of demonstrable proximal abnormalities, the distal anastomosis is generally explored first. Stenosis or dissection at the suture line should be corrected and thrombectomy of the graft limb accomplished from below with a Fogarty catheter. Compression of the contralateral femoral artery and graft limb should always be done when thrombectomizing one limb of a bifurcated graft. This produces a stagnant column of blood which decreases the possibility of contralateral embolization. If no obvious abnormality exists distally, thrombectomy and retrograde intraoperative arteriography may demonstrate proximal abnormalities, not evident on preoperative arteriograms.

Finally, if no evidence of poor inflow exists, the status of outflow vessels must be questioned. With superficial femoral artery obstruction, a patent profunda femoris is generally adequate to maintain patency of an aortofemoral graft. If the orifice of the profunda is stenotic or if it is diffusely diseased, outflow obstruction may occur causing limb occlusion. This may be revised by profundaplasty or extension of the femoral anastomosis down the profunda femoris artery, serving as a patch angioplasty.

If profunda reconstruction is not possible and distal collaterals are inadequate to handle flow from the aortofemoral graft, bypass from the femoral artery or limb of the graft to an open popliteal or tibial artery may be necessary to maintain patency of the aortic graft.

Although it has been demonstrated that lumbar sympathectomy will increase flow through aortofemoral grafts, we have not added it routinely to maintain early graft patency following a primary or re-do vascular procedure.

LATE GRAFT OCCLUSION

Aorto-iliac

Late graft occlusion may occur as a result of technical error, but most commonly is due to progression of the arteriosclerotic process proximal or distal to the graft. If due to technical error, it is corrected in a similar fashion to early graft occlusion, although correction is often more difficult due to difficulties with exposure and control of vessels scarred from the previous surgery.

Late total graft occlusion may occur as a result of proximal stenosis or kinking of the graft. This will require revision or replacement of the proximal segment of the graft. If the previous aortotomy is widely patent, it may be re-used. Another cause of late proximal graft occlusion is progression of arteriosclerosis, proximal to the aortic anastomosis. Grafts inserted far below the renal arteries are subject to this type of occlusion. This requires removal of the old graft and re-anastomosis just below the renal arteries, usually end to end. Exposure of the infra-renal aorta to gain proximal control may be difficult until the old graft has been detached. In this situation proximal aortic control may be gained at the diaphragm by external compression or clamping the aorta above the renal arteries. Exposure for clamping is achieved by dividing the gastrohepatic omentum at the oesophago-gastric junction and retracting the oesophagus to the left. The aorta will be found directly behind the oesophagus, lying on the spine. Once the infra-renal aorta is adequately exposed, proximal control may be gained by clamping below the renal arteries, minimizing the period of renal ischaemia. An alternative method of proximal control is to insert a large balloon catheter into the supra-renal aorta from below, using manual compression to the aorta, at the diaphragm, until the balloon is sufficiently inflated to provide intraluminal occlusion. This method is especially useful when the aortic lumen is inadvertently entered while sharply dissecting around the old graft. (Either way, one should be prepared to control quickly the brisk bleeding that ensues when the aorta is opened (*Fig. 7.1*).) When exposing the old graft and aorta, meticulous care should be given to atraumatic dissection of the duodenum, to prevent later aorto-enteric fistula.

Late limb occlusion of aortic bifurcation grafts is usually due to progression of distal disease. Aorto-iliac grafts may occlude as disease progresses in the external iliac and common femoral arteries. This requires replacement of the entire graft, with anastomoses distally in the groin. Occlusion of aortofemoral grafts may be due to progressive occlusion of the superficial femoral artery, profunda femoris or more distal collateral vessels. When exploring old graft limbs or tunnelling new limbs in the retroperitoneum, care should be taken to avoid damage to the ureters. If this cannot be done with confidence, a somewhat circuitous route for the new limb is preferable to risking damage to the ureter.

Although it is generally recognized that distal disease produces late occlusion of the graft limb, some controversy exists as to the best means to revise the graft limb. Crawford [7] reported a personal series, over 20

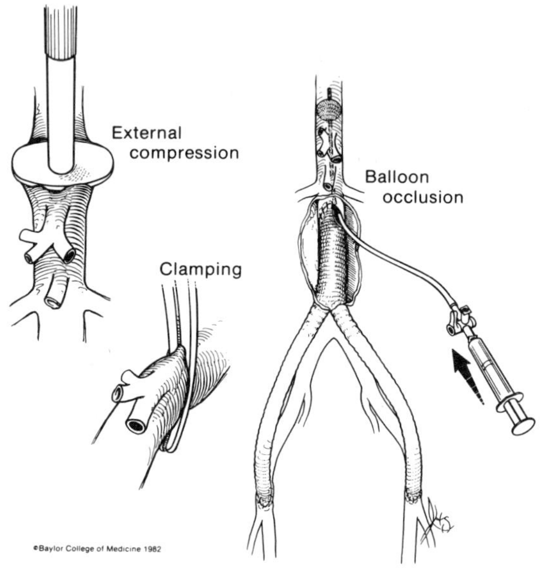

Fig. 7.1. Alternative methods for gaining proximal control of the aorta.

years, of 101 re-do operations. Of 17 patients who had a single limb operation for single limb occlusion (i.e. thrombectomy of single limb replacement), 14 had either recurrent thrombosis of that limb or occlusion of the opposite limb. This led Crawford to recommend total graft replacement for single limb occlusion.

Other authors, however [75–77], report high success rates with thrombectomy from below, combined with procedures to improve run-off, and this is our preferred approach. Mortality rates are lowest when the surgical procedure is confined to the leg. Careful attention to compression of the opposite femoral pulse will prevent contralateral embolization at the time of thrombectomy (*Fig. 7.2.*) Once the limb has been thrombectomized and brisk inflow is ensured, distal reconstruction is undertaken. Exposure of the femoral anastomosis is best accomplished with a scalpel. The graft is usually palpable even when occluded. The dense scar may be incised sharply down to the graft. No bleeding will occur even if the thrombosed graft is inadvertently lacerated. Once thrombectomized, bleeding from the native circulation is easily controlled with balloon catheters. This avoids unnecessary dissection of the native circulation and possible irreparable damage.

If profunda stenosis is the cause of distal obstruction, profundaplasty using a patch of autogenous saphenous vein or a section of

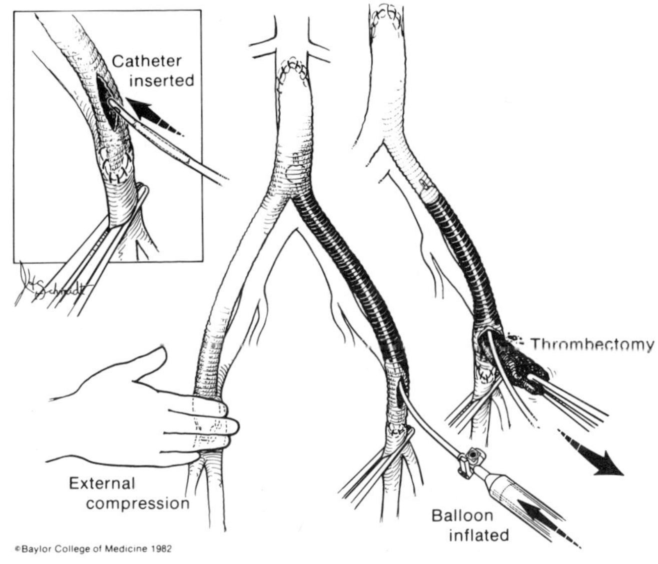

Fig. 7.2. Left limb thrombectomy with prevention of right limb embolism.

endarterectomized superficial femoral artery should be performed [77]. This may need to be quite extensive, past the third or fourth branches, but usually an open, relatively clear vessel will then be reached. If no stenosis is present or if arteriosclerotic involvement of the profunda is diffuse throughout its entire length, bypass to an open popliteal or tibial vessel may be necessary.

Failure of Femoral and/or Popliteal Reconstruction

Failure of these reconstructions falls into two categories: (*a*) failure to remain patent and (*b*) failure to relieve the symptoms for which the operation was undertaken. These reconstructions are often undertaken for limb salvage. Reoperation with further distal reconstruction is sometimes necessary even when technical success has been achieved with the first operation. The urgency for reoperation depends upon the symptoms and the threat to limb viability.

EARLY FAILURE

Failure of profundaplasty to relieve symptoms is rarely the result of thrombosis unless a technical error has occurred, in which case prompt re-exploration to correct the error is indicated. More often, if profundaplasty fails to relieve symptoms and produce an objective improvement in the distal circulation it is due to poor patient selection—no proximal obstruction of significance existed or profunda collaterals were inadequate to increase distal flow. In these cases distal reconstruction or bypass grafting should be employed early to prevent limb loss. As in primary operations, grafting is from the common femoral artery to a satisfactory distal vessel (popliteal or tibial), employing autogenous vein whenever possible below the knee.

Early failure to relieve symptoms in femoropopliteal or femorotibial grafts is usually due to graft occlusion. This may be due to a technical error such as kinking or twisting of the graft or stenosis or dissection at an anastomosis. Arteriography frequently will not demonstrate the technical error until the graft has been disobliterated at the time of re-exploration. If no technical error is demonstrated and inflow is adequate, failure of femoropopliteal and femoro-tibial grafts is usually due to inadequate run-off. Sympathectomy has been shown to increase flow in these grafts [56] and may be added to try to improve outflow in the graft by reducing peripheral resistance. It has the added advantage of improving cutaneous flow and may help sustain the limb even if graft occlusion recurs.

Finally, profundaplasty remains an option to improve collateral flow, if patency of the bypass graft cannot be maintained. This added blood supply may salvage an otherwise doomed extremity.

Late Failure of Femoropopliteal Reconstruction

Late failure may be due to progression of disease proximally or distally. Progressive disease in the aorto-iliac system may result in return of symptoms, even with a patent profundaplasty or femoropopliteal graft, and efforts to disobliterate distal bypass grafts without some procedure to improve inflow are invariably futile.

If progression of disease distally results in recurrent symptoms after profundaplasty, it may be possible to employ a bypass to the popliteal or distal tibial vessels to salvage the extremity. Progression of the disease to a bypass graft will often result in late thrombosis. If bypass more distally is feasible it may be tried. If no suitable vessel is identified distally on arteriography or exploration, profundaplasty may be tried to supply collateral flow in limb salvage attempts.

Finally, sympathectomy is all too often the last option after failure of femoropopliteal reconstructions and may relieve symptoms or salvage limbs in a small percentage of cases.

FALSE ANEURYSMS

False aneurysms occur in up to 5 per cent of cases of aortic reconstructive procedures. They occur most commonly in the groin and are rare after primary endarterectomy. False aneurysms may result from a variety of factors, such as inadequate bites of graft or arterial wall while suturing the anastomosis, excessive graft tension, fracture or disintegration of suture, graft degeneration, progressive arterial disease and infection. These complications were more common with nylon and homografts than in the present era of Dacron grafts. Also, many aneurysms were associated with the use of silk or polyethylene sutures. Presently, the most common aetiology is weakness in the native artery at the anastomosis [78].

False aneurysms can occur in the presence of graft infection and repair *in situ* invariably results in recurrence (*see below*).

Sterile false aneurysms at an aortic suture line may be due to deterioration of graft or suture. While we do not recommend prophylactic removal of grafts known to be subject to such deterioration, if in fact no such evidence exists; we do recommend whole graft replacement once deterioration is manifested in any portion of the graft. False aneurysms at the aortic suture line are frequently accompanied by another in the groin, and these should always be sought. If a false aneurysm of the aortic suture line is due to a local defect in the aortic wall with an otherwise intact suture line, reinforcement with interrupted sutures will often suffice. Assurance of proximal control must be established before exposure of the false aneurysm is attempted. This may necessitate clamping temporarily above the renal arteries. As soon as safely possible, the clamp should be moved to below the renal vessels to minimize renal ischaemia. Extensive disruption of the proximal suture line is best treated by detachment of the graft and replacement with a new segment of graft. The aortotomy may be 'freshened-up' and re-used if widely patent. The new graft may be attached to the trunk or limbs of the old graft, thus completing the operation intra-abdominally.

Sterile false aneurysms in the groin may be due to weakness in the native vessel with an otherwise intact suture line. This may be reinforced with interrupted mattress sutures. Frequently, however, total disruption of the suture line exists with distraction of the graft from the vessel. This is particularly common after deterioration of silk sutures or fracture of running polyethylene sutures. The old graft is rigidly fixed by old scar and would require extensive dissection to mobilize. Also, the tension which helped create the original false aneurysm would be re-established. Therefore, we prefer to repair this situation with interposition of a Dacron tube graft [71]. Exposure is often difficult owing to dense scarring, and dissection to control vessels may damage critical collaterals or major vessels. It is often safer to gain proximal and distal control intraluminally by ballon catheters. While manually compressing the graft and femoral artery proximally, the false aneurysm may be entered. Fogarty catheters are then inserted into the native vessels and graft limb, to control bleeding (*Fig. 7.3*). This may

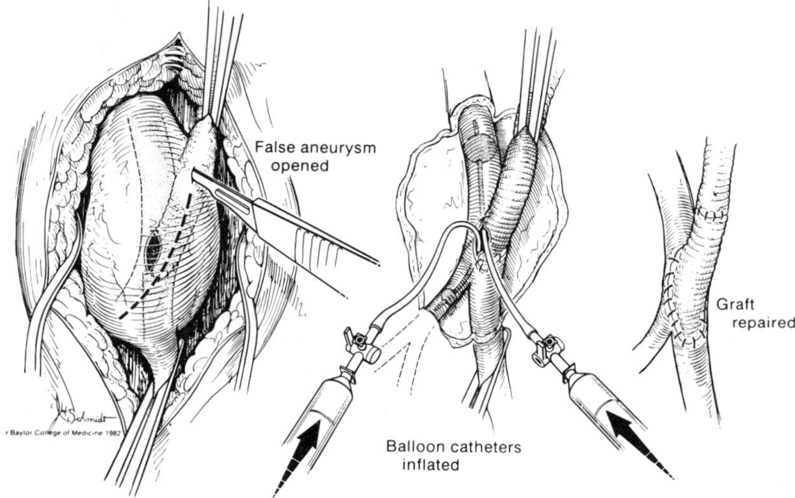

Fig. 7.3. The use of balloon catheters allowing safe dissection of a groin false aneurysm.

afford enough exposure and control to complete the graft interposition. If not, visualization of the lumina of the femoral vessels facilitates the exposure of their location and course.

GRAFT INFECTION

Graft infection following aorto-iliac and femoropopliteal reconstruction is fortunately infrequent, occurring in less than 2 per cent of cases. It is, however, the most difficult of complications because loss of life and limb are common, regardless of the treatment selected. Several general principles regarding pathogenesis and treatment have emerged and bear emphasis.

Before the dense fibrous sheath around a graft forms there is no barrier to the spread of suppuration along the entire course of a graft.

Early contamination of a prosthesis usually involves the entire graft, whereas late graft infection may be localized. Most authors agree that removal of an infected prosthesis is necessary in most instances to cure infection [79–81]. In the case of a localized infection, this may require removing only a portion of the graft. If the whole graft is involved, it must be removed entirely.

Another principle that has become evident is that some effort must be made to ensure adequate blood supply to the distal vascular bed after the graft is removed. Collective experience shows that efforts to treat graft infection without attempts to revascularize the lower extremities when significant ischaemia results, carry a higher mortality and incidence of limb loss than if revascularization is accomplished. Therefore, removal of all infected prostheses with revascularization of the lower extremities when necessary is the optimal treatment for graft infection.

Localized groin infections of aorto-bilateral femoral grafts may present as false aneurysms or as a chronic draining sinus. These frequently will swell, then drain spontaneously and present as brisk haemorrhage. Attempts to repair these locally are fruitless, and recurrent aneurysms should always be suspected of being infective in origin.

Sinograms of the graft should be performed, and if the evidence suggests a localized process, local treatment may be tried. If the native circulation is intact and promises to sustain the extremity, the proximal segment of the infected limb may be disconnected transabdominally or retroperitoneally. The distal tunnel is closed off from the abdomen and the graft limb is removed via the femoral incision. The native femoral vessel is closed primarily or with an autogenous patch or ligated depending upon the extent of the infection. If the native circulation is inadequate to sustain the extremity, an extra-anatomical bypass may be constructed at the time the infected limb is disconnected either through the obturator canal or from the ipsilateral axillary artery. The distal anastomosis is carried out in the distal superficial femoral, popliteal or profunda femoris artery, taking care not to enter any contaminated field with the new graft. The groin wound and graft tunnel are débrided locally and allowed to heal by secondary intention. Occlusion and thrombosis of a limb of an infected graft with later graft resection has also been practised [82].

If an entire aortic bifurcated prosthesis is infected, removal must be considered. It may present with evidence of infection in the groin, like a localized infection. Other presenting signs or symptoms may be more subtle, such as fever of unknown origin with retroperitoneal abscess or gastrointestinal bleeding with aorto-enteric fistula. Sinograms, computerized axial tomographic scans or ultrasound, however, will reveal spread of the infection up the graft to the aorta.

When time permits, an effort should be made to study the native circulation. If it promises to support the lower extremities, a bifurcated aortic graft with end-to-side anastomosis may simply be removed, closing the arteriotomies primarily or with autogenous patches. If the native circulation is inadequate and aortic reconstruction deemed unsafe, bilateral axillofemoral bypass should be constructed first and the infected graft removed afterwards.

In the case of aortoenteric fistula, prompt surgical intervention may be necessary to prevent exsanguination. After the graft has been removed and if local repair or graft replacement is not advisable, the abdomen should be closed and the extremities examined. If any uncertainty exists about the viability of the lower extremities, bilateral axillofemoral bypasses should be constructed at that time.

Ehrenfeld et al. [79] have reported the successful use of autogenous tissue reconstruction in the management of selected patients with graft infections. Endarterectomy combined with autogenous artery or vein grafts is used within the infected fields. Autogenous grafts seem to tolerate infection very well and the reported mortality (13 per cent) and amputation (18 per cent) rates are very promising.

In selected cases with chronic stable aortofemoral graft infection total graft resection is not performed. The graft to the femoral artery is partially resected in the groin and the femoral artery ligated. The groin wound is left open and maintained as a chronic draining sinus. Distal circulation is augmented with an extra-anatomical bypass if indicated. This procedure avoids or delays an intra-abdominal procedure and graft removal, which is frequently followed by aortic false aneurysms, rupture and death.

Foreign body reaction with sterile fluid collection sometimes develops around extra-anatomical bypasses when they are used in patients with infected grafts. The use of autogenous tissue or a prosthetic graft of a different material seems to diminish its occurrence.

AUTOTRANSFUSION

We have found autotransfusion to be particularly useful in re-do vascular surgery. Patients are generally anticoagulated with heparin. Control of bleeding both proximally and distally is sometimes less than optimal because of technical difficulties with safe exposure. Disobliteration of thrombosed grafts necessitates thorough flushing, often with considerably more blood loss than the initial operation. Use of autotransfusion conserves the resources of the blood bank and minimizes the risk of hepatitis and transfusion reactions attendant on the use of homologous blood [83].

TRANSLUMINAL ANGIOPLASTY

Occasionally, recurrent symptoms are produced by localized, stenotic areas in a vein graft or in the native circulation above or below a graft. If these are discovered before progression to total occlusion, they may be dealt with early, avoiding graft thrombosis. Transluminal angioplasty was originally described in 1964 by Dotter and Judkins [84] but evoked little general interest in the United States. Recently, popularization of the technique in the treatment of localized coronary artery stenosis by Gruntzig [85] has led to renewed interest in its use in aorto-iliac and femoropopliteal segments. We consider this technique particularly useful in two groups of patients: (*a*) poor risk patients threatened with limb loss who cannot tolerate definitive surgery or (*b*) patients with recurrent symptoms due to localized stenosis, which threatens graft patency. Beebe [86] showed that symptomatic improvement after dilatation depended upon distal run-off and correlated with an increase in ankle pressure indices.

In properly selected cases this technique has a role in the treatment of patients with previous vascular reconstruction. The decision to use this technique rather than reoperate involves consideration of the surgical options and is probably best left with the vascular surgeon. Gruntzig has reported success in 87 per cent of patients followed up to 2 years after aorto-iliac dilatation and in 72 per cent after dilatation in the femoropopliteal region [86].

THROMBOLYTIC THERAPY

Although not a new modality, thrombolytic therapy has undergone a resurgence of interest in the past decade. Perhaps stimulated by its utility in dissolving thrombus in the pulmonary and coronary circulations, systemic and local thrombolytic therapy has been used to treat acute vascular thrombosis. Success rates in the aorta and common iliac areas are in the range of 50–75 per cent [87, 88]. The rates for the femoral, popliteal and tibial areas, however, are considerably less. Authors stress the need for early intervention, i.e. within 2 weeks after thrombosis. After 6 weeks the thrombus is organized and no therapeutic benefit occurs.

Thrombolytic therapy of occluded grafts is also possible. Occluded autogenous vein grafts are ideal candidates and we have experienced success with thrombolytic therapy of PTFE grafts. A word of caution is warranted in regard to porous Dacron grafts. Dissolution of the clot in graft interstices can lead to significant bleeding. This possibility must be taken into consideration when contemplating thrombolytic therapy in newly inserted Dacron prostheses.

REFERENCES

1. Leriche R. (1923) Des obliterations artérielles heutes (obliteration de la termination de l'aorte). Comme causes des insuffisances circulatoires des membres inferieurs. *Bull. Mem. Soc. Chir. (Paris)* **49**, 1404.
2. Leriche R. (1940) De la resection du carrefour aorticoiliaque avec double sympathectomie lombaire pour thrombose artériteque de l'aorte: le syndrome de l'obliteration termino-aortique par artérite. *Presse Med.* **48**, 601.
3. Morris G. C., Edwards W., Cooley D. A. et al. (1961) Surgical importance of profunda femoris artery. *Arch. Surg.* **82**, 52.
4. Morris G. C., Beall A. C., Berry W. B. et al. (1960) Anatomic studies of the distal popliteal artery and its branches. *Surg. Forum* **10**, 498.
5. Thompson J. E. and Garrett W. V. (1980) Peripheral-arterial surgery. *N. Engl. J. Med.* **302**, 495.
6. Strandness D. E. and Bell J. W. (1965) Peripheral vascular disease, diagnosis and objective evaluation using a mercury strain gauge. *Ann. Surg.* Suppl. 161, 1.
7. Darling R. C., Raines J. K., Brener B. J. et al. (1972) Quantitative segmental pulse volume recorder: a clinical tool. *Surgery* **72**, 873.
8. Yao S. T., Hobbs J. T. and Irvine W. T. (1969) Ankle systolic pressure measurement in arterial disease affecting the lower extremities. *Br. J. Surg.* **56**, 676.
9. Bergan J. J. and Yao S. T. (1980) Invited overview: role of the vascular laboratory. *Surgery* **88**, 9.
10. Yao S. T., Needham T. N. and Gourmoss C. et al. (1972) A comparative study of strain-gauge plethysmography and Doppler ultrasound in the assessment of occlusive arterial disease of the lower extremities. *Surgery* **71**, 4.
11. dos Santos R., Lamas A. and Saldas J. (1949) Arteriografia de aorta e dos vasos abdominalis. *Med. Contemp.* **47**, 93.
12. Beall A. C., Henley W. S., Morris G. C. et al. (1963) Translumbar aortography: a simple, safe technique. *Ann. Surg.* **175**, 882.
13. Beall A. C., Morris G. C., Garrett H. E. et al. (1964) Translumbar aortography. present indications and techniques. *Ann. Intern. Med.* **60**, 843.
14. Seldinger S. I. (1953) Catheter replacement of needle in percutaneous arteriography: new technique. *Acta Radiol.* **39**, 368.
15. Beals J. W. M., Adcock F. A., Frawley J. E. et al. (1971) The radiologic assessment of disease of the profunda femoris artery. *Br. J. Radiol.* **44**, 854.
16. Sethi G. K., Scott S. M. and Takaro T. (1975) Multiple-plane angiography for more precise evaluation of aortoiliac disease. *Surgery* **78**, 154.
17. Domingo D. and Johnson K. W. (1981) Assessment of aorto-iliac disease by non-invasive quantitative Doppler waveform analysis. *Br. J. Surg.* **68**, 1979.
18. Boyd A. M. (1962) Natural causes of arteriosclerosis of the lower extremities. *Proc. R. Soc. Med.* **55**, 591.
19. Malone J. M., Moore W. S. and Goldstone J. (1977) Life expectancy following aortofemoral arterial grafting. *Surgery* **81**, 551.
20. Imparato A. M., Kim G., Davidson T. et al. (1975) Intermittent claudication: its natural course. *Surgery* **78**, 795.
21. McAllister F. F. (1976) The fate of patients with intermittent claudication managed non-operatively. *Am. J. Surg.* **132**, 593.
22. Dickinson P. H., McNeill I. F. and Morrison J. M. (1967) Aorto-iliac occlusion a review of 100 cases treated by direct arterial surgery. *Br. J. Surg.* **54**, 764.
23. Szilagyi D. E. (1964) Ten years experience with aortoiliac and femoropopliteal arterial reconstruction. *J. Cardiovasc. Surg.* **5**, 502.
24. Brewster D. C. and Darling R. C. (1978) Optimal methods of aortoiliac reconstruction. *Surgery* **84**, 739.

25. Malone J. M., Moore W. S. and Goldstone J. (1975) The natural history of bilateral aortofemoral bypass grafts for ischaemia of the lower extremities. *Arch. Surg.* **110**, 1300.
26. DeBakey M. E.: Unpublished data.
27. Wylie E. J., Olcott C. and String S. T. (1976) Aortoiliac thromboendarterectomy. In: Varco R. L. and Delaney J. P. (ed.) *Controversy in Surgery*. Philadelphia, Saunders, p. 443.
28. Humphries A. W., Young J. R. and McCormack L. J. (1969) Experiences with aortoiliac and femoropopliteal endarterectomy. *Surgery* **65**, 48.
29. Pilcher D. B., Barker W. F. and Cannon J. A. (1970) An aortoiliac case series followed ten years or more. *Surgery* **65**, 5.
30. Dean R. H. and Foster J. H. (1973) Aortoiliac occlusive disease; fifteen years' operative experience. *South. Med. J.* **66**, 813.
31. Duncan W. C., Linton R. R. and Darling R. C. (1971) Aortoiliofemoral atherosclerotic occlusive disease: comparative results of endarterectomy and Dacron bypass grafts. *Surgery* **70**, 974.
32. Sawyer P. N., Pasupathy C. E., Fitzgerald J. et al. (1972) Six-year follow-up study in the use of gas endarterectomy. *Surgery* **72,** 837.
33. Szilagyi D. E., Smith R. F., Elliot J. P. et al. (1965) Long-term behaviour of a Dacron arterial substitute. *Ann. Surg.* **162**, 453.
34. Butcher H. R. and Jaffee B. M. (1971) Treatment of aortoiliac arterial disease by endarterectomy. *Ann. Surg.* **173**, 925.
35. Kouchoukos N. T., Levy J. F., Balfour J. F. et al. (1968) Operative therapy for aortoiliac arterial occlusive disease. *Arch. Surg.* **96**, 628.
36. Szilagyi D. E., Smith R. F. and Whitney D. G. (1964) The durability of aorto-iliac endarterectomy. *Arch. Surg.* **89**, 827.
37. Waibel P. P. and Dunant J. H. (1973) Late results of aorto-iliac reconstructive surgery. *J. Cardiovasc. Surg.* **14**, 492.
38. Healey S. J., Wheeler H. B., Crane C. et al. (1964) Reconstructive operations for aortoiliac obliterative disease. *N. Engl. J. Med.* **271**, 1386.
39. Inahara T. (1972) Endarterectomy for occlusive disease of the aortoiliac and common femoral arteries. *Am. J. Surg.* **124**, 235.
40. Crawford E. S., Banberger R. A., Glaeser D. H. et al. (1981) Aortoiliac occlusive disease; factors influencing survival and function following reconstructive operation over a twenty-five year period. *Surgery* **90**, 1055.
41. Nevelsteen A., Suy R., Daenen W. et al (1980) Aortofemoral grafting: factors influencing late results. *Surgery* **88**, 642.
42. Mozersky D. J., Summer D. S. and Strandness D. E. (1972) Long-term results of reconstructive aortoiliac surgery. *Am. J. Surg.* **123**, 503.
43. Malone J., Moore W. S. and Goldstone J. (1975) The natural history of bilateral aortofemoral bypass grafts for ischaemia of the lower extremities. *Arch. Surg.* **110**, 1300.
44. Liddicoat J. E., Bekassy S. M. and DeBakey M. E. (1975) Intraoperative arteriography during femoral-popliteal bypass. *Arch. Surg.* **110**, 839.
45. Johnson W. C. (1979) Preliminary experience with expanded polytetrafluoroethylene grafts. *Surgery* **85**, 173.
46. Gupta S. K. and Veith F. J. (1980) Three-year experience with expanded polytetrafluoroethylene arterial grafts for limb salvage. *Am. J. Surg.* **140**, 214.
47. Campell D. R., Hoar C. S. and Gibbons G. W. (1979) The use of arm veins in femoropopliteal bypass grafts. *Ann. Surg.* **190**, 740.
48. Edwards W. H. and Mulherin J. L. (1980) The role of graft material in femorotibial bypass grafts. *Ann. Surg.* **191**, 721.

49. Lee B. Y., Trainor F. S., Kauvner D. et al. (1978) Evaluation of modified human umbilical vein as an arterial substitute in femoropopliteal reconstructive surgical procedures. *Surg. Gynecol. Obstet.* **147**, 721.
50. Reichle F. A., Martinson M. W. and Rankin K. P. (1980) Infra-popliteal arterial reconstruction in the severely ischaemic lower extremity. *Ann. Surg.* **191**, 59.
51. Collins G. J., Rich N. M. and Anderson C. A. (1976) Limb salvage procedures for lower extremity ischemia. *Am. J. Surg.* **132**, 707.
52. Edwards W. H. and Wright R. S. (1976) Tibial and peroneal bypass in severe occlusive disease of the lower extremities. *Ann. Surg.* **183**, 710.
53. Dardik H., Ibrahim I. M. and Dardik I. I. (1979) The role of the peroneal artery for limb salvage. *Ann. Surg.* **189**, 189.
54. Potts J. R., Wendelken J. R., Elkins R. C. et al (1979) Lower extremity amputation; review of 110 cases. *Am. J. Surg.* **138**, 924.
55. Kazmers M., Satiani B. and Evans W. E. (1980) Amputation level following unsuccessful distal limb salvage operations. *Surgery* **87**, 683.
56. Collins G. J., Rich N. M., Auduson C. A. et al. (1978) Acute hemodynamic effects of lumbar sympathectomy. *Am. J. Surg.* **136**, 714.
57. Masvoka S. and Shimomuna T. (1978) Lumbar sympathectomy and blood flow in the lower extremity. *Am. J. Surg.* **136**, 369.
58. Shanik G. D., Ford J., Hayes A. C. et al. (1976) Pedal vasomotor tone following aortofemoral reconstruction. *Ann. Surg.* **183**, 136.
59. Leeds F. H. and Gilfillan R. S. (1961) Revascularization of the ischaemiac limb; importance of the profunda femoris artery. *Arch. Surg.* **82**, 25.
60. Welsh P. and Repetto R. (1975) Revascularization of the profunda femoris artery in aortoiliac occlusive disease. *Surgery* **78**, 389.
61. Mitchell R. A., Bome G. E., Bridges R. et al. (1979) Patient selection for isolated profundaplasty. *Am. J. Surg.* **138**, 912.
62. David T. E. and Drezner A. D. (1978) Extended profundaplasty for limb salvage. *Surgery* **84**, 758.
63. Leather R. P., Shah D. M. and Karmody A. M. (1978) The use of extended profundaplasty in limb salvage. *Am. J. Surg.* **136**, 359.
64. Sladen J. G. and Burgess J. J. (1980) Profundaplasty; expectations and ominous signs. *Am. J. Surg.* **140**, 242.
65. Boren C. H., Towne J. B. and Bernhard V. M. (1980) Profundapopliteal collateral index. *Arch. Surg.* **115**, 1368.
66. Dick L. S., Brief D. K., Alpert J. et al. (1980) A 12-year experience with femorofemoral crossover grafts. *Arch Surg.* **115**, 1359.
67. LoGerfo F. W., Johnson W. C., Corson J. D. et al. (1977) A comparison of the late patency rates of axillobilateral femoral and axillo-unilateral femoral grafts. *Surgery* **81**, 33.
68. Plecha F. R. and Pories W. J. (1976) Extra-anatomic bypasses for aortoiliac disease in the high-risk patients. *Surgery* **80**, 480.
69. Mannick J. A., Williams L. E. and Nabseth D. C. (1970) The late results of axillofemoral grafts. *Surgery* **68**, 1038.
70. DeLaurentis D. A., Sala L. E., Russell E. et al (1978) A twelve-year experience with axillofemoral and femorofemoral bypass operations. *Surg. Gynecol. Obstet.* **147**, 881.
71. Crawford E. S., Manning L. G. and Kelly T. F. (1979) 'Re-do' surgery of the operations for aneurysm and occlusion of the abdominal aorta. *Surgery* **81**, 41.
72. Davis J. H. (1975) Complications of surgery of the abdominal aorta. *Am. J. Surg.* **130**, 523.
73. Thompson W. M., Johnsrude I. S., Jackson D. C. et al. (1977) Late complications of abdominal aortic reconstructive surgery. *Ann. Surg.* **185**, 3.

74. Crawford E. S., DeBakey M. E., Morris G. C. et al. (1960) Evaluation of late failures after reconstructive operations for the aorta, iliac, femoral and popliteal arteries. *Surgery* **47**, 79.
75. Szilagyi D. E., Elliot J. P., Smith R. F. et al. (1975) Secondary arterial repair. *Arch. Surg.* **110**, 485.
76. Bernhard V. M., Ray L. I. and Towne J. B. (1977) The reoperation of choice for aortofemoral graft occlusion. *Surgery* **82**, 867.
77. Malone J. M., Goldstone J. and Moore W. S. (1978) Autogenous profundaplasty, the key to long term patency in secondary repair of aortofemoral graft occlusion. *Ann. Surg.* **188**, 817.
78. Szilagyi D. E., Smith R. F., Elliot J. R. et al. (1975) Anastomotic aneurysms after vascular reconstruction: problems of incidence, etiology and treatment. *Surgery* **78**, 800.
79. Ehrenfeld W. K., Wilbur B. G., Olcott C. N. et al. (1979) Autogenous tissue reconstruction in the management of infected prosthetic grafts. *Surgery* **85**, 82.
80. Spanos P. K., Gilsdorf R. B., Sakio Y. et al. (1976) The management of infected abdominal aortic grafts and graft-enteric fistulas. *Ann. Surg.* **183**, 397.
81. Liekweg W. G. and Greenfield L. J. (1977) Vascular prosthetic infections: collected experience and results of treatment. *Surgery* **81**, 335.
82. Diethrich E. B., Noon G. P., Liddicoat J. E. et al. (1970) Treatment of infected aortofemoral arterial prosthesis. *Surgery* **68**, 1044.
83. Noon G. P. (1978) Intraoperative autotransfusion. *Surgery* **84**, 719.
84. Dotter C. T. and Judkins M. P. (1964) Transluminal treatment of atherosclerotic obstruction: description of a technique and preliminary report of its application. *Circulation* **30**, 654.
85. Gruntzig A. R., Senning A. and Siegenthaler W. E. (1979) Nonoperative dilatation of coronary artery stenosis. *N. Engl. J. Med.* **301**, 61.
86. Beebe H. G., Stark R. and Freeny P. C. (1980) Indications for transluminal angioplasty: a surgical view. *Am. J. Surg.* **140**, 31.
87. Martin M., Schoop W. and Zeiflu E. (1970) Streptokinase in chronic arterial occlusive disease. *JAMA* **211**, 1169.
88. Martin M. (1979) Thrombolytic therapy in arterial thromboembolism. *Prog. Cardiovasc. Dis.* **21**, 351.

Crawford Jamieson and Martin Thomas

8 Limb Salvage

DEFINITION OF LIMB SALVAGE

Limb salvage may be simply defined as 'treatment which improves the circulation of an ischaemic limb to an extent which saves it from amputation and restores it to useful function.' It is not easy to decide which limbs will progress to severe irreversible ischaemia [1]. Clinically, a limb is considered to be in danger when the patient suffers from rest pain or when there is evidence of distal pre-gangrene or gangrene. Rest pain is, however, subjective and does not necessarily herald progression of ischaemia to gangrene and amputation. Furthermore, pre-gangrene and gangrene themselves may not cause inevitable loss of the limb. Gangrene may be due to a local cause, such as a small embolus into a digital artery, and this gangrenous area may separate and heal spontaneously. Rest pain or gangrene with loss of distal pulses is also not invariably associated with the loss of a limb because local causes can co-exist with lesser degrees of proximal arterial stenosis sufficient to cause loss of pulses, but not sufficient to jeopardize the limb.

An exact clinical definition is probably impossible. Attempts have been made to render the definition of limb salvage more precise by measuring ankle systolic pressure. Ankle pressure is measured with a Doppler probe and ankle cuff and the ankle/brachial pressure index has been found to correlate with the degree of ischaemia [2, 3]. Yao showed that a pressure index below 0·26 accompanied ischaemic rest pain. This has been confirmed by others; Marston's study, for instance, quoted a pressure index of 0·28 in limbs with pain at rest [4]. According to Carter, when ischaemic ulceration occurs the ankle pressure is near 30 mmHg [2]. Using a pulse volume recorder, Raines found the mean ankle systolic pressure was 33 mmHg in limbs with rest pain and 28 mmHg with ischaemic skin lesions [5].

In general, an ankle systolic blood pressure which is less than 25 per cent of the brachial pressure or less than 50 mmHg is associated with a high incidence of limb loss unless the pressure subsequently rises. The converse is not necessarily true for it is possible, particularly in Buerger's disease, to have a normal ankle blood pressure but an arterial occlusion in the foot which results in loss of the foot and possibly the lower limb as well [6, 7]. In addition, calcification in the posterior tibial or dorsalis pedis artery can cause an artificially high pressure to be recorded when blood pressure is assessed using an inflatable cuff because the vessel is incompressible. Such calcified vessels are relatively common in diabetics and are occasionally found in other patients with vascular disease [8–10]. Therefore, a low pressure indicates that the limb will be lost, but a high pressure does not guarantee that the limb will not be lost.

This lack of a precise definition of limb salvage is most unfortunate as it makes comparison of published series of patients treated in different ways very difficult, and the natural history of individual patients difficult to forecast. Mean levels of ankle blood pressure in a series of patients are of some value, but exact documentation of the lesions present in each patient, and in particular the number of patients in a series with an ankle pressure of less than 50 mmHg systolic, would be of greater value.

CAUSES OF LIMB-THREATENING ISCHAEMIA

Embolism

The commonest source of an embolus to a lower limb is the heart, either from the fibrillating atrial appendage or from ventricular mural thrombus after myocardial infarction [11–15]. Among a long list of rarer causes, atheromatous and cholesterol emboli have recently stimulated interest [16], but the great majority of emboli which occlude a major vessel come from the heart. The patients present with acute ischaemia of one or both lower limbs accompanied by loss of pulses and the degree of ischaemia parallels the loss of pulses, as there is no collateral formation. The treatment is systemic anticoagulation followed by emergency embolectomy [15].

Atheroma

Although atheromatous arterial disease usually presents with gradual onset of ischaemia, it may present suddenly, particularly in patients who are not ambulant and have not therefore been warned of its presence by the onset of intermittent claudication. Acute thrombosis of a diseased artery is often the cause [1, 17]. The diagnosis can usually be distinguished from that of embolism by the presence of arterial disease elsewhere, by the relatively small area of severe ischaemia compared with the loss of pulses because of the previously formed collateral circulation and by the lack of either atrial fibrillation or recent myocardial infarction to suggest an embolus. The treatment may be complicated and requires accurate arteriographic information on the exact extent of arterial occlusive disease. It is therefore most important, when there is any doubt, that an emergency arteriogram is performed before operative treatment on an acutely ischaemic limb [17, 18]. This may in itself distinguish the smooth artery ending in sudden occlusion of a patient with embolism from the diseased arteries and collaterals of a patient with atheromatous disease, and it allows a definitive vascular reconstruction to be planned. It is not infrequent for an embolus to lodge in an atheromatously diseased arterial tree, and this creates a very complex problem of surgical diagnosis and management.

Trauma

Acute arterial ischaemia produced by arterial trauma is often complicated by venous injury, fractures and by damaged nerves and muscle. Immediate arterial, and frequently venous reconstruction are necessary if the limb is to be saved [19]. A preoperative arteriogram may be unnecessary if there is nothing in the history or examination to suggest pre-existent vascular disease. In cases of penetrating injury, especially gunshot wounds, angiography is advisable. All these patients are at risk from gas gangrene and must be covered with prophylactic penicillin [20, 21].

Thrombosed aneurysm

Thrombosed popliteal aneurysm and very occasionally common femoral and aortic aneurysm are causes of acute ischaemia. Thrombosis of a popliteal aneurysm is associated with an incidence of amputation of up to 30 per cent [22, 23]. Thrombosed aneurysm may be diagnosed by the presence of a non-pulsatile, possibly tender, swelling in the popliteal fossa, and by the 60 per cent incidence of a pulsatile swelling on the contralateral popliteal fossa [23] or the 50 per cent incidence of aortic aneurysm [24]. These patients have a poor prognosis as there has usually been embolization into the distal arterial tree, before final thrombosis of the aneurysm, causing chronic occlusion of the distal arteries [25, 26]. A popliteal aneurysm is best treated while it is asymptomatic before it thromboses, although some question this policy [22, 27].

Dissecting Aneurysm

Aortic dissection is a rare, but well recognized, cause of ischaemia of the lower limb [28]. It should be evident in a patient with a history of chest or back pain followed by acute ischaemia, but the pain may be slight and this part of the history is not uncommonly missed. The symptoms may be confused with myocardial infarction followed by embolism of mural thrombus. Patients with aortic dissection suffer from occlusion of vessels, due to the dissection, but also have a risk of sudden fatal haemorrhage due to rupture of the dissection through the outer layer of the aorta. Dissection occurs in younger patients with Marfan's syndrome [29] or Ehlers–Danlos syndrome [30] and in middle-aged hypertensive patients [31]. If the diagnosis has been missed until the artery is explored, it becomes obvious when the typical appearance of a dissection is seen, or—if the dissection is confined to the iliac artery—because an embolectomy catheter will pass up the artery and down it quite freely but is not followed by either clot or down-flow, as it merely compresses the dissection during its passage. No other pathology except a dissection produces this extraordinary finding during exploration of an artery.

Thromboangiitis Obliterans

The exact definition and nature of this disease has been open to a good deal of debate over the years [32, 33]. It is common in young men who smoke heavily and consists of distal occlusion of the arteries of the lower limb and to a lesser extent of the upper limb. Arterial insufficiency is frequently associated with thrombophlebitis and has characteristic angiographic appearances with spiral corkscrew collateral vessels, no distal patent vessels, and smooth, apparently normal proximal arteries [34]. The treatment consists of persuading the patient to stop smoking completely, plus supportive measures and possibly sympathectomy. The place of steroids is not clear.

Arteritis

Polyarteritis nodosa [35], disseminated lupus erythematosus [36, 37], giant cells arteritis [38], rheumatic vasculitis [39, 40], Takayasu's disease [41, 42], and others may all cause loss of a limb. Their treatment is discussed in general below but the patients usually present with diffuse evidence of small vessel disease, which is often associated with rashes, systemic illness and characteristic alterations in their serum protein and erythrocyte sedimentation rate.

Ergotism

St Antony's Fire is fortunately now rare. Ischaemia of digits due to ergot ingestion is occasionally seen in patients with migraine who overdose themselves with ergotamine tartrate [43]. Withdrawal of the drug, combined with lumbar sympathectomy, gives very good results.

Accidental Intra-arterial Injection

This catastrophic complication of intravenous therapy or more recently of radial artery pressure recording during surgery is followed by a high incidence of local amputation [44, 45]. As soon as the accident is recognized a further injection of heparin together with local anaesthetic or papaverine should be made, preferably through the same needle as was used for the accidental injection, although evidence that these or other supportive measures have any beneficial effect is scanty.

AGGRAVATING FACTORS IN LIMB-THREATENING ISCHAEMIA

Polycythaemia and Thrombocythaemia

Both true polycythaemia rubra vera and false polycythaemia, in which the packed cell volume is raised but the patient's red cell mass is normal because plasma volume is decreased, are associated with a high incidence of thrombosis [46], and haemorrhage [47]. This high haematocrit can be the sole cause of primary arterial occlusion, but is more frequently seen in combination with some other cause of arterial occlusive disease. The viscosity of polycythaemic blood does, however, limit tissue perfusion and control of polycythaemia, or thrombocythaemia may be beneficial to any patient with severe ischaemia [46].

Oral Contraceptive Agents

There is a well-established incidence of venous thrombosis [48] and definite but rare cases of arterial occlusion [49] associated with the use of oral contraceptives. It is likely, therefore, that these drugs are a risk factor associated with other causes of arterial occlusion, and they should not be prescribed for these patients.

Control of Hypertension

The circulation of an ischaemic foot relates both to the resistance to arterial flow to the extremity and the blood pressure. Occasionally control of hypertension results in distal perfusion falling to a level which is insufficient to sustain the tissues at rest—in which instance rest pain or gangrene may occur. This can be reversed by allowing the hypertension to be uncontrolled, and indeed artificially induced hypertension has been proposed as a treatment of severe ischaemia [50]. Both naturally induced and artificially induced hypertension, however, carry similar risks of heart failure and cerebrovascular accident, and other methods of improving the arterial flow to the limb are preferred to allowing hypertension to continue.

Congestive Cardiac Failure

Congestive cardiac failure lowers tissue perfusion and may therefore accentuate any existing deficit and produce limb ischaemia [51]. Control of cardiac failure may lift arterial flow out of the range of rest pain and pre-gangrene and save a limb.

Sepsis and Trauma

Damage to an extremity, either by sepsis, trauma or pressure, may cause tissue necrosis which requires repair. Higher blood flow and tissue perfusion are needed to repair tissue than to maintain viability of undamaged tissue. Thus trauma or sepsis may be the precipitating factors which result in loss of a limb in a patient with chronic ischaemia. Such damage is more likely in patients with impaired pain sensation as the protective effect of pain is lost. This is particularly common in diabetics where neuropathy, sepsis and relatively trivial trauma combine to cause gangrene of a foot [52].

TREATMENT OF LIMB-THREATENING ISCHAEMIA

Non-operative Treatment

Anti-coagulation

Acute ischaemia causes distal arterial and venous stasis which is followed by arterial and venous thrombosis; these conspire to accentuate the orginal ischaemic episode. Thrombosis can be postponed by the immediate use of effective doses of intravenous heparin, a standard regimen being 5000 i.u. stat. followed by 10 000 i.u. 6 hourly by continuous intravenous infusion [53]. Occasionally even this dose is inadequate and heparin must always be controlled by regular monitoring of the clotting time which should be maintained at twice control values. Anticoagulants do not dissolve arterial thrombus although there is some evidence that larger doses may augment fibrinolysis. There is no good evidence that intravenous fibrinolytic activating agents, such as streptokinase or urokinase, have any effect on arterial occlusion. Even intra-arterial injection of fibrinolytic activators does not seem to have stood the test of time and has been generally abandoned.

In many circumstances thrombosis of an artery is merely a reflection of poor flow through it, and even if the thrombus were to be completely dissolved it is likely to recur because the same flow characteristics will obtain until the arterial circulation is improved by reconstructive vascular surgery.

Arteriography

Arteriography is indicated in the acutely ischaemic limb when the cause is not clinically apparent. This may be possible preoperatively but there are frequent circumstances in which the cause of ischaemia is not clear even when a vessel is explored and in this situation operative arteriography is invaluable [54].

Supportive Treatment

There is very little objective evidence that any supportive treatment alters the natural history of severe ischaemia of the lower limb. In the past claims have been made for the efficacy of hyperbaric-oxygen [55], rhythmic compression and massage of the ischaemic limb and a variety of pharmacological agents [56]. Intra-arterial reserpine has been shown to produce increases in distal flow which may last for several days after its administration; other vasodilator agents may have similar effects. Intra-arterial solcoseryl enjoyed some enthusiastic support but is no longer used. These effects may be equally well obtained in the lower limb by sympathectomy. It has been claimed that the agent naftidrofuryl (Praxilene) may relieve the pain of ischaemia and clinical impression is that it may have some beneficial effect in relieving symptoms [57, 58], although there is no evidence that it actually saves any limb in the long run. Recently encouraging, but totally uncontrolled, claims have been made for the use of prostaglandins administered intra-arterially or intravenously [56, 59]. These last agents possibly do have some clinical value, but we must await controlled trials of their use before their exact position in therapy is clear.

In arteritis, plasmapheresis, which lowers viscosity and may also have a beneficial effect of removing immune complexes, has been claimed to have some value [60, 61]. Systemic steroid therapy has a beneficial effect in polyarteritis nodosa, disseminated lupus erythematosus and rheumatic vasculitis [62], but no apparent benefit in scleroderma. It must be emphasized that uncontrolled trials of drugs and other treatments in the management of severe ischaemia are useless as the natural history of this disease is so extremely variable. This variation makes balanced controlled trials difficult as spontaneous dramatic improvement is common.

Operative Treatment

Amputation

Amputation rather than limb salvage is indicated where there is irreversible ischaemia. Evidence of muscle induration and fixed skin mottling which does not blanch on pressure indicates death rather than reversible anoxia of tissues [63, 64]. Some patients with traumatized limbs have such gross damage to muscles, bones and nerves that it is quite clear the limb will never be useful. Gas gangrene and crush syndrome [65, 66] may develop in such limbs and are a serious danger to the patient. A joint decision by an orthopaedic and vascular surgeon that immediate amputation is required will save the patient from these dangers and from the disappointment of having a useless limb which will eventually require amputation.

There is no point in making vigorous efforts to save a limb of a patient who is not ambulant. Many geriatric patients fall into this category and they are best treated by immediate amputation rather than being subjected to the discomfort and risk of arteriography and reconstructive vascular surgery.

It is inadvisable to perform an amputation through a level at which there is gross sensory neuropathy with impaired pain sensation. Such patients are unable to use a prosthesis without damaging their anaesthetic stumps, and soon return with painful trophic ulcers that require revision of the amputation to a higher level at which sensation is better. Finally, gas gangrene is an ever-present but rare threat which may necessitate urgent amputation in a patient who otherwise was progressing favourably even after a successful reconstruction.

Fasciotomy

Muscle that has been ischaemic and is revascularized becomes oedematous. The muscles of the lower limb are enclosed within a rigid sleeve of deep fascia and the oedema causes a rise in pressure in the fascial compartments of the leg which soon embarrasses the circulation [67]. The anterior tibial compartment of the leg is most commonly affected but any of the fascial compartments of the leg, or even the thigh, may be similarly damaged, particularly when ischaemia is associated with muscle trauma. The only method whereby this damage can be avoided, particularly after reconstructive surgery, is adequate division of the investing deep fascia to allow the muscle to expand. Semi-closed fasciotomy, in which one or more small incisions in the skin are made and then a knife or scissors passed blindly down the limb to divide the deep fascia, may be sufficient [66]. If the skin is contributing to the constricting process, skin and deep fascia must be divided if muscle is to survive. The most effective decompression of the whole leg is obtained by an extraperiosteal excision of the shaft of the fibula and this may be required in the presence of massive swelling which may occur after trauma. Each of the fascial sheets enclosing the various compartments of the leg is attached to the fibula and the excision of this bone opens them all. The signs of impending muscle death are tenderness, induration and erythema over the affected compartment, but these are all signs that muscle damage has already started, and is probably already irreversible. Fasciotomy should not be postponed until these signs appear, but is indicated in any revascularization after acute ischaemia, especially when there is evidence of previous muscle injury, such as weak foot movements.

Sympathectomy

The effect of sympathectomy is to increase blood flow to the limb, redistribute this flow so that there is a relative increase in distal perfusion (i.e. into hand or foot) over proximal perfusion and augment flow to skin and bone rather than to muscle [68]. This measured increase in flow may represent mainly useless arteriovenous shunting [69, 70] and is significantly diminished in the presence of either proximal or distal arterial stenosis or occlusion [71]. Sympathectomy has better long term effects in the lower limb [72] than in the upper limb. Experimentally significant increases in flow have been shown to persist for nearly 3 years. The restoration of vascular tone and the recurrence of vasospastic disorders is definitely slower in the lower limb than in the arm, where the mean duration of remission of symptoms following sympathectomy is probably less than 12 months [73].

The indications for sympathectomy in limb salvage are: (*a*) as an adjunct to reconstructive surgery—an attempt to revascularize a limb may achieve a less-than-perfect result, in which case sympathectomy might supplement skin blood flow and there is some evidence that a simultaneous sympathectomy may help by increasing blood flow through a reconstructed segment [74] to maintain patency; and (*b*) to increase skin blood flow when reconstructive vascular surgery is impossible [68].

This operation is widely performed in patients with ischaemic limbs for a variety of reasons and it is so established in surgical management that no controlled trial in limb salvage is now possible as most clinicians would consider it unethical. There is, however, little evidence that lumbar sympathectomy has any effect on distal circulation which is sufficient to save a limb, except in those patients with vasospastic disease or an element of vasospasm plus arterial occlusion. Many uncontrolled studies have claimed improvement in skin blood flow [68] following lumbar sympathectomy but animal studies have shown that most of the increase in blood flow is diverted into the venous system via arteriovenous shunts, with no beneficial effect upon tissue perfusion [69, 70].

There is also evidence that lumbar sympathectomy seldom saves a very ischaemic limb [72, 75, 76]. In a study of 92 patients receiving lumbar sympathectomy alone for limb salvage it was found that of 50 patients with an ankle/brachial pressure index less than 0·25, all but 6 lost their leg; and of those 6, 4 patients' limbs were saved by subsequent arterial reconstruction [76]. Only 4 of the 42 patients with a higher ankle pressure came to amputation. This study has been amply confirmed [73, 75] and it is clear that there is no point in performing a lumbar sympathectomy without arterial reconstruction in a patient whose pressure index is less than 0·2. If those cases with severe pain requiring narcotic analgesia and prolonged dependency for control or with extensive ischaemic lesions are excluded, then sympathectomy can have a beneficial effect in about 60 per cent of patients [77–79]. Sympathectomy alone should be reserved for those patients who have no proximal lesion amenable to reconstruction, with peripherally distributed lesions from atherosclerosis, thromboangiitis obliterans or diabetes mellitus. This last group may have already undergone an autosympathectomy [80], but even so, operative sympathectomy may be of benefit since it may be more complete. It is more accurate and complete than phenol sympathectomy [81].

It has also, by convention, been advocated that removal of the lumbar sympathetic chain should at least include the second lumbar ganglion. The nerve/skin supply by the fourth lumbar ganglion includes all of the skin of the foot, and a variable amount of skin of the leg. The third lumbar ganglion supplies the leg and the lower thigh. The second lumbar ganglion supplies most of the thigh. There is possibly a more rapid restoration of sympathetic tone following sympathectomy above L3 due to variations in anatomy and to regeneration of sympathetic fibres [82]. There is also a theoretical chance of making ischaemia worse by a high lumbar sympathectomy, particularly in a patient who has inflow obstruction of the limb, from iliac arterial disease. In such circumstances where inflow cannot rise, sympathectomy may shunt blood into the skin of the thigh and decrease the share of blood to the foot, making ischaemia worse [83–85]. Worsening ischaemia following sympathectomy has been well documented in a minority of patients, and is either due to this 'steal' or to embolization of a plaque or thrombus from the aorta or iliac artery during retraction at operation [86–88]. Thus there is no good evidence that a high lumbar sympathectomy has any value over a low lumbar sympathectomy, and it may have positive disadvantages. Removal of the fourth and possibly the third lumbar ganglion is all that is required to obtain the maximum beneficial effect.

It has been claimed that bilateral lumbar sympathectomy may result in impotence but the sympathetic nerve supply to the genitalia is mostly from the level of T10 down to L1. It has been stated that 50 per cent of men who undergo removal of L1 ganglion become impotent [89], but most recorded cases of impotence following sympathectomy occurred after thoraco-abdominal operations for hypertension in which an extensive division of the sympathetic chain was made [85]. Recent objective methods have cast new light on this confused subject [90, 91] and there is no evidence that a sympathectomy below the level of L2, even if bilateral, has any effect on potency.

The lumbar sympathectomy may be performed by an expert using an injection of 7 per cent phenol in water, controlled by image intensifier [92, 93]. There are relatively few complications of this procedure compared with even the few complications of operative sympathectomy, but there is some evidence that its effect is less complete [81], particularly if the clinician is not experienced in its use. Operative sympathectomy may be more difficult following a failed attempt at phenol ablation.

Upper thoracic sympathectomy may be approached by transaxillary [94], cervical [95] or posterior [96] routes. Injection of the chain by phenol is not sufficiently precise to avoid damage to the stellate ganglion, with a consequent risk of Horner's syndrome. Recently, small series have been described in which the second and third thoracic ganglion have been ablated via a laparoscope passed through a small incision in the axilla [97]. The chain is apparently easily identified and may be ablated with cautery. This technique holds great promise.

Sympathectomy reduces excess vascular tone in both the lower and the upper limb, but its effect in the upper limb may be very transient, lasting less than 6 months, whereas in the lower limb it is more permanent [72]. The reason for this restoration of vascular tone has been hotly debated, most surgeons believe it to be due to inadequate sympathectomy [98, 99], residual sympathetic pathways allowing cross-over renervation [100], or to nerve regeneration [101]. Operations have been devised to divide these regenerated fibres and good results have been claimed. It is interesting, however, that sudomotor activity, which depends on sympathetic nerve supply, is permanently lost following successful sympathectomy. This sudomotor activity does not return when vascular tone is restored, suggesting that the mechanism is not one of regeneration of nerves but the escape of vascular tone from sympathetic control, unless the sweat glands atrophy during the period of denervation.

Embolectomy

Invention of the balloon embolectomy catheter has revolutionized the surgical technique of thrombo-embolectomy both in the arterial and the venous system [15], although the perioperative mortality of these patients remains depressingly high. Embolectomy is an absolute surgical emergency and must be performed as early as possible. The femoral artery may be explored under local infiltrative anaesthesia in a patient unfit for general anaesthesia. The surgeon may find that the occlusion is not due solely to an embolus but to a thrombosis or embolism in an atheromatous limb, when a more complex procedure will be required. The definitive arterial reconstruction must be planned by operative aeteriography and performed immediately if it is to have any value in this complex and desperate situation. Patients with an embolus must also be treated with preoperative heparin to minimize propagated thrombus whilst they are being prepared for operation, and should be maintained on anticoagulants following operation if their embolus came from a site which could embolize again. Techniques of this operation have been fully described [15] and its complications are related to those of the embolus itself and to damage of the arterial tree by the balloon catheter, either by loosening an atheromatous plaque or by perforation of a distal artery [102].

Femoropopliteal Vein Bypass

This must include bypasses distal to the popliteal artery which are now regularly performed with results that are only slightly inferior to those of femoropopliteal bypass [103]. Limb salvage rates after reversed femoropopliteal vein bypass are between 60 and 80 per cent [104, 105].

Most surgeons agree that autogenous vein graft bypasses are superior to artificial bypasses [106], although recent claims have been made for velour Dacron [107], expanded PTFE [108] and human umbilical vein [109]. Autogenous vein has a better documented long term follow-up than any other material and its results, though less than ideal, have stood the test of time. It remains the standard by which other grafts must be measured [110]. Overall patency figures for femoropopliteal bypass are approximately 40 per cent at 5 years, and for distal bypass, slightly less.

In severe limb ischaemia, salvage rates are higher than patency rates at 5 years. Sometimes the graft may stay open sufficiently long to 'heal' and preserve the limb which then survives when the graft subsequently blocks. Thus, Taylor found a 5-year salvage rate of 65 per cent after femoropopliteal bypass in severe ischaemia, but a 40 per cent patency rate [104]. Similar results at 5 years have been reported in North America; in one series 47 per cent of grafts were patent among the surviving patients while 70 per cent of limbs were salvaged. Bypass with autogenous vein to the proximal popliteal artery gives only a slightly superior 2–5-year salvage rate (80 per cent) than bypass to the distal popliteal artery. The distal tibial and peroneal bypasses have slightly less good results. Salvage rates in a series of 364 limbs showed a 10-year limb survival rate of 60 per cent for femoropopliteal bypass as against 40 per cent for femoro-tibial bypass [103]. Many authors now claim acceptable limb salvage rates from distal bypass on to tibial arteries or the dorsalis pedis artery [99].

Most surgeons favour reversed vein bypass after initial enthusiastic reports of *in situ* vein bypass were not fulfilled in practice [111, 112]. The difficulties associated with *in situ* vein bypass are mainly related to those of inadequate destruction of valves, as there are theoretical reasons why it should be superior to reverse vein bypass. With the *in situ* vein bypass technique the larger extremity of the vein is sutured to the larger artery and *vice versa*. It is easier to prevent twisting and kinking of an *in situ* bypass than reverse bypass and there is some evidence that the lessened trauma and better blood supply of an *in situ* bypass gives a lower incidence of subintimal fibrosis, which is a common cause of late failure of reversed vein bypass. Recently a variation of the *in situ* vein bypass technique has been reported which appears to give better results in ablation of valves than any previous reported method [113]. The saphenous vein is dissected free at both its extremities and the distal vein and artery assessed as being suitable for bypass. The proximal extremity of the vein is then sutured end to side to the common femoral artery and the clamps are removed so that the vein is distended by arterial blood under full arterial blood pressure, down to the first valve. A small instrument, the Cartier vein valve stripper, is then passed up the vein and withdrawn through the tense valve cusps which are ruptured. The other valves are then ruptured in sequence as the vein distends with arterial blood until good pulsatile down-flow is obtained at the distal end. This minor modification of technique, in which the valves that are to be ablated are tense and distended by the pulsing arterial blood, may have overcome many of the practical disadvantages of *in situ* bypass and warrants further clinical trials. In many patients, however, the saphenous vein has either been previously removed or is not suitable for a long bypass, in which case there is no alternative but to use some other form of material. Debate still rages over which is the most suitable material to use in these circumstances.

Dacron Bypass

Woven Dacron femoropopliteal bypasses were used many years ago with apparently successful results. Later reports suggested that they were inadequate in the long term and their use has generally been abandoned. Knitted and, more recently, velour Dacron prostheses, associated with special techniques of pre-clotting, have been claimed to have better results [107]. Patency rates of 76 per cent at 2 years have been reported [107]. In general, however, the use of Dacron tubes below the inguinal ligament and particularly when traversing the knee joint is still unsatisfactory.

PTFE Bypass

This graft of fibrillary expanded polytetrafluoroethylene has been widely publicised and popularly acclaimed in the past 5 years. It is negatively charged, inert and seems to be a suitable graft material for large vessels. There is, however, still doubt over its value in long bypasses where flow is poor. The initial short term results of this material were encouraging, some claiming it to be as good as autogenous vein [108]. The mean follow-up period in this study was less than a year in both groups. Longer term results are slightly less encouraging. In a series of 144 Gore-Tex grafts placed below the knee patency was 62 per cent after only 18 months [114]. Controlled trials of this material versus vein are in progress. Gore-Tex has different physical properties and handling qualities from Dacron. It is non-porous, non-elastic, comes uncrimped and must be cut to the exact length and size required. A tight Gore-Tex graft is doomed to fail.

Umbilical Vein Graft

The gluteraldehyde-stabilized human umbilical cord vein is expensive but has given encouraging early results. The graft is surrounded by a Dacron mesh to prevent the aneurysm formation that was so common with bovine heterografts, although even without the mesh aneurysm formation is rare [115].

The handling properties of this graft are again quite different from either Dacron or Gore-Tex and at first it is not technically easy to use. Current reports suggest that about three-quarters of femoropopliteal biografts are patent at 2–3 years [116]. Five-year results are not yet available. Surgeons may yet be disappointed by these new grafts, as they have been by so many before.

Superficial Femoral Endarterectomy

This operation was widely practised in the early years of vascular surgery [117] but it has generally fallen from favour as its results were inferior to those of reversed vein bypass. The published results from those days, however, are not inferior to those of the modern synthetic bypasses [118]. With modern techniques of intraoperative arteriography, intraoperative monitoring of flow and fibreoptic systems to inspect the interior of an endarterectomized vessel [118], it is possible that long endarterectomy may return to favour. Some recent uncontrolled studies suggest that modern results are not inferior to reversed vein bypass.

Profundaplasty

The surgical importance of the profunda femoris artery was first recognized two decades ago [119, 120]. Direct surgical reconstruction is best reserved for those patients with an occluded superficial femoral artery and a definite tight profunda stenosis of moderate length. In these circumstances an initial limb salvage rate of 80 per cent can be expected [76, 121], although this falls to below 50 per cent at 4 years [122]. Opening up an unstenosed profunda origin has been suggested but appears to have little to recommend it. Simple profundaplasty seldom elevates ankle blood pressure much [76, 121], and is therefore of little use in claudicants. Reconstruction of the stenosed profunda femoris artery is a safe but limited operation with limited but definite benefit. It is to be recommended for the salvage of limbs of patients who do not have either the vein or the run-off to allow a long bypass. The results of long artificial bypasses remain unproved and profundaplasty, in suitable cases, is probably preferable in the first instance.

Proximal Reconstruction

A patient with a superficial femoral arterial occlusion may be tipped into a state of rest pain or gangrene by subsequent stenosis or occlusion of an iliac vessel or aorta. Good results can be obtained by a proximal arterial reconstruction into the profunda femoris artery, ignoring the distal occlusion in the superficial femoral artery. Traditionally, aorto-iliac occlusion was treated by aorto-iliac endarterectomy [123, 124], but more recently bypass from the aorta to the femoral artery has gained favour as the operation is simpler and there are fewer early re-occlusions [125–127]. The results of aorto-iliac endarterectomy and bypass are comparable; in a European series of 1071 patients with aorto-iliac disease, patency rates at 5 and 10 years were identical [128]. Endarterectomy is usually performed in the more favourable patients with more localized disease and it is therefore likely that the results of bypass are slightly superior. Endarterectomy requires special skill that many modern surgeons do not possess [63]. Bypass, however, is accompanied by a higher incidence of false aneurysm formation [129, 130], and sepsis [131] than is endarterectomy. These two procedures should really be considered not as surgical alternatives but rather complementary procedures allowing the surgeon to offer his patient the optimal vascular repair.

In poor risk patients extra-anatomical bypass from the other femoral artery [132, 133], or from the axillary artery [134–136] to one or both femoral arteries has been widely performed. The results have been surprisingly good in selected cases. It is clearly vital that a bypass must not be taken from a diseased femoral artery or one with proximal iliac stenosis or the good limb may be in danger. Many of these proximal reconstructions, both aortic and extra-anatomical, are combined with profundaplasty to improve the distal run-off. It has been suggested that failure to open up the profunda orifice is the commonest cause of aortofemoral graft thrombosis [137, 138].

It is difficult to be certain of the results of aorto-iliac reconstructions for limb salvage. Most series mix claudicant and limb salvage patients and contain a preponderance of the former. Often a distal procedure or sympathectomy is added. Results are expressed as patency rates rather than limb salvage rates. The European experience is that the overall amputation rate (14 per cent) can be halved [139].

RESULTS AND MORTALITY

The natural history of these patients and the long term results of operations for limb salvage are not well reported. This account of the graft materials and vascular procedures used in limb salvage must necessarily be inconclusive as it is extremely difficult to evaluate the true results from published studies. The difficulties in definition of the degree of ischaemia suffered by patients into whom the grafts are inserted has already been outlined in the first part of this chapter, and the definition of limb salvage itself is open to debate. Most series include patients who suffered from intermittent claudication rather than rest pain or pre-gangrene, and the percentage of patients in each category is often not mentioned. Objective data such as mean ankle blood pressure is seldom recorded and even the follow-up may be obscured by various forms of statistical analysis. No good controlled trials of the use of graft materials against autogenous vein have yet been published. It is encouraging to note that several trials are now in progress and within 2 years much harder data may be available on the true merits of these various procedures. There is no doubt, however, that the ideal vascular bypass material has yet to be found and both vascular and cardiac surgeons await its discovery.

Mortality, particularly late mortality, has also been poorly reported. In a typical case series it is often stated that so many patients were studied of whom this many were available for study at 4 years. What happened to the rest is not usually made clear, probably because most of them die. Mortality amongst patients undergoing limb salvage procedures is frighteningly high. Hospital mortality rates are about 5 per cent with a 5-year mortality around 50 per cent [140]; these figures are higher than those more usually quoted for these operations. Limb salvage saves a leg, but it does not affect the coronary artery disease, cerebrovascular disease, respiratory disease, or the incidence of cancer, all of which kill these patients. The high mortality of patients following successful limb salvage renders the long term results of operations of mostly academic value. The patients often die of systemic disease before losing their leg. Patients having embolectomy have at least a 15 per cent mortality, which is associated more with their simultaneous life-threatening disease than the dangers of the operation. The mortality of primary amputation remains even higher than that of arterial reconstruction. Hospital mortality for above-knee amputation is 15 per cent [141, 142]. Approximately a further 15 per cent will suffer delayed stump healing or require re-amputation [141]. A quarter of amputees will have died at 2 years [142] and an astonishing 75 per cent at 5 years [141]. The primary operation of limb salvage is less dangerous than amputation and the quality of life is better, although it may not be lengthened.

Really worth-while results can be obtained in patients with advanced ischaemia in whom the only alternative is amputation [143]. It must be a useful limb that is salvaged, not one that is still the seat of rest pain and ulceration. Increasing cynicism of some claims from studies of limb salvage has led eminent surgeons to suggest that limb salvage is a waste of time [144]. We consider that what is necessary is not to abandon attempts at limb salvage, but to investigate it more scientifically and assess the patients more accurately before operation. In this way those patients who will truly benefit can be selected for vascular surgery and those who will not can be treated by primary amputation. We have a long way to go to this end.

REFERENCES

1. Eastcott H. H. G. (1974) *Arterial Surgery,* 2nd ed. London, Pitman Medical, pp. 30–40.
2. Carter S. A. (1978) Role of pressure measurements in vascular disease. In: Bernstein E. F. (ed.) *Non-invasive Diagnostic Techniques in Vascular Disease.* St Louis, Mosby, p. 275.
3. Yao J. S. T., Hobbs J. T. and Irvine W. T. (1969) Ankle systolic pressure measurements in arterial disease affecting the lower extremities. *Br. J. Surg.* **56**, 676–9.
4. Cutajar C. L., Marston A. and Newcombe J. F. (1973) Value of cuff occlusion pressures in assessment of peripheral vascular disease. *Br. Med. J.* **2**, 392.
5. Raines J. K., Darling R. C., Buth J. et al. (1976) Vascular laboratory criteria for the management of peripheral vascular disease of the lower extremities. *Surgery* **79**, 21.
6. Carter S. A. and Lezack J. D. (1971) Digital systolic pressures in the lower limb in arterial disease. *Circulation* **43**, 905.
7. Schatz I. J., Fine G. and Gyler W. R. (1966) Thromboangiitis obliterans. *Br. Heart J.* **28**, 84.
8. Conrad M. C. (1967) Large and small artery occlusion in diabetics and non-diabetics with severe vascuiar disease. *Circulation* **36**, 83.
9. Gensler S. W., Haimovici H., Hoffert P. et al. (1965) Study of vascular lesions in diabetic, non-diabetic patients. *Arch Surg.* **91**, 617.
10. Strandness D. E., Priest R. E. and Gibbons G. E. (1964) Combined clinical and pathologic study of diabetic and non-diabetic peripheral arterial disease. *Diabetes* **13**, 366.
11. Jacobs A. L. (1959) *Arterial Embolism in the Limbs.* Edinburgh, Livingstone.
12. Somerville W. and Chambers R. J. (1964) Systemic embolism in mitral stenosis: relation to the size of the left atrial appendix. *Br. Med. J.* **2**, 1167.
13. Cranley J. J., Krause R. J., Strasser E. S. et al. (1964) Peripheral arterial embolism: changing concepts. *Surgery* **55**, 57.

14. Darling R. C., Austen W. G. and Linton R. R. (1967) Arterial embolism. *Surg. Gynecol. Obstet.* **124**, 106.
15. Fogarty T. J., Daily P. O., Shumway N. E. et al. (1971) Experience with balloon catheter technique for arterial embolectomy. *Am. J. Surg.* **122**, 231.
16. Edwards W. S. (1978) Lower limb ischaemia from atheromatous emboli. In: Bergan J. J. and Yao J. S. T. (ed.) *Gangrene and Severe Ischaemia of the Lower Extremities*. New York, Grune & Stratton, pp. 157–68.
17. Perry M. O. (1977) Acute arterial insufficiency. In: Rutherford R. B. (ed.) *Vascular Surgery*. Philadelphia, Saunders, p. 417.
18. Nieman H. L. (1978) Angiography in patients with severe peripheral ischaemia. In: Bergan J. J. and Yao J. S. T. (ed.) *Gangrene and Severe Ischaemia of the Lower Extremities*. New York, Grune & Stratton, pp. 63–83.
19. Rutherford R. B. (1973) *Peripheral Vascular Injuries. The Management of Trauma*. Philadelphia, Saunders.
20. Parker M. T. (1969) Postoperative clostridial infections in Britain. *Br. Med. J.* **3**, 671.
21. Hall H. R. and Shucksmith H. S. (1971) The above-knee amputation for ischaemia. *Br. J. Surg.* **58**, 656.
22. Evans W. E. and Steele G. (1977) Peripheral artery aneurysms. In: Rutherford R. B. (ed.) *Vascular Surgery*. Philadelphia, Saunders, p. 692.
23. Wychulis A. R., Spittell J. A. and Wallace R. B. (1970) Popliteal aneurysms. *Surgery* **68**, 942.
24. Evans W. E. and Steele G. (1977) Peripheral artery aneurysms. In: Rutherford R. B. (ed.) *Vascular Surgery*. Philadelphia, Saunders, p. 688.
25. Leading Article (1966) Popliteal aneurysms. *Br. Med. J.* **1**, 625.
26. Woodruff M. (1966) Popliteal aneurysms. *Br. Med. J.* **1**, 918.
27. Eastcott H. H. G. (1966) Popliteal aneurysms. *Br. Med. J.* **1**, 799.
28. Eastcott H. H. G. (1973) Aortic and peripheral aneurysms. In: *Arterial Surgery*, 2nd ed. London, Pitman Medical, p. 319.
29. McKusick V. A. (1955) The cardiovascular aspects of Marfan's syndrome: a hereditable disorder of connective tissue. **11**, 321.
30. Barabas A. P. (1972) Vascular complications of the Ehlers–Danlos syndrome: with special reference to the 'arterial type' or Sack's syndrome. *J. Cardiovasc. Surg.* **13**, 160.
31. Hirst A. E., Johns V. J. and Kime S.W. (1958) Dissecting aneurysms of the aorta: a review of 505 cases. *Medicine (Baltimore)* **37**, 217.
32. Greenhalgh R. M. and Mills S. P. (1978) On Buerger's disease: a recognisable syndrome. In: Bergan J. J. and Yao J. S. T. (ed.) *Gangrene and Severe Ischaemia of the Lower Extremities*. New York, Grune & Stratton, pp. 139–55.
33. Nielubowicz J. (1980) Buerger's disease. *J. Cardiovasc. Surg.* **21**, 529–36.
34. Eastcott H. H. G. (1973) Buerger's disease. In: *Arterial Surgery*, 2nd ed. London, Pitman Medical, p. 103.
35. Bron K. M., Strott C. A. and Shapiro A. P. (1965) The diagnostic value of angiographic observations in polyarteritis nodosa. A case of multiple aneurysms in the visceral organs. *Arch. Intern. Med.* **116**, 450.
36. Dubois E. L. and Arterberry J. D. (1964) Gangrene as a manifestation of systemic lupus erythematosus. *Am. Heart J.* **68**, 119.
37. Miller G. A. H., Thomas M. L. and Medd W. E. (1962) Aortic arch syndrome and polymyositis with LE cells in peripheral blood. *Br. Med. J.* **1**, 771.
38. Hauser W. A., Ferguson R. H., Holley K. E. et al. (1971) Temporal arteritis in Rochester, Minnesota, 1951 to 1967. *Mayo Clin. Proc.* **46**, 597.
39. Bywaters E. G. L. (1957) Peripheral vascular obstruction in rheumatoid arthritis and its relationship to other vascular lesions. *Ann. Rheum. Dis.* **16**, 84.
40. Scott J. T., Hourihane D. O., Doyle F. H. et al. (1961) Digital arteritis in rheumatoid disease. *Ann. Rheum. Dis.* **20**, 224.

41. McCusick V. A. (1962) A form of vascular disease relatively frequent in the Orient. *Am. Heart J.* **63**, 57.
42. Bonventre M. V. (1974) Takayasu's disease revisited. *NY State J. Med.* **74**, 1960.
43. Cranley J. J., Krause R. J., Strasser E. S. et al. (1963) Impending gangrene of four extremities secondary to ergotism. *N. Engl. J. Med.* **269**, 727.
44. Cohen S. M. (1948) Accidental intra-arterial injection of drugs. *Lancet* **2**, 361, 409.
45. Gagnon R. (1966) Superficial arteries of the cubital fossa with reference to accidental intra-arterial injections. *Can. J. Surg.* **9**, 57.
46. Perkins J., Israels M. C. G. and Wilkinson J. F. (1964) Polycythaemia vera. Clinical studies on a series of 127 patients managed without radiation therapy. *Q. J. Med.* **33**, 499.
47. Wasserman L. R. and Gilbert H. S. (1963) Surgery in polycythaemia vera. *N. Engl. J. Med.* **269**, 1226.
48. Inman W. H. W., Vessey M. P., Westerholm B. et al. (1970) Thromboembolic disease and the steroidal content of oral contraceptives. *Br. Med. J.* **2**, 203.
49. Keown D. (1969) Review of arterial thrombosis in association with oral contraceptives. *Br. J. Surg.* **56**, 486–8.
50. Dahn I., Hallböök T., Larsen O. A. et al. (1969) Treatment of acute ischaemic pain in the leg by induced hypertension. *Acta Chir. Scand.* **135**, 391.
51. Wade O. L. and Bishop J. M. (1962) *Cardiac Output and Regional Blood Flow*. Oxford, Blackwell.
52. Levin M. E. and O'Neal L. W. *The Diabetic Foot*. St Louis, Mosby.
53. Bauer G. (1964) Clinical experiences of a surgeon in the use of heparin. *Am. J. Cardiol.* **14**, 29.
54. Margolies M. N., Ring E. J., Waltman A. C. et al. (1972) Arteriography in the management of hemorrhage from pelvic fractures. *N. Engl. J. Med.* **287**, 317.
55. Illingworth C. (1962) Treatment of arterial occlusion under oxygen at two-atmospheres pressure. *Br. Med. J.* **2**, 1271.
56. Pardy B. J., Eastcott H. H. G. and Miles C. (1980) Preliminary experience with prostaglandin E1 in extremity ischaemia. *Br. J. Surg.* **67**, 824.
57. Greenhalgh R. M. (1981) Naftidrofuryl for ischaemic rest pain: a controlled trial. *Br. J. Surg.* **68**, 265.
58. Clyne C. A. C., Galland R. B., Fox M. J. et al. (1980) A controlled trial of naftidrofuryl (Praxilene) in the treatment of intermittent claudication. *Br. J. Surg.* **67**, 347–8.
59. Baird R. N. (1980) Treatment of vasospastic disease with prostaglandin E1. *Br. Med. J.* **281**, 1031.
60. Talpos G., Horrocks M., White J. M. et al. (1978) Plasmapheresis in Raynaud's disease. *Lancet* **1**, 416.
61. Dodds A. J., O'Reilly M. J. G., Yates C. J. P. et al. (1979) Haemorheological response to plasma exchange in Raynaud's phenomenon. *Br. Med. J.* **2**, 1186.
62. Eastcott H. H. G. (1973) Arteritis. In: *Arterial Surgery*, 2nd ed. London, Pitman Medical, p. 143.
63. Stoney R. J. (1978) Ultimate salvage for the patient with limb threatening ischaemia. In: Bergan J. J. and Yao J. S. T. (ed.) *Gangrene and Severe Ischaemia of the Lower Extremities*. New York, Grune & Stratton, pp. 383–92.
64. Thompson R. G. (1978) Performance of major amputations for severe ischaemia. In: Bergan J. J. and Yao J. S. T. (ed.) *Gangrene and Severe Ischaemia of the Lower Extremities*. New York, Grune & Stratton, pp. 407–17.
65. Leading Article (1977) *Br. Med. J.* **2**, 1244.
66. Brown A. A. and Nicholls R. J. (1977) Crush syndrome: a report of 2 cases and a review of the literature. *Br. J. Surg.* **64**, 397–402.
67. Patman R. D. and Thompson J. E. (1970) Fasciotomy in peripheral vascular surgery. *Arch Surg.* **101**, 663.

68. Rutherford R. B. and Valenta J. (1971) Extremity blood flow and distribution: the effects of arterial occlusion, sympathectomy and exercise. *Surgery* **69**, 332.
69. Rutherford R. B. (1980) Complications of sympathectomy. In: Bernhard V. M. and Towne J. B. (ed.) *Complications in Vascular Surgery*. New York, Grune & Stratton, p. 134.
70. Cronenwett J. L. and Lindenauer S. M. (1980) Haemodynamic effects of sympathectomy in ischaemic canine hindlimbs. *Surgery* **87**, 417.
71. May A. G., De Weese J. A. and Rob C. G. (1968) Effect of sympathectomy on blood flow in arterial stenosis. *Ann. Surg.* **158**, 182.
72. Gillespie J. A. (1960) Late effects of lumbar sympathectomy on blood flow in the foot in obliterative vascular disease. *Lancet* **1**, 891.
73. Yao J. S. T. and Bergan J. J. (1973) Predictability of vascular reactivity relative to sympathetic ablation. *Arch. Surg.* **107**, 676.
74. Terry H. J., Allan J. S. and Taylor G. W. (1970) The effect of adding lumbar sympathectomy to reconstructive arterial surgery in the lower limb. *Br. J. Surg.* **57**, 51.
75. Seeger J. M., Lazarus H. M. and Aho D. (1977) Pre-operative selection of patients for lumbar sympathectomy by use of Doppler index. *Am. J. Surg.* **134**, 749.
76. Lewis J. D. and Jamieson C. W. (1972) Pressure and flow in blood vessels. *Proc. R. Soc. Med.* **65**, 1121–3.
77. Kim G. E., Ibrahim L. M. and Imparato A. M. (1976) Lumbar sympathectomy in end-stage arterial occlusive disease. *Ann Surg.* **183**, 157–60.
78. Taylor G. W. and Calo A. R. (1962) Atherosclerosis of arteries of lower limbs. *Br. Med. J.* **1**, 507.
79. Strand L. (1969) Lumbar sympathectomy in the treatment of peripheral obliterative arterial disease. *Acta Chir. Scand.* **135**, 597.
80. Ozeran R. S., Wagner G. R. and Reimer T. R. (1970) Neuropathy of the sympathetic nervous system associated with diabetes mellitus. *Surgery* **68**, 953.
81. Lemberger R. J., Hopkinson B. R. and Makin G. S. (1980) An assessment of the completeness of phenol lumbar sympathectomy. Paper read to the Vascular Surgical Society of Great Britain and Ireland, London, 1980.
82. Yeager G. H. and Cowley R. A. (1948) Anatomical observations on the lumbar sympathetic with evaluation of sympathectomies in organic peripheral disease. *Ann. Surg.* **127**, 953.
83. Szilagyi D. E., Smith R. F., Scerpella J. R. et al. (1967) Lumbar sympathectomy; current role in the treatment of arteriosclerotic occlusive disease. *Arch. Surg.* **95**, 753.
84. Fulton R. L. and Blakeley W. R. (1968) Lumbar sympathectomy. A procedure of questionable value in the treatment of arteriosclerosis obliterans of the legs. *Am. J. Surg.* **116**, 735.
85. Gillespie J. A. (1960) Further place of lumbar sympathectomy in obliterative vascular disease of lower limbs. *Br. Med. J.* **2**, 1640.
86. Key J. A. (1960) Silent thrombosis in major limb arteries: a post-operative hazard. *Surgery* **47**, 734.
87. Bergan N. J. and Trippel D. H. (1962) Arteriograms in ischaemic limbs worsened after lumbar sympathectomy. *Arch Surg.* **85**, 643.
88. Eastcott H. H. G. (1973) Sympathectomy. In: *Arterial Surgery*, 2nd ed. London, Pitman Medical, p. 196.
89. Whitelaw G. P. and Smithwick R. H. (1951) Some secondary effects of sympathectomy, with particular reference to disturbance of sexual dysfunction. *N. Engl. J. Med.* **245**, 22.
90. Queral L. A., Whitehouse W. M. and Flinn W. R. (1979) Pelvic haemodynamics after aortoiliac reconstruction. *Surgery* **86**, 799.
91. Engel G., Burnham S. and Carter M. F. (1978) Penile blood pressure in the evaluation of erectile impotence. *Fertil. Steril.* **30**, 687.

92. Haxton H. A. (1949) Chemical sympathectomy. *Br. Med. J.* **1**, 1026.
93. Reid W., Watt J. K. and Gray T. G. (1970) Phenol injection of the sympathetic chain. *Br. J. Surg.* **57**, 45.
94. Atkins H. J. B. (1954) Sympathectomy by the axillary approach. *Lancet* **1**, 538.
95. Telford E. D. (1935) The technique of sympathectomy. *Br. J. Surg.* **23**, 448.
96. Smithwick R. H. (1940) The rationale and technic of sympathectomy for the relief of vascular spasm of the extremities. *N. Engl. J. Med.* **222**, 699.
97. Weale F. E. (1980) Upper thoracic sympathectomy by transthoracic electrocoagulation. *Br. J. Surg.* **67**, 71–3.
98. Pratt G. H. (1955) Amputation after surgical sympathectomy for obliterative vascular disease. *Surg. Gynecol. Obstet.* **100**, 43.
99. Popkin R. J. (1957) Sympathectomies in peripheral vascular diseases: follow-up studies in twenty years. *Angiology* **8**, 156.
100. Ray B. S. and Console A. D. (1948) Residual sympathetic pathways after paravertebral sympathectomy. *J. Neurosurg.* **5**, 23.
101. Murray J. C. and Thompson J. W. (1957) Collateral sprouting in response to injury of the autonomic nervous system and its consequence. *Br. Med. Bull.* **13**, 213.
102. Foster J. H. (1970) Arterial injuries secondary to the use of the Fogarty catheter. *Ann. Surg.* **171**, 971.
103. Reichle F. A. (1978) Long and short term results of autogenous vein bypass in the severely ischaemic lower extremity. In: Bergan J. J. and Yao J. S. T. (ed.) *Gangrene and Severe Ischaemia of the Lower Extremities*. New York, Grune & Stratton, p. 250.
104. Taylor G. W. (1973) Chronic arterial occlusion. In: Birnsting M. (ed.) *Peripheral Vascular Surgery*. London, Heinemann Medical, p. 231.
105. De Weese J. A. and Rob C. G. (1971) Autogenous vein bypass: 5 years later. *Ann. Surg.* **174**, 346.
106. Szilagyi D. E., Smith R. F., Elliot J. P. et al. (1965) Long-term behaviour of a Dacron arterial substitute. Clinical, roentgenologic and histologic correlations. *Ann. Surg.* **162**, 453.
107. Yates S. G., Barros D'Sa A. A. B., Berger K. et al. (1978) The preclotting of porous arterial prostheses. *Ann. Surg.* **188**, 611–22.
108. Veith F. J., Moss C. M., Fell S. C. et al. (1978) Comparison of expanded polytetrafluoroethylene and autologous saphenous vein grafts in high risk arterial reconstructions for limb salvage. *Surg. Gynecol. Obstet.* **147**, 749–52.
109. Dardik H., Ibrahim I. M., Dardik I. (1978) Experience with infrageniculate vascular reconstructions using glutaraldehyde-stabilized umbilical vein prosthesis. In: Bergan J. J. and Yao J. S. T. (ed.) *Gangrene and Severe Ischemia of the Lower Extremities*. New York, Grune & Stratton, pp. 285–302.
110. Linton R. R. (1971) Long term results of femoropopliteal autogenous vein grafts. In: Dale A. W. (ed.) *Management of Arterial Occlusive Disease*. Chicago, Year Book, pp. 97–117.
111. Rostad H., Hall K. V. and Dundas P. (1979) The great saphenous vein used in situ after vein valve extirpation. Long term results. *J. Cardiovasc. Surg.* **20**, 545–52.
112. Rob C. G. (1963) Autogenous in situ saphenous vein bypass for femoropopliteal occlusive disease. *Surgery* **55**, 114.
113. Galland R. B., Young A. E. and Jamieson C. W. (1981) In situ bypass: a modified technique. *Ann. R. Coll. Surg. Engl.* **63**, 186.
114. Raithel D. and Groitl H. (1980) Small artery reconstruction with a new vascular prosthesis. *World J. Surg.* **4**, 223–30.
115. Baier R. E., Akers C. K., Natiella J. R. et al. (1980) The physiochemical properties of the stabilised umbilical vein. *Vasc. Surg.* **14**, 145–57.
116. Dardik H., Ibrahim I. M., Jarrah M. et al. (1980) Three year experience with glutaraldehyde-stabilized umbilical vein for limb salvage. *Br. J. Surg.* **67**, 229–32.

117. Cockett F. B. and Maurice B. A. (1963) Evolution of direct arterial surgery for claudication and ischaemia of legs: a nine years' survey. *Br. Med. J.* **1**, 353–60.
118. Vollmar J., Trede M., Laubach K. et al. (1968) Principles of reconstructive procedures for chronic femoropopliteal occlusions. Report on 546 operations. *Ann. Surg.* **168**, 215.
119. Morris C. G., Edwards W. and Cooley D. A. (1961) Surgical importance of the profunda femoris artery. *Arch. Surg.* **82**, 32–9.
120. Natali J. (1962) Les pontages utilisant l'artere-femorale profunde. Techniques et indications. *J. Chir.* **83**, 565–80.
121. Hill D. A. and Jamieson C. W. (1977) The results of arterial reconstruction using the profunda femoris artery in the treatment of rest pain and gangrene. *Br. J. Surg.* **64**, 359–62.
122. Ward A. S. and Morris-Jones W. (1977) The long term results of profundaplasty for femoropopliteal occlusion. *Br. J. Surg.* **64**, 365–7.
123. Inhara T. (1972) Endarterectomy for occlusive disease of the aortoiliac and common femoral arteries. *Am. J. Surg.* **124**, 235.
124. Pilcher D. B., Barker W. F. and Cannon J. A. (1970) An aortoiliac endarterectomy case series followed 10 years or more. *Surgery* **67**, 5.
125. Malone J. M., Moore W. S. and Goldstone J. (1975) The natural history of bilateral aortofemoral bypass grafts for ischaemia of the lower extremities. *Arch. Surg.* **110**, 1300.
126. Malone J. M., Moore W. S. and Goldstone J. (1977) Life expectancy following aortofemoral arterial grafting. *Surgery* **81**, 551.
127. Garpard et al. (1972) Aorto-ilio femoral thromboendarterectomy versus bypass grafts. *Arch. Surg.* **105**, 898.
128. Schulz Z., Laubach K. and Preissler P. (1977) Zur wahl des operationsver fahrens im aorto-iliacalen. *Langenbecks Arch. Chir.* **344**, 41–52.
129. Szilagyi D. E., Smith R. F., Elliott J. P. et al. (1976) Anastomotic false aneurysms and vascular reconstruction: problems of incidence, etiology and treatment. *J. Cardiovasc. Surg.* **17**, 100.
130. Christensen R. D. and Bernatz P. E. (1972) Anastomotic aneurysms involving the femoral artery. *Mayo Clin. Proc.* **47**, 313.
131. Szilagyi E. D., Smith R. F., Elliott J. P. et al. (1972) Infection in arterial reconstruction with synthetic grafts. *Ann. Surg.* **176**, 321.
132. Brief D. K., Brener B. J. and Parsonnet V. (1975) Crossover femoro-femoral grafts followed up five years or more. *Arch. Surg.* **110**, 294.
133. Sethi G. K., Crawford F. A., Scott S. M. et al. (1975) Femoro-femoral bypass graft: choice or compromise? *Am. Surg.* **41**, 61.
134. Johnson W. C., Logerfo F. W., Vallman R. W. et al. (1977) Is axillo-bilateral femoral graft an effective substitute for aortic-bilateral iliac-femoral graft? *Ann. Surg.* **186**, 123.
135. Plecha F. R. and Pories W. J. (1976) Extra-anatomic bypasses for aorto-iliac disease in high risk patients. *Surgery* **80**, 480.
136. Mannick J. A. et al. (1970) The late results of axillo-femoral grafts. *Surgery* **68**, 1038.
137. Bernhard V. M., Ray L. I. and Towne J. B. (1977) The reoperation of choice for aortofemoral graft occlusion. *Surgery* **82**, 867–74.
138. Boren C. H., Towne J. B. and Bernhard V. M. (1980) Femoro-popliteal collateral index: a guide to successful profundaplasty. *Arch. Surg.* **115**, 1366.
139. Vollmar J. F. and Heyden B. (1979) Experiences with reconstructive surgery of the aorto-iliac segment. In: Bergan J. J. and Yao J. S. T. (ed.) *Surgery of the Aorta and its Body Branches*. New York, Grune & Stratton, p. 260.
140. Leading Article (1980) *Lancet* **1**, 23.
141. Finch D. R. A., MacDougal M., Tibbs D. J. et al. (1980) Amputation for vascular disease: the experience of a peripheral vascular unit. *Br. J. Surg.* **67**, 233–7.

142. Huston C. C., Bivins B. A., Ernst C. B. et al. (1980) Morbid implications of above knee amputations. *Arch. Surg.* **115**, 165–7.
143. Eastcott H. H. G. (1973) The contribution of arterial reconstruction to limb salvage. In: *Arterial Surgery*, 2nd ed. London, Pitman Medical, p. 90.
144. Stoney R. J. (1978) Ultimate salvage for the patient with limb threatening ischaemia. Realistic goals and surgical considerations. *Am. J. Surg.* **136**, 228.

G. D. O. Lowe and C. R. M. Prentice

9 Medical Management of Peripheral Arterial Disease

In this chapter we shall discuss the medical management of peripheral arterial disease in three parts—chronic lower limb ischaemia, Raynaud's syndrome and peripheral thromboembolism. In conclusion, we attempt to place the role of medical management in its proper perspective.

CHRONIC LOWER LIMB ISCHAEMIA

Symptomatic peripheral arterial disease of the lower limbs is a malignant condition with a 5-year survival rate of about 50 per cent [1] —a prognosis similar to colonic cancer. The basic cause is athero-sclerosis, often complicated by arterial thromboembolism: the relative importance of these pathological entities to clinical events in the lower limbs is not well understood [2]. The exact nature of 'Buerger's disease' remains controversial. Significant arterial disease of the lower limbs is usually accompanied by comparable disease of the coronary and carotid arteries [3]. This accounts for the high incidence of clinical symptoms and signs of coronary and cerebral disease in patients with chronic limb ischaemia, and also for their poor prognosis. The majority will die of ischaemic heart disease; stroke is the next commonest killer, and about 5 claudicants out of 6 die from vascular disease [4, 5].

The prevalence of intermittent claudication in patients aged 45–69 years from two general practices in Oxfordshire was 2 per cent in men and 1 per cent in women [6]. The prevalence in those aged over 70 is not known: the provocative suggestion has been made that 'perhaps almost every person over the age of 70 would claudicate, if unhampered by physical or social constraints' [7]. Epidemiological studies show that intermittent claudication is associated with smoking, male sex, high blood pressure, glucose intolerance and increased plasma levels of cholesterol, triglyceride, uric acid and fibrinogen; but not with obesity [4, 6, 8, 9].

The initial presentation of chronic occlusion of lower limb arteries is often intermittent claudication. The natural history of the disease, obscured by an enthusiastic wave of reconstructive vascular surgery in the 1960s [7], is becoming clearer. The majority of patients improve their walking ability over a few months—this is attributed to development of collateral vessels. However, progressive occlusion in some patients leads to reduction in walking ability, progression of unilateral symptoms to bilateral, and development of coldness, numbness, rest pain and gangrene. A heart attack or stroke may occur at any time and kill the patient, or render his claudication irrelevant due to limitation of walking by angina, hemiparesis, or the tiredness and breathlessness of heart failure. Chronic bronchitis may also disable the smoker before claudication occurs. There is no doubt that patients who continue to smoke have a worse prognosis, with or without surgery [1, 4, 10–13]. Other factors associated with poor prognosis are age, clinical evidence of coronary or cerebral artery disease and diabetes [1, 4]. On the other hand, levels of blood pressure, plasma lipids and plasma glucose do not appear to be related to prognosis [1, 4]. We have reviewed studies relating various haemostatic and haemorheological factors to prognosis (*see* Chapter 2) and concluded that these relationships could arise from mutual associations of blood tests and prognosis with other variables, such as smoking. Juergens et al. [4] associated poor prognosis with aorto-iliac disease compared to femoral disease; and Lassen and Tønnesen [14] have suggested that low resting distal blood pressure may be an adverse factor.

General Management of Lower Limb Ischaemia

In view of the high frequency of co-existing coronary and cerebral arterial disease and chronic bronchitis, an overall assessment of the patient's general condition and prognosis should be made in planning treatment. At the time of initial assessment, patients with mild or moderate *claudication* should be given an explanation of their symptoms in simple terms, and told of the possibility of some spontaneous improvement. After a reasonable period of observation to see if this occurs, say 3 months, patients should be referred to the vascular surgery clinic for consideration for reconstructive surgery. Patients with disabling claudication, *rest pain,* or *pre-gangrene* require more urgent referral to the surgeon. They should be advised to avoid injury to the feet from tight footwear, hot water bottles or inexpert cutting of the nails. The services of a chiropodist should be arranged, especially for diabetics, who commonly have peripheral neuropathy and poor vision for cutting their own toenails. Unremitting nocturnal pain, insomnia and fear of amputation may lead to depression: sympathetic communication, adequate analgesia and judicious use of hypnotics and antidepressants are important. Infection should be treated with appropriate antimicrobials in doses large enough to achieve adequate levels in ischaemic tissue.

Smoking

As discussed above, there is now abundant evidence that continued smoking is associated with poor prognosis for life and for limb, with or without surgery. The mechanisms by which smoking exerts these effects are not fully understood, but may include vasoconstriction, endothelial injury, increased levels of carboxyhaemoglobin causing tissue hypoxia [15] and a variety of changes in haemostatic and haemorheological factors (Chapter 2). All patients must be strongly advised to give up smoking completely, but doctors must realize how difficult withdrawal is for the nicotine addict, even when motivated by his gangrenous foot. Few patients can stop smoking at once. The logical approach is the standard method of withdrawing any addictive drug—gradual dose reduction while the patient tries to change his lifestyle. A recently introduced aid to nicotine withdrawal is nicotine chewing-gum (Nicorette), which has shown promising initial results. During nicotine withdrawal, continuous counselling is required to support and motivate the patient. Hughson et al. [1] found it helpful to show their patients a life table from their article, which graphically demonstrated the difference in prognosis between patients who stopped smoking and patients who did not.

Exercise

It appears reasonable to encourage patients with intermittent claudication to exercise daily up to the point of pain: it should be explained that reducing the speed of walking allows increased claudication distance. Following regular exercise, walking capacity improves [16–18], but the mechanisms are not understood [19]. Some centres use supervised exercise classes to supplement patients' own daily activities [19], but their value requires assessment in controlled studies.

Obesity

While it would seem sensible to encourage weight reduction and reduce the load on calf muscles, especially in the obese and in diabetics, it is well recognized that smokers are thinner than non-smokers and put on weight when they stop smoking. Since smoking is associated with arterial disease and its prognosis, whereas obesity is associated with neither, reduction in smoking must take precedence over reduction in weight.

Diabetes

All patients with peripheral arterial disease must be screened for diabetes with random tests of urine and blood. It is reasonable to attempt good control of blood glucose levels, but the effect of glycaemia control on atherosclerosis is still uncertain, and other 'risk factors' in diabetics should not be ignored [20].

Hyperlipidaemia

Elevated plasma levels of cholesterol and triglyceride are associated with peripheral arterial disease. Whether they play a causal role is not established. The benefits of lowering raised lipid levels are not known. There is some evidence that lipid reduction may prevent progression of peripheral arterial disease [21–23], but long-term controlled studies with clinically meaningful end points are required. In a primary prevention trial of blood lipid reduction using clofibrate, treatment did not reduce fatal heart attacks, angina or clinical peripheral arterial disease: furthermore, total mortality was increased [24].

Hypertension

Elevated levels of systolic and diastolic blood pressure are associated with peripheral arterial disease. Treatment of hypertension has been shown to reduce the incidence of stroke, heart failure and renal failure and is, therefore, justified: however, there is as yet little evidence of benefit in terms of peripheral or coronary arterial disease [25–27].

Beta-adrenergic Blocker Drugs

These drugs are commonly prescribed for hypertension and/or angina in patients with peripheral arterial disease. A careful watch should be kept for symptoms of cold extremities, which are frequent in patients taking beta-blockers and which are probably related to reduced peripheral blood flow. Cardioselective beta-blockers have been advocated, as they may be less likely to cause peripheral vascular symptoms, bronchospasm in patients with chronic obstructive airways disease and masking of hypoglycaemic symptoms in diabetics. There are occasional reports of peripheral skin necrosis on beta-blocker therapy [28] but the mechanism is not understood.

Anaemia and Polycythaemia

A blood count should be routinely performed in patients with arterial disease. Anaemia increases tissue hypoxia and should be investigated and appropriately treated. Polycythaemia increases blood viscosity, may present as a peripheral vascular episode and should also be investigated and treated. Men with a haematocrit over 0·54, and women with a haematocrit over 0·50, should be referred to a haematologist. A fall in haematocrit may follow reduction in smoking habit [29]. Blood volume studies differentiate true polycythaemia (increased red cell mass) from pseudo-polycythaemia (decreased plasma volume): however, both these groups are at increased risk of vascular events [30, 31], and in both groups the haematocrit can be reduced by venesection [32]. Current practice in polycythaemia vera is to maintain the venous haematocrit in the low–normal range (below 0·45) by venesection or ^{32}P therapy [31]. However, in patients with claudication there is no evidence of benefit in walking ability after venesection from a high or high–normal haematocrit to a low or low–normal haematocrit [33 and unpublished personal observations]. While thrombotic and haemorrhagic complications after vascular surgery are related to high preoperative haemoglobin levels [34], there is as yet no evidence that preoperative venesection reduces such complications. Controlled trials of preoperative haematocrit reduction would certainly be of interest.

Haemodilution

The deliberate induction of anaemia by venesection combined with fluid infusion to maintain blood volume (isovolaemic haemodilution) has been advocated in peripheral arterial disease. The rationale is that improved blood flow from viscosity reduction will outweigh decreased oxygen carriage from reduced haemoglobin concentration, and hence tissue oxygen delivery (blood flow × oxygen content) will increase. Uncontrolled studies have reported improvement in claudication [35] and ischaemic skin ulceration [36]. In view of the expense of this therapy, as well as the possible risks of coronary and cerebral events (from anaemia, hypovolaemia and reactive thrombocytosis) in patients with diseased coronary and cerebral arteries, controlled studies are indicated.

The observation of Bailey et al. [37] that diabetics undergoing limited amputations fared better if their haemoglobin level was low (< 12 g/dl) suggests that similar controlled studies would also be worth while in this situation.

Dextran

Intravenous infusion of dextran has been advocated in the treatment of rest pain or pre-gangrene. Contrary to popular belief, dextrans have no specific effect on blood viscosity. In fact, the high molecular weight dextran molecules increase the viscosity of plasma. This effect is counterbalanced by a fall in haematocrit and hence in whole blood viscosity due to the diluting effect of the infused fluid, and also to a further increase in plasma volume as the hyperosmolar dextran draws in further fluid from the extravascular space. Thus, dextran reduces blood viscosity by haemodilution [38]. In low-flow states, the increase in blood volume may increase blood flow: at the same time hypervolaemia may induce acute pulmonary oedema in patients with impaired cardiac reserve. Other adverse effects include anaphylaxis, bleeding and renal failure.

Peripheral blood flow increases acutely following dextran infusion: this is probably a consequence of hypervolaemia rather than reduction in blood viscosity [39, 40], and nutritional blood flow is not increased [41]. Clinical benefit from dextran infusion has yet to be assessed by double-blind controlled trials.

Defibrinating Agents

Venesection and fluid infusion lower blood viscosity by reducing the haematocrit. A second approach to viscosity reduction is lowering the plasma fibrinogen level. As discussed previously (Chapter 2), fibrinogen reduction causes decreased plasma viscosity and also decreased red cell aggregation: these two effects cause reduction in blood viscosity, particularly at the low shear rates which favour red cell aggregation. Two defibrinating agents, derived from snake venoms, have been used in the treatment of peripheral arterial disease: ancrod (Arvin) is available in the United Kingdom and batroxobin (Defibrase) is also available in Europe. Both these agents cause a rapid fall in fibrinogen and viscosity when given by intravenous or subcutaneous injection. They appear to be reasonably safe, but bleeding is sometimes encountered after trauma or from lesions with bleeding potential. Treatment is possible for about 6 weeks, after which antibodies usually develop and neutralize the defibrinating effects. Several uncontrolled studies have reported clinical benefit in claudication [42] and rest pain [43]. However, three double-blind controlled trials have shown no benefit of defibrination over placebo in either claudication [44] or rest pain [45, 46].

Other Drugs Altering Blood Viscosity

Clofibrate reduces plasma fibrinogen and hence blood viscosity [47] as well as blood lipid levels. Postlethwaite and Dormandy [48] reported benefit in claudication, but this has not been confirmed by double-blind trials. As previously noted, clofibrate increases mortality [24] and should therefore be reserved for treatment of diabetic retinopathy only. In recent years several vasodilator drugs, both old and new, have been claimed to reduce blood viscosity, to increase red cell deformability, and to increase walking ability. At present we, like Mashiah et al. [49] and Dormandy, who has recently reviewed this topic [50], reserve judgement on these claims. Further studies are required—laboratory studies using improved rheological techniques and clinical studies which should be double-blind controlled trials.

Vasodilator Drugs

Vasodilators are of no proved value in peripheral arterial disease [51–53] but millions of pounds are spent each year in prescribing them, presumably because of their placebo effect. This money could be better spent if cheap placebos were prescribed. In severe ischaemia vasodilatation is already maximal due to hypoxia: drug-induced vasodilatation in other tissues may then divert blood away from areas of critical ischaemia, to their detriment. Recently infusions of the potent vasodilators, prostaglandin E_1 and prostaglandin I_2 have been reported to benefit patients with severe ischaemia in uncontrolled studies [54, 55]. These reports await confirmation in controlled trials.

Antiplatelet Agents

Blakely and Pogoriler [56] found no benefit from sulphinpyrazone in preventing occlusion of arterial grafts. Although several other trials of antiplatelet drugs in peripheral arterial disease are being performed, there is as yet no convincing evidence that they alter the natural history of the disease. However, a syndrome of recurrent attacks of pain and cyanosis in the fingers and toes has been associated with thrombocytosis and evidence of increased platelet activity *in vitro*. The digital pulses are normal and it is thought that microvascular ischaemia may arise from platelet aggregation *in vivo*, a hypothesis supported by the beneficial clinical response to aspirin [57–59]. It seems worth while therefore to check the platelet count in all patients with small vessel ischaemia and to consider a trial of aspirin if platelets are increased.

Anticoagulants

There is no benefit from long term anticoagulant therapy in peripheral arterial disease as regards life expectancy, further arterial events, or graft patency [60–62].

Fibrinolytic Agents

Oral drugs enhancing endogenous fibrinolytic activity, such as the anabolic steroid stanozolol, have shown promising results in Raynaud's syndrome (*see below*), but have yet to be evaluated in lower limb arterial disease.

Infusions of the exogenous plasminogen activators, streptokinase or urokinase, have been evaluated in the past decade. Sadly, no randomized controlled studies have been reported. The largest series of patients treated with streptokinase was reported by Martin [63]. In this series lysis of arteriographic occlusions and stenoses was most frequently achieved when occlusions were recent, proximal and shaped like thrombi rather than atheromatous stenoses ('short, irregular and crumbly'). Even with favourable lesions, patency was achieved in only half the patients. The total morbidity and mortality of streptokinase therapy in this series was not reported, but the incidence of fatal cerebral vascular accidents reported (0·7 per cent) is worrying, especially as the elderly and patients with a history of neurological symptoms of hypertension were excluded from the study. It seems likely that the mortality of streptokinase therapy approaches that of reconstructive surgery (1–2 per cent). The recent successes reported for percutaneous transluminal dilatation of short stenoses suggest that this form of therapy may be preferred to streptokinase in patients unfit for major surgery.

Human tissue plasminogen activator, which only activates plasminogen associated with fibrin thrombi, has recently been produced from tissue culture. This material was used successfully in the treatment of extensive venous thrombosis, without systemic activation of fibrinolysis or bleeding [64]. It is to be hoped that mass production of such human activators might in the future allow safer and more widely available thrombolysis than has been achieved in the past with streptokinase.

Other Proteases

Verhaeghe et al. [65] reported a controlled trial of brinolase (Brinase), a protease from Aspergillus spp. which directly lyses blood clots. Clinical results, and pressure indices at 6 months, were significantly better in the treated group. Hyaluronidase of bovine origin has also given encouraging results in a pilot study [66]. Further experience with these proteases is required to assess their place as alternatives to surgery.

RAYNAUD'S SYNDROME

Conventional management of Raynaud's syndrome comprises informed advice on prevention, e.g. keeping the hands warm, and exclusion of secondary causes. These include cervical rib, use of vibratory tools, phaeochromocytoma, hypotensive drugs (clonidine, beta-adrenergic blockers), ergotism, cryoglobulinaemia and connective tissue diseases such as scleroderma. The latter two causes are suggested by elevated erythrocyte sedimentation rates (over 50 mm/h). The role of vasoactive drugs is not well defined. Cervical sympathectomy may produce transient improvement but relapse is common and the patient is left with dry hands.

Recently three medical measures have been reported to benefit patients with severe Raynaud's syndrome resistant to conventional measures—stanozolol, plasma exchange and prostaglandin infusion.

Stanozolol

Stanozolol (Stromba) is an anabolic steroid which, when given orally, enhances endogenous fibrinolysis and lowers plasma fibrinogen levels. In an open trial, Jarrett et al. [67] reported increased hand blood flow, improvement in symptoms and healing of digital ulcers. They suggested that these effects might be due to lysis of fibrin in digital arteries, or to reduction of plasma viscosity caused by the fall in plasma fibrinogen levels. In a further study, Ayres et al. [68] confirmed the increase in hand blood flow, but demonstrated no change in blood viscosity—the fall in plasma fibrinogen being balanced by an increase in haematocrit. (Increase in red cell production from the bone-marrow is a recognized effect of anabolic steroids.) The authors suggested therefore that lysis of arterial fibrin was the more likely explanation for the increased blood flow.

Plasma Exchange

Plasma exchange involves the intermittent removal of plasma by a cell separator, and its replacement by plasma protein fraction or albumin. It has been used to remove immunoglobulins and correct the increased plasma viscosity in macroglobulinaemia or myeloma, to remove lipoproteins in hyperlipidaemia and to remove immune complexes and mediators of inflammation in various inflammatory or auto-immune diseases. In a controlled trial, O'Reilly et al. [69] reported clinical benefit from plasma exchange in severe Raynaud's syndrome, supported by improved digital artery patency measured by Doppler ultrasound. The mechanisms by which these effects occur are poorly understood, but may involve changes in platelet function [70] or blood rheology [71].

Prostaglandin Infusion

Intermittent infusions of prostaglandin E_1 [72] or prostaglandin I_2 (prostacyclin) [73] have been reported in pilot studies to produce clinical improvement and increased hand blood flow in severe Raynaud's syndrome. Interestingly, benefit has been reported to persist for several months after therapy: possibly these potent vasodilators break a vicious cycle of vascular and tissue changes produced by vasoconstriction. The effects of prostacyclin occurred without any change in platelet behaviour [73], suggesting that the vasodilator effects are a more likely mechanism for increased blood flow than the anti-platelet effects.

Further controlled, double-blind studies are required to evaluate the place of these three approaches to therapy, but the initial reports offer some hope in the management of intractable digital ischaemia.

THROMBOEMBOLISM

The management of acute limb ischaemia due to thromboembolism is primarily the surgical removal of thrombus or embolus. Immediate anticoagulation with heparin [74, 75] is logical, to prevent secondary thrombosis propagating from the embolus, and to prevent further embolism from the parent thrombus. However, no controlled trials have been reported to document the benefit of heparin. Intravenous dextran has also been advocated [74], but again there are no controlled trials.

Fibrinolytic Agents

While streptokinase infusions produce thrombolysis in the majority of patients with recent occlusions [63], the risk of bleeding is an important problem, as discussed above. Since embolectomy by balloon catheter can be performed under local or regional anaesthesia even in severely ill patients, streptokinase or urokinase are usually reserved for surgical failures. Unfortunately, bleeding from the arterial puncture sites is then common. There is little evidence that direct infusion into the blocked artery is superior to systemic infusion via a distant vein. Human tissue plasminogen activator [64] merits future evaluation in this difficult situation.

Prevention of Further Thromboembolism

Long term anticoagulant therapy is commonly given to patients with diseased or prosthetic heart valves, especially if the mitral valve is involved. This treatment is logical and difficult to resist in patients who have already suffered an embolic episode. However, no adequately controlled studies of anticoagulation have been reported. Sullivan et al. [76] found that the addition of the antiplatelet agent, dipyridamole, to oral anticoagulant therapy reduced embolic events in patients with prosthetic valves. Dale [77] found that the addition of aspirin to oral anticoagulant therapy also reduced embolic events in patients with aortic valve prosthesis.

CONCLUSIONS

Prior to 1955, before the development of Dacron arterial prostheses, a clinician had no alternative but to treat peripheral vascular disease medically. There followed a period of enthusiastic application of vascular surgery. We have now arrived at the stage where the pendulum is swinging so that a balance between medical and surgical management is being sought. The modern clinician must be aware of the changes that can be brought about by disease and by drugs in relation to blood flow.

All patients being considered for vascular reconstructon must have a thorough medical assessment, to allow recognition and, if possible, correction, of the risk factors highlighted above.

While main vessel reconstruction can now be performed in many patients with gratifying results, there are certain conditions (e.g. secondary Raynaud's) which do not have long-lasting benefit from surgery. It is particularly in these areas that the correct use of modern drugs (e.g. prostacyclin) may find widespread application. The results of controlled trials are awaited with interest. In the treatment of arterial embolism, surgery is clearly indicated. However, when thrombosis occurs in diseased vessels, early results with the new plasminogen activators are encouraging and offer a potential improvement in the management of these difficult problems.

REFERENCES

1. Hughson W. G., Mann J. I., Tibbs D. J. et al. (1978) Intermittent claudication: factors determining outcome. *Br. Med. J.* **1**, 1377–9.
2. Mitchell J. R. A. (1978) Clinical events resulting from thrombus formation. *Br. Med. Bull.* **34**, 103–6.
3. Mitchell J. R. A. and Schwartz C. J. (1965) *Arterial Disease*. Oxford, Blackwell Scientific.
4. Juergens J. L., Barker M. W. and Hines E. A. (1960) Arteriosclerosis obliterans: review of 520 cases with special reference to pathogenic and prognostic factors. *Circulation*, **21**, 188–95.
5. Richards R. L. (1970) Peripheral Arterial Disease. A Physician's Approach. Edinburgh, Livingstone.
6. Hughson W. G., Mann J. I. and Garrod I. (1978) Intermittent claudication: prevalence and risk factors. *Br. Med. J.* **1**, 179–81.
7. Editorial (1980) Management of intermittent claudication. *Lancet* **1**, 404–5.
8. Taylor G. W. and Calo A. R. (1962) Atherosclerosis of arteries of lower limbs. *Br. Med. J.* **1**, 507–10.
9. Gordon T. and Kannel W. B. (1972) Predisposition to atherosclerosis in the head, heart and legs. The Framingham Study. *JAMA* **221**, 661–6.

10. Silbert S. and Zazeela H. (1958) Prognosis in arteriosclerotic peripheral vascular disease. *JAMA 166*, 1816–21.
11. Wray R., de Palma R. G. and Hubay C. H. (1971) Late occlusion of aortofemoral bypass grafts; influence of cigarette smoking. *Surgery* **70**, 969–73.
12. Robicsek F., Daugherty H. K., Mullen D. C. et al. (1975) The effect of continued cigarette smoking on the patency of synthetic vascular grafts in Leriche syndrome. *J. Thorac. Cardiovasc. Surg.* **70**, 107–12.
13. Myers K. A., King R. B., Scott D. F. et al. (1978) The effect of smoking on the late patency of arterial reconstruction in the legs. *Br. J. Surg.* **65**, 267–271.
14. Lassen N. A. and Tønnesen K. H. (1980) Management of intermittent claudication (Letter). *Lancet* **1**, 594.
15. Sagone A. L. jun., Lawrence T. and Balcerzak S. P. (1973) Effects of smoking on tissue oxygen supply. *Blood* **41**, 845–51.
16. Foley W. T. (1957) Treatment of gangrene of the feet and legs by walking. *Circulation* **15**, 689–700.
17. Larsen O. A. and Lassen N. A. (1966) Effect of daily muscular exercise in patients with intermittent claudication. *Lancet* **2**, 1093–6.
18. Skinner J. S. and Strandness D. E. jun. (1967) Exercise and intermittent claudication. II. Effect of physical training. *Circulation* **36**, 23–9.
19. Clifford P. C., Davies P. W., Hayne J. A. et al. (1980) Intermittent claudication: is a supervised exercise class worth while? *Br. Med. J.* **1**, 1503–5.
20. Stowers J. M. (1975) Complications in relation to diabetic control—general review. In: Keen H. and Jarrett R. J. (ed.) *Complications of Diabetes*. London, Arnold, pp. 1–5.
21. O'Connor J., Ballantyne D., Pollock J. G. et al. (1977) Limb blood flow in treated hyperlipoproteinaemic patients with peripheral vascular disease. A preliminary report. *Atherosclerosis* **27**, 325–31.
22. Barndt R., Blankehorn D. H., Crawford D. W., et al. (1977) Regression and progression of early femoral atherosclerosis in treated hyperlipoproteinaemic patients. *Ann. Intern. Med.* **86**, 139–46.
23. Kuo P. T., Hayase K., Kostis J. B. et al. (1979) Use of combined diet and colestipol in long-term (7–7½ years) treatment of patients with Type II hyperlipoproteinaemia. *Circulation* **59**, 199–211.
24. Oliver M. F., Heady J. A., Morris J. N. et al. (1978) A co-operative trial in the primary prevention of ischaemic heart disease using clofibrate. *Br. Heart J.* **40**, 1069–118.
25. Veterans Administration Cooperative Study Group on Anti-hypertensive Agents (1967) Effects of treatment on morbidity in hypertension. I. *JAMA* **202**, 1028–34.
26. Veterans Administration Cooperative Study Group on Anti-hypertensive Agents (1970) Effects of treatment of morbidity in hypertension. II. *JAMA* **213**, 1143–52.
27. Breckenridge A., Dollery C. T. and Parry E. H. O. (1970) Prognosis of treated hypertension. *Q. J. Med.* **39**, 411–29.
28. Gokal R., Dornan T. L. and Ledingham J. G. G. (1979) Peripheral skin necrosis complicating beta-blockage. *Br. Med. J.* **1**, 721–2.
29. Sagone A. L. jun. and Balcerzak S. P. (1975) Smoking as a cause of erythrocytosis. *Ann. Intern. Med.* **82**, 512–15.
30. Burge P. S., Johnson W. S. and Prankerd T. A. J. (1975) Morbidity and mortality in pseudopolycythaemia. *Lancet*, **1**, 1266–9.
31. Pearson T. C. and Wetherley-Mein C. (1978) Vascular occlusive episodes and venous haematocrit in primary proliferative polycythaemia. *Lancet* **2**, 1219–22.
32. Humphrey P. R. D., Michael J. and Pearson T. C. (1980) Management of relative polycythaemia: studies of cerebral blood flow and viscosity. *Br. J. Haematol.* **46**, 427–33.
33. Ford T. F., Berent A., Speed K. et al. (1978) Symptomatic and objective effects of venesection on patients with intermittent claudication. *Br. Med. J.* **1**, 1189.

34. Bouhoutsos J., Morris T., Chavatzas D. et al. (1974) The influence of haemoglobin and platelet levels on the results of arterial surgery. *Br. J. Surg.* **51**, 984–6.
35. Yates C. J. P., Andrews V., Berent A. et al. (1979) Increase in leg blood-flow by normovolaemic haemodilution in intermittent claudication. *Lancet* **2**, 166–8.
36. Rieger H., Kohler M., Schoop W. et al. (1979) Hemodilution (HD) in patients with ischaemic skin ulcers. *Klin. Wochenschr.* **57**, 1153–61.
37. Bailey M. J., Yates C. J. P., Johnston C. L. W. et al. (1979) Preoperative haemoglobulin as predictor of outcome of diabetic amputations. *Lancet* **2**, 168–70.
38. Dormandy J. A. (1971) Influence of blood viscosity on blood flow and the effect of low molecular weight dextran. *Br. Med. J.* **4**, 716–19.
39. Collins G. M. and Ludbrook J. (1966) The intrinsic effect of low molecular weight dextran on resistance to blood flow in man. *Surg. Gynecol. Obstet.* **123**, 774–8.
40. Humphreys W. V., Walker A., Cave F. D. et al. (1976) The effect of an infusion of low molecular weight dextran on peripheral resistance in patients with arteriosclerosis. *Br. J. Surg.* **63**, 691–3.
41. Groth C. G. and Löfström E. (1966) The effect of infused high and low molecular weight dextrans on tissue oxygen tension. An experimental study on the rabbit. *Acta Chir. Scand.* **131**, 275–289.
42. Dormandy J. A., Goyle K. B. and Reid H. L. (1977) Treatment of severe intermittent claudication by controlled defibrination. *Lancet* **1**, 625–6.
43. Gerber T. and Safer A. (1978) Retrospektive Beobachtuingstudie uber die Dauer des Behandlungserfolges nach der Arwin-Therapie bei chronischer arterieller Verschlusskrankheit. *Fol. Angiol.* **26**, 21–8.
44. Martin M., Hirdes E and Auel H. (1976) Defibrinogenation treatment in patients suffering from severe intermittent claudicaton—a controlled study. *Thromb. Res.* **9**, 47–57.
45. Tonneson K. H., Sager P. and Gormsen J. (1978) Treatment of severe foot ischaemia by defibrination with ancrod: a randomised blind study. *Scand. J. Clin. Lab. Invest.* **38**, 431–5.
46. Lowe G. D. O., Dunlop D., Lawson D. H. et al. (1982) Double-blind controlled clinical trial of ancrod in the relief of ischaemic rest pain of the leg. *Angiology* **33**, 46–50.
47. Dormandy J. A., Gutteridge J. M. C., Hoare E. et al. (1974) Effect of clofibrate on blood viscosity in intermittent claudication. *Br. Med. J.* **4**, 259–62.
48. Postlethwaite J. C. and Dormandy J. A. (1975) Results of ankle systolic pressure measurements in patients with intermittent claudication being treated with clofibrate. *Ann. Surg.* **181**, 799–802.
49. Mashiah A., Patel P., Schraibman I. G. et al. (1978) Drug therapy in intermittent claudication: an objective assessment of the effects of three drugs on patients with intermittent claudication. *Br. J. Surg.* **65**, 342–5.
50. Dormandy J. A. (1981) Drug modification of erythrocyte deformability. In: Lowe G. D. O., Barbenel J. C. and Forbes C. D. (ed.) *Clinical Aspects of Blood Viscosity and Cell Deformability*. Berlin, Springer-Verlag, pp. 251–6.
51. Taylor G. W. (1973) Chronic arterial occlusion. In: Birnstingl M. (ed.) *Peripheral Vascular Surgery*, London, Heinemann, pp. 211–34.
52. Strandness D. E. jun. and Sumner D. S. (1975) *Hemodynamics for Surgeons*. New York, Grune & Stratton.
53. Coffman J. D. (1979) Vasodilator drugs in peripheral vascular disease. *N. Engl. J. Med.* **300**, 713–17.
54. Carlson L. A. and Olsson A. (1976) Intravenous prostaglandin E1 in severe peripheral vascular disease. *Lancet* **2**, 810.
55. Szczeklik A., Nizankowski R., Skawinski S. et al. (1979) Successful therapy of advanced arteriosclerosis obliterans with prostacyclin. *Lancet* **1**, 1111–14.

56. Blakely J. A. and Pogoriler G. (1977) Prospective trial of sulphinpyrazone in the maintenance of patency following peripheral vascular surgery. *Thromb. Haem.* **38**, 238.
57. Vreeken J. and van Aken W. G. (1971) Spontaneous aggregation of blood platelets as a cause of idiopathic thrombosis and recurrent painful toes and fingers. *Lancet* **2**, 1394–7.
58. Bierme R., Boneu B., Guirand B. et al. (1972) Aspirin and recurrent painful toes and fingers in thrombocythaemia. *Lancet* **1**, 432.
59. Preston F. E., Emmanuel I. G., Winfield D. A. et al. (1974) Essential thrombocythaemia and peripheral gangrene. *Br. Med. J.* **3**, 548–52.
60. Selvaag O. (1962) Long-term anticoagulant treatment in atherosclerosis obliterans of the lower extremities. *J. Oslo City Hosp.* **12**, 89–107.
61. Evans G. and Irvine W. T. (1966) Long-term arterial-graft patency in relation to platelet adhesiveness, biochemical factors, and anticoagulant therapy. *Lancet* **2**, 353–5.
62. Richards R. L. and Begg T. B. (1967) Long-term anticoagulant therapy in atherosclerotic peripheral arterial disease. *Vasc. Dis.* **4**, 27–35.
63. Martin M. (1979) Thrombolytic therapy in arterial thromboembolism. *Progr. Cardiovasc. Dis.* **21**, 351–74.
64. Weimar W., Stibbe J., van Seyen A. J. et al. (1981) Specific lysis of an iliofemoral thrombus by administration of extrinsic (tissue-type) plasminogen activator. *Lancet* **2**, 1018–20.
65. Verhaeghe R., Verstraete M., Schetz J. et al. (1979) Clinical trial of Brinase and anticoagulants as a method of treatment for advanced limb ischaemia. *Eur. J. Clin. Pharmacol.* **16**, 165–70.
66. Elder J. B., Raftery A. J. and Cope V. (1980) Intra-arterial hyaluronidase in severe peripheral arterial disease. *Lancet* **1**, 648–9.
67. Jarrett P. E. M., Morland M. and Browse N. L. (1978) Treatment of Raynaud's phenomenon by fibrinolytic enhancement. *Br. Med. J.* **1**, 523–5.
68. Ayres M. L., Jarret P. E. M. and Browse M. L. (1981) Blood viscosity, Raynaud's phenomenon and the effect of fibrinolytic enhancement. *Br. J. Surg.* **68**, 51–4.
69. O'Reilly M. J. G., Talpos G., Roberts V. C. et al. (1979) Controlled trial of plasma exchange in the treatment of Raynaud's syndrome. *Br. Med. J.* **1**, 1113–15.
70. Zahavi J., Hamilton W. A. P., O'Reilly M. J. G. et al. (1980) Plasma exchange and platelet function in Raynaud's phenomenon. *Thromb. Res.* **19**, 85–93.
71. Dodds A. J., O'Reilly M. J. G., Yates C. J. P. et al. (1979) Haemorheological response to plasma exchange in Raynaud's syndrome. *Br. Med. J.* **4**, 1186–7.
72. Clifford P. C., Martin M. F. R., Sheddon E. J. et al. (1980) Treatment of vasospastic disease with prostaglandin E1. *Br. Med. J.* **2**, 1031–4.
73. Belch J. J. F., Newman P., Drury J. K. et al. (1981) Successful treatment of Raynaud's syndrome with prostacyclin. *Thromb. Haem.* **45**, 255–6.
74. Slaney G. and Hamer J. D. (1973) Arterial embolism. In: Birnstingl M. (ed.) *Peripheral Vascular Surgery*. London, Heinemann, pp. 189–210.
75. Wessler S. (1974) Anticoagulant therapy—1974. *JAMA* **228**, 757–61.
76. Sullivan J. M., Harken D. E. and Gorlin R. (1971) Pharmacologic control of thromboembolic complications of cardiac valve replacement. II. Conclusions. *N. Engl. J. Med.* **284**, 1391–4.
77. Dale J. (1977) Prevention of arterial thrombosis with acetylsalicylic acid in patients with prosthetic heart valves. *Thromb. Haem.* **38**, 66.

Index

age
  and aortic surgery, 156
  and intermittent claudication, 212
amputation
  in limb ischaemia, 14–15, (*Fig. 3.12*) 73, 74, 188 194–5; risk factors, 164, 169
  mortality in, 203–4
anaesthesia in cerebrovascular surgery, 119
analgesia
  in ischaemia, 212
  postoperative, 152
aneurysm
  aortic, 20–1, 92, 135–58, 190–1
  brachiocephalic, 114
  carotid artery, 130
  cerebral artery, surgery for, 105
  false, after bypass surgery, 74, 171–2, 179–80
  in ischaemia, 190–1
  popliteal, bypass surgery in, 64
angiography
  of carotids, 97, 118
  coronary, before aneurysm surgery, 142
  intraoperative, 149
  in thromboangiitis obliterans, 191
  of umbilical vein grafts, 76–7
angioplasty, transluminal, 183
antibiotics
  in aneurysm surgery, 142–3
  in arterial reconstruction, 165; after penetrating injury, 190
  in ischaemia, 212
anticoagulant(s)
  action, 30
  and platelet adhesion, 26
  therapy, 193, 217, 220
antiplatelet agents, 217, 220
aorta
  anatomy, 89
  disorders of, 92, 97, 99–101
  in reoperation for arterial occlusive disease, 175
aortic aneurysm, 20–1, 92, 135–58, 190–1
aortic arch branches
  anatomy, 88–91
  disorders, 91–4: diagnosis of, 96–7; haemodynamics in, 94–6; surgery for, 97–111
aortic dissection, 92, 190–1
aortic stenosis, 3
aortography, (*Fig. 1.2*) 2, 97, 138–40, 163; *see also* arteriography
arterial reconstruction
  in aortic aneurysm, 144–54, 157–8
  in arterial occlusive disease, 161
  see also bypass surgery, endarterectomy, profundaplasty
arteriography, 1–3, 9, 97–8, *see also* aortography
  intraoperative, 22–3, 66, 150, 169
  in ischaemia, 189–90, 193–4
  in umbilical vein grafts, 76–7
  in vascular occlusive disease, 163–4, 168–9, 173–4
arteritis, 92–3, 191, 194

beta-blockers, 214
bleeding, prevention and cessation of
  coagulation factors and, 29–32
  platelets and, 26–9
  vessel wall and, 25–6, (*Fig. 2.1*) 27
blood flow
  Doppler probe measurement of, 5–8, 11–14; in aortic aneurysm surgery, 150; in carotids, 16–18, 117; intraoperative, 22; scanning, 19–20
  electromotive force meter measurements of, 148
  in prostheses, 83–4
  rate: and platelet adhesion, 26–8; and viscosity, 39–40, 41–4
  and sympathectomy, 196
blood gas analysis, 144, 151
blood lipids, 9, 214
blood pressure
  in aortic aneurysm surgery, 144, 152
  catheter measurements of, 10–12
  differential, 96, 104
  Doppler measurements of, 3–5, 14–15; in arterial occlusive disease, 162–3, 172–3; in ischaemia, 188
bypass surgery
  in aortic arch vessels, 98–111
  aorto-coronary, 141–2.
  in arterial occlusive disease, 10, 165–71; reoperation following, 171–83

bypass surgery (*cont.*):
  Dacron grafts in, 49–50, 53–5
  extra–intracranial, 124–6, 128–30
  Gore-Tex (PTFE) grafts in, 51, 57–62
  in limb salvage, 64, 188, 199–202
  umbilical vein grafts in. 64–80
calcification, 70, 138, 188–9
carotid arteries
  anatomy, 89–91
  disorders, 93–4, 94–5, 114, 116–18
  surgery on, 103, 107–11; for stroke syndrome, 112–13, 118–30
cerebrovascular disease, 15–20, 113–16, 118–30
cerebrovascular insufficiency, 96, 105
claudication
  and arterial reconstruction, 162, 164–5
clotting
  factors, 28, 29–32; and arterial lesions, 35–6; deficiency, 34–5; Factor VIII, 26, 33
  and platelets, 26–9
  pre-, of prostheses, 52, 146
  and vessel wall injury, 25–6, (*Fig. 2.1*) 27
collagen and clotting, 25–6, (*Fig. 2.1*) 27
computerized tomography and aneurysm, 21, (*Fig. 1.19*) 22, 138
critical surface tension, 75,

Dacron grafts, 49–50, 51–4
  in aortic aneurysm, 146–8, 158
  in bypass surgery, 54–5, 169, 179–80, 200
  mechanical properties of, 82–3
defibrinating agents, 216
defibrination syndrome, 34–5
dextran, intravenous, 215–16
diabetes
  and arterial grafts, 68–71
  and blood viscosity, 44
  and lower limb ischaemia, 193, 212, 213–14
diagnosis
  of aortic aneurysm, 136–41, 154–6
  of aortic arch vessel lesions, 96–7
  of carotid artery disease, 116–18
disseminated intravascular coagulation, 34
Doppler probe measurement
  of blood flow, 5–8, 11–14; in aortic aneurysm surgery, 150; in carotids, 16–18, 117; intra-operative, 22; scanning, 19–20
Doppler probe measurement (*cont.*):
  of blood pressure, 3–5, 14–15: in arterial occlusive disease, 162–3, 172–3; in ischaemia, 188
  see also ultrasound

Ehlers–Danlos syndrome, 191
electrocardiogram
  exercise, 142
  intraoperative, 143
embolism and lower limb ischaemia, 189–90, 198–9, 220
endarterectomy
  in arterial occlusive disease, 10, 165–7
  in carotids, 109, 112–13, 119–24, 127–8, 129
  in graft infection, 182
  in limb salvage, 201, 202
exercise testing, 4–5, 142

Fahreus–Lindqvist effect, 42
fasciotomy in limb salvage, 195–6
fibrin
  and clotting, 26, (*Fig. 2.1*) 27, 29–31
  in fibrinolysis, 32, (*Fig. 2.3*) 33
fibrinolysis, 32, (*Fig. 2.3*) 33, 34–5
  and arterial disease, 37, 217–18, 219, 220
  of arterial thrombus, 193
fibrinolytic agents, 217–18, 219, 220
fluid balance in aortic aneurysm surgery, 144, 152, 158

gangrene
  gas, 190, 194–5
  incipient, 4
  in ischaemia, 212
  and limb loss, 188
  and vascular reconstruction, 64–5, 162
Gore-Tex (PTFE) grafts, 50–1
  in bypass surgery, 57–62, 169, 200–1
  mechanical properties of, 82–3

haematocrit
  and blood viscosity, 41, 42–4
  and lower limb ischaemia, 192, 214–15
  and platelet adhesion, 28

haemodilution, 42–3, 215–16
haemodynamics
  in aortic arch disorders, 94–6
  in arterial occlusive disease, 164
  in carotid disorders, 117
  in prostheses, 83–4
haemoglobin and blood viscosity, 43–4
haemorheology
  in arterial disease, 43–4, 192, 214–17, 219
  in ischaemia, 9, 39–43
  in prostheses, 83
haemostasis
  and arterial disease, 25–32, 35–8
  defects of, 32–5
  postoperative, 111
heparin
  action of, 30
  in ischaemia, 193, 220
hyperlipidaemia, 9, 214
hypertension
  in aortic dissection, 92, 191
  and cerebrovascular disease, 114
  induced: in ischaemia, 192; in surgery, 119–20
  in ischaemia, 192, 214
  postoperative, 111, 126
hypotension and aortic aneurysm surgery, 148, 157

ileus, 152–3
infection
  in arterial grafts, 70, (*Fig. 3.11*) 72, 80, 171–2, 180–2
  in ischaemia, 212
  prevention, 143, 165
innominate artery
  anatomy, 89
  disorders, 93, 94, 96; surgery for, 101–2
internal reflection spectroscopy, 75–7
intestinal ileus, 152–3
intraoperative monitoring, 21–3, 66
  in aneurysm, 143–4, 149–50, 157–8
  in carotid endarterectomy, 124
ischaemia
  cerebral, 112–16, 118–30
  and haemostasis, 35
  and limb salvage, 188–204
  lower limb: amputations in, 14–15, (*Fig. 3.12*) 73, 74, 188; arterial reconstruction in, 10, 64–5, 165, 170, 171–2; blood lipids in, 9;

ischaemia, lower limb (*cont.*):
    haemorheology in, 9; management of chronic, 211–18; measurements in, 3–8, 9–10, 11–14, 163

Javid shunt, 121

limb salvage, 10, 169, 177–8, 188–204
  Dacron grafts in, 54–5
  Gore-Tex (PTFE) grafts in, 57–62
  umbilical vein graft in, 64–80
lipid deposition in umbilical vein grafts, 75–6, 80
'Liverpool' graft, mechanical properties of, 86

management of peripheral arterial disease, 211–21
Marfan's syndrome, 191
monitoring, intraoperative, 21–3, 66
  in aneurysm, 143–4, 147–50, 157–8
  in carotid endarterectomy, 124

obesity and ischaemia, 9, 213
occlusion
  of aorta, 155, 202
  of aortic arch vessels, 93, 94, 97–111
  fibrinolysis of, 218
  of grafts, 38, 70, 169, 171, 173–7
occlusive disease, arterial, 211–12
  assessment in, 161–5, 171–3
  surgery for, 161, 165–71, 173–83
oculoplethysmography, 18–19, 96, 117–18

paraesthesia and claudication, 3
paraproteinaemia, 43
patency
  of Gore-Tex grafts, 58–9, 60–2
rates: after aorto-iliac surgery, 166–7; in limb salvage, 199
  of umbilical vein grafts, 68–70
patent ductus arteriosus, 91–2
peripheral vascular laboratory, 162–3, 172–3

pharmacological treatment of peripheral arterial disease, 194, 214–21
phonoangiography of carotids, 18, 96
plasma exchange in Raynaud's syndrome, 219
plasma proteins and blood viscosity, 41, 43, 219
platelets
  and arterial disease, 36–8, 217, 219–20
  and haemostasis, 32–3
  in prevention of bleeding, 26–9
polycythaemia, 43–4, 192, 214–15
polyethyleneterephthalate grafts, *see* Dacron
polytetrafluoroethylene grafts, *see* Gore-Tex
popliteal entrapment syndrome, 4
pre-clotting of prostheses, 52, 146
profundaplasty
  in arterial occlusive disease, 166–7, 170, 177, 178
  in limb salvage, 201–2
prostacyclin
  in arterial disease, 36, 220
  and clotting, 25–6, (*Fig 2.1*) 27
prostaglandins in Raynaud's syndrome, 219–20
prostheses (*see also* vein grafts)
  Dacron, 49–50, 51–4; in aortic aneurysm, 146–8, 158; in bypass surgery, 54–5, 169, 179–80, 200; mechanical properties of, 82–3
  deterioration of, 179
  Gore-Tex (PTFE), 50–1; in bypass surgery, 57–62, 169, 200–1
  and haemostatic factors, 37–8
  infection in, 70, (*Fig. 3.11*) 72, 80, 171–2, 180–2
  mechanical properties of, 82–6
  occlusion of, 38, 70, 169, 171, 173–7
  thrombolytic therapy in, 183
pulmonary artery anomalies, 92
pulmonary function tests, preoperative, 142
pulsatility index, Doppler measurement of, 5–8, 12–13, 117
pulse volume recording
  in arterial occlusive disease, 162–3
  intraoperative use, 22, 150
  in ischaemia, 188

Raynaud's syndrome
  and blood viscosity, 44
Raynaud's syndrome (*cont.*):
  and haemostatic factors, 38
  management of, 218–19
red cells
  and blood viscosity, 40–4
  and platelet adhesion, 28
renal function
  and aortic aneurysm surgery, 142, 145, 153
rest pain, ischaemic, 188, 212
  bypass surgery in, 64–5, 168
  pressure measurements and, 4, 163
run-off
  and Dacron grafts, 54
  and Gore-Tex (PTFE) grafts, 57–8
  and graft failure, 178
  and umbilical vein grafts, 68–71

saphenous vein grafts, 49–50, 62, 169
serotonin and platelets, 28–9
shunting in carotid endarterectomy, 121, 123–4, 127
smoking
  and blood viscosity, 43–4
  and fibrinolysis, 37
  and graft occlusion, 38
  and intermittent claudication, 8, 211–12, 213
  and thromboangiitis obliterans, 191
Sparks Mandril graft, 50
stanozolol in Raynaud's syndrome, 219
steals, vascular
  subclavian, 95–6, 103, 105
  vertebral artery, 104
stenosis
  aortic arch vessel, 96, 97–111
  and arterial reconstruction, 172, 174, 183
  carotid artery, 16–18, 117–18, 128, 130
  cerebral artery, 115
  fibrinolysis of, 218
  iliac, 4, 10–12
  limb salvage in, 201–2
stroke syndrome, 113–16
  carotid artery surgery in, 112–13, 118–30
subclavian arteries
  anatomy, 89–91, 92
  disorders, 93, 94–6
  surgery for, 98, 102–11
sympathectomy
  in arterial occlusive disease, 170, 178
  in ischaemia, 164, 196–8

sympathectomy (*cont.*):
for rest pain, 65

Takayasu's arteritis, 92–3, 191
thrombectomy
in arterial grafts, 66–8, 70, (*Fig. 3.10*) 72, 174, 176–7
in carotids, 110
in ruptured aortic aneurysm, 158
thromboangiitis obliterans, 191
thrombocythaemia, 192
thrombocytopenia, 32–3
thromboembolism, 220–1, *see also* thrombosis, embolism
thrombolytic therapy, 183, 218, 220
thromboplastin and clotting, 26, (*Fig. 2.1*) 27, 30–2
thrombosis
in grafts, 50, 55, 66–8, 70, 172
and haemostasis, 35–7
and ischaemia, 189–90, 193, 220
thromboxane A_2, (*Fig. 2.1*) 27, 29
thrombus formation, 28, 29
in grafts, 38, 83–4
transient ischaemic attacks, 114–16
trauma and limb salvage, 190

ultrasound investigations
of aorta, 20–1
ultrasound investigations (*cont.*):
in aortic aneurysm, 138, 150
of carotids, 96–7, 117
see also Doppler
umbilical vein graft, 63–4
in bypass surgery, 64–80, 201

vascular insufficiency
in arterial occlusive disease, 161
vasodilators, 216–17, 220
vein grafts
in limb salvage, 199–200
saphenous, 49–50, 62, 169
umbilical, 63–80
ventilation, postoperative, 151, 158–9
vertebral arteries
anatomy, 91
disorders, 95–6, 98–9
vessel wall
defects: and arterial disease, 36; and haemostasis, 32–4
factors in prevention of bleeding, 25–6, (*Fig. 2.1*) 27
viscosity, blood, 39–44
and ischaemia, 192, 215–16
and Raynaud's syndrome, 219

white cells and blood viscosity, 41, 43